Persevering during the Pandemic

LEXINGTON STUDIES IN COMMUNICATION AND STORYTELLING

Series Editors

Kathleen M. Ryan and Deborah A. Macey

Lexington Studies in Communication and Storytelling engages scholarship in mediated storytelling, be it the traditional book or television program, the performed oral narrative, or the emerging media platform. Interdisciplinary in scope, this series looks at the myriad theoretical and practical approaches to the story. From the audience member-turned creator to new narrative, this series explores what storytelling means in the twenty-first century.

Recent Titles in This Series

Persevering during the Pandemic: Stories of Resilience, Creativity, and Connection Edited by Deborah A. Macey, Michelle Napierski-Prancl, and David Staton

*The Digital Closet: LGBT*Q Identities and Affective Politics in a Social Media Age* by Patrick M. Johnson

The Audience and Business of YouTube and Online Videos Edited by Louisa Shu Ying Ha

Friends, Lovers, Co-Workers, and Community: Everything I Know about Relationships I Learned from Television Edited by Kathleen M. Ryan and Deborah A. Macey

Mothers Work: Confronting the Mommy Wars, Raising Children, and Working for Social Change by Michelle Napierski-Prancl

Persevering during the Pandemic

Stories of Resilience, Creativity, and Connection

Edited by

Deborah A. Macey,
Michelle Napierski-Prancl, and David Staton

LEXINGTON BOOKS
Lanham • Boulder • New York • London

Published by Lexington Books
An imprint of The Rowman & Littlefield Publishing Group, Inc.
4501 Forbes Boulevard, Suite 200, Lanham, Maryland 20706
www.rowman.com
86-90 Paul Street, London EC2A 4NE

British Library Cataloguing in Publication Information Available

Library of Congress Cataloging-in-Publication Data

Names: Macey, Deborah A., 1970- editor. | Napierski-Prancl, Michelle, editor. | Staton, David (College teacher), editor.
Title: Persevering during the pandemic : stories of resilience, creativity, and connection / edited by Deborah A. Macey, Michelle Napierski-Prancl, and David Staton.
Description: Lanham : Lexington Books, [2022] | Series: Lexington studies in communication and storytelling | Includes bibliographical references and index.
Identifiers: LCCN 2022020314 (print) | LCCN 2022020315 (ebook) | ISBN 9781666901153 (cloth) | ISBN 9781666901160 (ebook)
Subjects: LCSH: COVID-19 Pandemic, 2020---Social aspects. | Interpersonal relations. | Resilience (Personality trait) | Creation (Literary, artistic, etc.)
Classification: LCC RA644.C67 P474 2022 (print) | LCC RA644.C67 (ebook) | DDC 362.1962/414--dc23/eng/20220610
LC record available at https://lccn.loc.gov/2022020314
LC ebook record available at https://lccn.loc.gov/2022020315

Dedication

To my niece, Macey, who demonstrated grace and maturity in a time of great upheaval and brought joy to our favorite pandemic pastime—picnics at the park.

-Deborah A. Macey

This book is for the Class of 2020 and is dedicated to my father, Eugene E. Napierski.

-Michelle Napierski-Prancl

Dedicated to everyone who kept playing music and kept the music playing. Thank you.

-David Staton

Contents

Acknowledgments

We, the editors, would like to thank each of the contributing authors who shared their research and stories of persistence and perseverance during the COVID-19 global pandemic. We understand the complex intersection of personal and scholarly lives as together we explored resiliency, creativity, productivity, connection, and comfort. Thank you for your dedication to this project. We would also like to thank all those involved at Lexington Books and Rowman & Littlefield Publishers, Inc., specifically Nicolette Amstutz and Sierra Apaliski for their help in bringing this anthology to publication. Finally, and most importantly, we would like to acknowledge our gratitude to essential workers who helped us in many known and unknown ways persevere during this pandemic. Thank you.

Chapter One

Introduction

Documenting Pandemic Stories

Michelle Napierski-Prancl, David Staton,
and Deborah A. Macey

While each historical period in time is important, every once in a while, an event (natural or human created) occurs that shapes a generation. We, the editors, have seen this from both a scholarly perspective and a personal one. Our parents told stories with great detail about where they were when they heard the news that President John F. Kennedy had been assassinated. In return, we find ourselves sharing our own stories about the space shuttle *Challenger* explosion and the terrorist attacks of September 11, 2001. Often an event occurs that serves as a significant marker and functions as a point of reference for a generation or for a larger population of people who will recount happenings as "before" or "after" such event. Our grandparents' generation may have shared stories about what life was like before the Second World War; in the same way, we will reference time as pre- or post-COVID-19.

When a population shares a common experience, whether it be a natural disaster, a war, or some type of significant cultural change, it can have a lasting effect on those who lived through and share this common history. Social researchers term such significant circumstances and social forces as period effects (Doherty, Kiley, Tyson & Jameson, 2015). Undoubtedly, since March 2020, we have been living through the ongoing period effect of COVID-19. As individuals, we started to take note of the historical and global significance of our community and individual responses to the global pandemic, contentious elections, school closings, protests for racial justice, and a growing political divide. We knew in our bones and brains 2020 was a challenging year: science proves us correct. Neuroscientist Sophie Scott emphasizes how "almost all perception is based on the detection of change" (Storr, 2020, p. 11). How we respond to such alterations is made manifest in myriad ways. Do we create or do we collapse? As witnesses, we started to recognize the ways activists, politicians, educators, families, and individuals approached the year in a variety of positive (and not-so-positive) ways to persevere during this unprecedented period. We decided that we needed to begin documenting this time and preserving the stories as we were living it and not wait for historians to reflect back on it as a past event or time period. As scholars, perhaps we even felt a responsibility to collect stories from those of us living through this tumultuous and uncertain time. It's a human compulsion to ascribe sense-making models in the face of change and challenge—to assign some vessel to contain cause and effect. And, too, notes Storr (2020), for all of its resultant alterations and adaptations, change can offer opportunity. "Change is hope. Change is promise. It's our winding path toward a more successful tomorrow. When unexpected change strikes, we want to know, what does it mean?" (p. 13). Subsequently, we did what many people did during the pandemic; we "Zoomed." While we come from different disciplinary perspectives, regions of the country, and even different time zones, Zoom, a newly embraced video conferencing technology whose popularity skyrocketed during the lockdown, allowed us to meet virtually to discuss our shared concerns. This anthology is the final product of those early editorial discussions. Together with the contributing authors, we put together an anthology of resiliency, which we believe will offer the reader the opportunity to process what we are experiencing, what we have learned, and how to move forward.

The stories in this book help us to see how we, as individuals and as communities, persevered during the pandemic. Storr's (2020) *The Science of Storytelling* notes that storytellers are attuned to the moments of unexpected change and channel such storms of information. And, if at times, you've felt all these challenges akin to being in a nightmare, you're not wrong, says Storr, "The cure for the horror is our story. Our brains distract us from this terrible truth by filling our lives with hopeful goals and encouraging us to strive for them" (p. 1). In this edited volume, we are sharing some of those stories because stories shape who we are. Stories offer organization amid dissonance, giving light in the darkness. This collection provides various forms of storytelling, and by extension, understanding, of a very tumultuous time. This assemblage brings together a diverse set of authors, methodologies, theoretical frameworks, and ultimately stories to reflect on how people responded, coped, survived, and perhaps even thrived during this unique period. In the future, when we refer to pre- and post-COVID-19 periods, this book will serve as a snapshot in time and a marker of what life was like during the global pandemic. It will document the important role of communication, creativity, and connection during this time, and it will underscore the additional themes of resilience, productivity, and comfort. As a whole, the chapters in this book serve as an anthology of resiliency, although it's certainly not complete. Its three sections—communication and resilience, creativity and productivity, and connection and comfort—address profound changes in our relationships to one another, to our communities, and to how we navigated an extraordinary time.

PART 1: COMMUNICATION AND RESILIENCE

In the first two chapters of Part 1, we revisit the early days of the lockdown period with a particular focus on academic life. In *"Don't worry, we're gonna figure this out": Exploring Resilient Pedagogy during the COVID-19 Pandemic,* Matthew J. Manierre, Jan DeWaters, Seema Rivera, and Martha Whalen interview professors who had to pivot midway through the spring 2020 semester. Their students left for spring break not knowing they would not be able to return to campus or to in-person classes to complete the semester. Through a series of interviews with faculty from four universities in Northern New York, the authors share with us the "Don't worry, we're gonna figure this out" moments that transpired between students and faculty in the early days of virtual classrooms. In their discussion of resilient pedagogy, we see how professors worked to foster learning as they learned to navigate the unfamiliar waters of distance learning. And for those of us in academia, the interviews validate our suspicions that we were not unique in applying what has come to be termed the "Corona Curve."

Lest we forget, faculty need empathy and respite too. Sarah Symonds LeBlanc, Elizabeth Spradley, Heather Olson Beal, Lauren Burrow, and Chrissy Cross remind us of this in chapter 3. In the same way, the students and professors in chapter 2 reassured one another that they were "gonna figure this out," the MotherScholars in *COVID-19 Moments: The Photographic Narratives of Resilience and Productivity among MotherScholars* create a support system to help one another negotiate the new work and life balance brought on by stay-at-home orders. This chapter takes us behind the scenes of their professional selves to show how MotherScholars coped during this time. One of the authors unsuccessfully attempted to establish a private workspace in her closet only to be interrupted a short time later by her toddler. Identifying as the blended identity of MotherScholar, which is recognizing how one's role as a mother informs one's scholarship and how one's scholarly identity informs one's mothering, the stories shared by these authors feature themes of support and resilience.

Chapter 4 shifts our focus from work done remotely to work done in remote locations. Derek Moscato's chapter, *Ritual of the Bering Sea:*

Commodity, Country, and Mortality in The Deadliest Catch, brings us into the intimate spaces of the crab fishing vessels; Cornelia Marie, Time Bandit, and Northwestern. The episodes showcase new and updated narratives of longstanding family dynamics both on and off the fishing boats. The sixteenth season of the *Discovery Channel* program documents the onset of COVID-19, a Cold War-esque trade war between the United States and Russia, and the tragic sinking of the F/V *Scandies Rose*. All of these real-world storylines provide an opportunity for viewers to consider the influence of the global pandemic on the fishing industry, reality television, and their own relationship to work, family, ecology, and supply-chain economics.

Chapter 5 moves out of the realm of reality television and into the realm of presidential press conferences. Alana Nicastro and Shelly Valdez's chapter, *Developing Voice Resilience: Building on Spiral of Silence Theory*, theorizes the ways Dr. Deborah Birx used verbal and nonverbal communication during and after her position on the coronavirus task force. The case study brings us back to the press briefing when then President Donald Trump thought out loud about the possibility of injecting disinfectant as a way to combat COVID-19 and Dr. Birx sat on the sidelines as a silent witness. Dr. Birx maintained her silence until leaving her role as coordinator of the White House's coronavirus task force. Nicastro and Valdez employ and expand upon the Spiral of Silence theory to analyze the interviews Dr. Birx gave on *Face the Nation* and with CNN's Dr. Sanjay Gupta when she addressed her role and her decision to remain silent.

Part 1 ends with Laurie Naranch's chapter, *What Reassurances? What Reality?: Governor Cuomo, COVID-19, and the Politics of Masculine Protection,* a chapter that went through multiple revisions as the status of Andrew Cuomo's governorship was in a constant state of flux during the period in which she was writing. As such, Naranch's chapter traces the rise and fall of now former New York State Governor Andrew Cuomo, who achieved almost hero status during the early stages of the lockdown period. Naranch suggests Cuomo's governing style provided a striking contrast to the leadership style of President Donald Trump, yet a strikingly similar need to be the hero in control. Cuomo offered a more typical executive masculine persona that combined familial stories with rhetoric of being New York tough, and for a while, it resonated well with his audience. However, before Naranch would complete her chapter, the trajectory of Cuomo's rise would take a dramatic turn, ultimately resulting in his resignation after New York Attorney General Letitia James's report that found credible evidence of abuse, sexual harassment, and a toxic workplace environment was published. Naranch's chapter guides us through these events, carefully dissecting Cuomo's signature press conferences, as they unfold, demonstrating the juxtaposition of the comforting crush of Cuomo's leadership—a blend of dominance and humor in his performance of care during the pandemic.

PART 2: CREATIVITY AND PRODUCTIVITY

We begin Part 2 with one of our editor's chapters. David Staton's *Being There and Not: Slippery Simulacrums of Song* speaks to the transformative ability of live music performance to allow us moments of being there and arriving, whether it be a concert venue or a house of worship from the cozy, but disconnected comfort of our rec-room couches. The simulated events are almost like being there. But, for Staton, almost isn't "there."

Chapter 8 by Izabela Derda, *Theater Doesn't Work: (Co-)Creation in Pandemic Theater-Making*, transports us to "being there" on the streets of Poland where we can watch an actor simply sit on a chair in a theater storefront window. The dramatic statement is clear: When a pandemic shuts down a theater, there is little else work that actors can do. Derda's chapter outlines the creative strategies theaters used when audiences and actors could no longer gather in the same physical space. Through the method of digital ethnography, Derda's chapter focuses on four theater case studies. It addresses the new ways theaters found to engage with their audiences and the role of technology in that creative process. While Dedra outlines the challenges and opportunities faced by theaters that could not allow audiences to enter their doors, Alicia Corts's chapter, *Projecting through the Mask: Theatre Techniques in the Hybrid Classroom*, brings elements of the theatre into the hybrid classroom. Corts suggests professors should see mask wearing not as an obstacle but as an opportunity to express their true character in the classroom. Corts introduces us to *Commedia dell'Arte and Commedia* methods of performance, challenging faculty to express their creativity through the act of wearing a mask. The mask can be a useful prop that will afford professors an opportunity to present an extension of their own personality through performance, physicality, and nonverbal gestures.

Corts challenges faculty to express their creativity while Heather Hether's chapter challenges students. The chapter *Cultivating Student Creativity during the Pandemic: Short-term Remedy with Long-term Value* connects coping with creativity and public health with resiliency. In it, Hether details how a classroom seminar can help foster creative expressions. It describes creative learning opportunities that worked to create a sense of community and connection among students, which was much needed during this period of pandemic-induced isolation and online instruction.

We conclude Part 2 by shifting gears a bit with Lauren Kelly and Sarah Royal's chapter, *Creativity and Consolation in The Golden Girls: How*

Revisiting an Old Show Was a Balm for the New Hard Times. Kelly and Royal describe how the creation of their podcast "Enough Wicker: Intellectualizing *The Golden Girls*" brought them comfort and purpose. Through a discussion of comfort viewing and academic analysis, this chapter provides a dose of nostalgia for the 1980s delivered from a fresh 2020 podcast perspective. The authors describe their delightful parasocial relationships with Dorothy, Blanche, Rose, and Sophia but are careful to offer criticism as well as adulation. While illustrating the ways *The Golden Girls* continues to provide life lessons and inspiration, particularly during difficult times, the authors pause much like a commercial break to interject hypothetical dialog between the characters, illuminating how they imagine the quartet might respond to 2020.

PART 3: CONNECTION AND COMFORT

The third section of the anthology begins with an invitation from author Therese Conefrey to join her as she embarks on her new pandemic ritual of walking through her neighborhood. In *Walking My Way to Community and Connection during the COVID-19 Pandemic: Theory and Practice,* Conefrey describes listening to her favorite podcasts and, as a result, you can envision the people and dogs she passes as well as the fruit she picks from the trees along the way. The new connection she makes to her neighborhood and her neighbors deepens her sense of community and benefits her physical and mental health. During the course of her walks, Conefrey comes across many artifacts specific to 2020 such as posters thanking essential workers, political and Black Lives Matter signage, and decorations saluting the Class of 2020. It is this cohort, the Class of 2020, that is the focus of the second chapter in this section and the second chapter written by one of the editors. As a parent of a Class of 2020 high school senior, Michelle Napierski-Prancl felt a need to document what happened in the absence of traditional ritual celebrations for the Class of 2020 as she watched the emotional impact school closings had on her son and his classmates. *The Class of 2020: Parents' Perspectives of the Pomp and Terrible Circumstance* tells the stories of parents from around the country who, with (or sometimes without) the support of their community and schools, worked to comfort their seniors when schools shut down. They share profound stories of both grief and joy as well as their feelings of powerlessness. They also acknowledge their own sense of loss in not being able to celebrate the traditional milestones with their children. Ultimately, Napierski-Prancl found that when communities tried to re-create or replace the lost rituals and ceremonies, it made a difference and provided comfort to parents and students.

In chapter 14, *Bridging Social Distancing Boundaries: Food Consumption and Community during Quarantine,* Edith Ritt-Coulter discusses the embodied and sensory experiences of cooking while re-creating recipes of loved ones she was unable to visit during the lockdown period. In the act of cooking, she finds comfort and a sense of belonging during an uncertain time. Much like Conefrey's chapter that takes us on a walk with her, Ritt-Coulter's chapter transports the reader to her kitchen table where one can envision themselves sitting with her and her father as they discuss oral histories and palate memory. Your mouth may water as she describes the smells of her great-grandmother's potato soup, and you can almost hear the onion burgers sizzling in the pan as she prepares them for her father. This chapter, with a focus on embodied food experiences, provides a recipe for finding comfort during uncertain times.

No doubt many found solace in binge watching during the pandemic and thus, the final two chapters in Part 3 take a critical look at two new shows that became synonymous with the act of pandemic binge watching: *Tiger King,* a Netflix sensation, and the feel-good comedy, *Ted Lasso*, from Apple TV+. In the chapter *The Escapism and Social Bond of Pandemic Binge Watching,* Gwendelyn Nisbett, Stephanie Schartel Dunn, and Newly Paul provide a critical look at the Netflix program with real-life characters but unreal storylines that made Joe Exotic and Carole Baskin household names. Through interviews with viewers, the chapter helps us better understand pandemic binge watching as a coping mechanism and as a collective experience while also exploring the appeal of *Tiger King* in and of itself.

The final chapter of Part 3, and the anthology, is written by Mary P. Erickson and the last remaining editor of the text, Deborah A. Macey. The two authors explore how the Apple TV+ *Ted Lasso* series charms audiences and critics alike, particularly two gender and media scholars. The authors explore how the humor of the series brought them smiles and comfort when they didn't feel comforted or much like smiling. Macey and Erickson detail how the characters—created by a talented group of writers and brought to life by remarkable actors in a new era of television—challenge media stereotypes. They describe how the male characters transcend traditional masculinity, contrasting those representations with the toxic masculinity of the political moment. In addition, Macey and Erickson show how the female characters are positive and powerful representations of female solidarity. Yet, the series isn't all feel-good, and the authors show how the characters' struggles resonate with the complex human difficulties we are all experiencing during this global pandemic.

This anthology was thoughtful and deliberate in selecting a range, but in no way exhaustive list, of chapter topics to include in what we see as a time capsule from the COVID-19 pandemic period. The chapters move us from pedagogy to politics to palate memory and offer contrasts as dramatic as those found in *The Golden Girls* and *Tiger King*. Ultimately, the objective is to illustrate the scope of the strategies employed by those living in and persevering through the pandemic. Along the way, the authors learned things and, often, these were things they didn't know they needed to learn. The small stuff became ever so much more important and some of the "big stuff" we found we can do without. That is one of many takeaways from living through a pandemic; we learn to think and live anew, altered but very extraordinarily human.

REFERENCES

Doherty, C., Kiley, J., Tyson, A., & Jameson, B. September 2015. *The whys and hows of generations research*. Pew Research Center. https://www.pewresearch.org/politics/2015/09/03/the-whys-and-hows-of-generations-research/.

Storr, W. (2020). *The Science of Storytelling: Why Stories Make Us Human and How to Tell Them Better.* New York, NY: Abrams.

PART 1

Communication and Resilience

Chapter Two

"Don't worry, we're gonna figure this out"

Exploring Resilient Pedagogy during the COVID-19 Pandemic

Matthew J. Manierre, Jan DeWaters, Seema Rivera, and Martha Whalen

In the spring 2020 semester, many university faculty were forced to reinvent their courses whilst simultaneously navigating a public health crisis. Some had family upheavals, others suffered COVID-related health complications, and some were tasked with the care of others. Meanwhile, students faced their own varied and complex challenges. Despite this, some faculty managed to stay positive and effective. One such professor, David, was subject to a mid-semester surgery that left him fatigued and in pain for several weeks thereafter. Meanwhile, his mortuary science students missed class because they served on the front line, helping to handle bodies of the numerous victims of the COVID-19 virus. However, he managed to 'figure it out' throughout the pandemic, retaining a strong support network and positively engaging his students, exhibiting resilience in the face of challenge and uncertainty. When he notified students of his surgery, they reached out, telling him: "Professor, don't worry . . . even if you can't teach, we know the PowerPoint slides are there, we'll go over it together. [I'll] form study groups. I can help you." This study explores the stories of faculty such as David to better understand the ways in which faculty overcame hurdles and excelled in terms of establishing a sense of community, redesigning their courses, and ultimately promoting student learning.

Our study was guided by the Community of Inquiry model (Garrison, 2017; Garrison et al., 1999), which provides a lens to identify the dimensions along which faculty adapted. It fits into a broader collection of discussions about the nature of resilient pedagogy in the context of the pandemic (Chow et al., 2020; Quintana & DeVaney, 2020). Our work adds to these conversations by documenting the difficult decisions which professors handled during the COVID-19 pandemic, complicating the picture of faculty resilience by considering the importance of fostering supportive and collaborative learning communities alongside curricular adaptations.

RESILIENCE AND PEDAGOGY

Resilience generally implies successful adaptation following exposure to an adverse event (Herrman et al., 2011; Southwick et al., 2014). As a discrete outcome, resilience bestows an individual with a strong ability to bounce back from setbacks (Herrman et al., 2011). Alternatively, resilience can be framed as a process of successful continual adjustment, selection of priorities, and pivoting in the face of change and loss (Southwick et al., 2014). Resilience results from a variety of factors ranging from personality traits (e.g., self-efficacy, optimism), biological/genetic traits, and social factors such as peer support, stable relationships, and access to institutionalized support systems (Herrman et al., 2011).

The idea of resilience can also be applied to pedagogical strategies (Chow et al., 2020; Quintana & DeVaney, 2020), especially with respect to the ability to adapt to unexpected disruptions, both personally and professionally. Quintana and Devaney (2020) conceptualize resilient pedagogy in terms of implementing course designs that are flexible and adaptable upfront, emphasizing that preemptive preparation is, in itself, an important aspect of resilience. In contrast, Chow and colleagues' (2020) framework for Crisis Resilience Pedagogy (CRP) emphasizes how faculty, students, and administrators successfully pivot following an emergency. In this model, success requires a joint effort—even a highly adaptable faculty member can experience course failure due to a lack of institutional support or student disengagement. CRP considers resilience as a multidimensional construct encompassing five elements, which also serve as measurable benchmarks: 1) adaptability to change; 2) creativity in overcoming challenges; 3) connectivity via shared resources; 4) employment of diverse teaching strategies; and 5) endurance/stress management.

Given the pandemic's effect on higher education, understanding resilience will help us discuss the ways that faculty have managed to overcome the challenges they faced. While these models of resilience largely center on rethinking and redesigning syllabi and assignments, equally important are the ways in which faculty seek to create a sense of community and maintain continued investment in the course (Garrison, 2017). The Community of Inquiry (CoI) model sensitizes us to a broader array of factors that may contribute to resilient pedagogy, particularly in an online setting.

The CoI model has been widely used as a theoretical framework for understanding key aspects of an effective online learning experience (Garrison, 2017; Garrison et al., 1999), recognizing the importance of a community of learners to support such higher-order learning skills as critical thinking, inquiry, analysis, and discourse. The framework structure includes three core elements: social presence, teaching presence, and cognitive presence (Garrison et al., 1999). The model posits that an effective learning community is supported through the interaction among these three elements, as shown in Figure 2.1.

Social presence refers to the ability of learners to identify themselves as part of a trusting community, and is created in an online community through collaboration, discourse, and communication among and between students and their instructor. Emotions are a component of this dimension; fostering students' emotional management can improve their emotional flexibility and/or resilience (Siegel, 2010). This promotes a sense of safety, belonging, or cohesiveness in a learning community (Moore & Mamiseishvili, 2012), which can help facilitate resilience by reducing feelings of isolation and attrition (Barber et al., 2019).

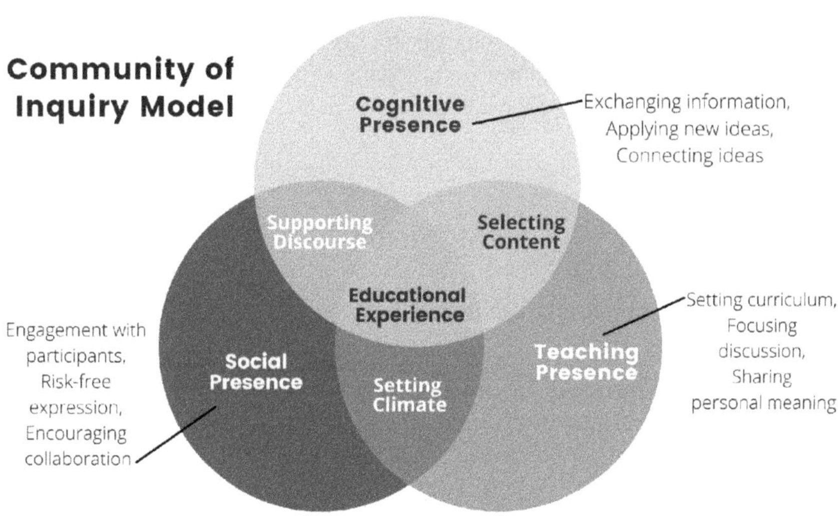

Figure 2.1 The Community of Inquiry Model.
Adapted from Garrison et al., 1999.

Teaching presence encompasses course design, facilitation, and instruction (Beck, 2015; Garrison et al., 1999). Achieved through robust course structure and active instructor leadership, a strong teaching presence is the binding element that enables cognitive and social activities necessary for achieving deep and meaningful learning experiences. This can positively impact students' participation and engagement (Kurek & Müller-Hartmann, 2019), provide relevance and a sense of meaning and purpose, and ultimately contribute to student resilience and flexible, resilient pedagogies (Irvin, 2012).

Cognitive presence is interdependent with teaching and social presence and, as such, is the ultimate goal of achieving a community of inquiry in the classroom (Beck, 2015; Garrison, 2017). A strong social presence paves the way for cognitive presence, which is further enabled by teaching strategies that shift the emphasis away from the information-delivery mode and empower students with skills to apply course content in a meaningful way. This is facilitated with inquiry-based learning that employs critical thinking and discourse, and illustrates connections between the course content and students' lives. These evidence-based pedagogies align with a strong teaching presence and have been shown to motivate student learning and improve retention (Lazonder & Harmsen, 2016).

In summary, the CoI invites instructors to approach teaching and learning with an emphasis on (1) building relationships with and among students; (2) including opportunities for discourse; (3) creating meaningful learning activities that require students to apply what they learn; and (4) empowering students to develop lifelong learning skills based on the course topic (Broda, 2018). While CRP frames faculty resilience largely in terms of course redesign, the CoI approaches the concept from multiple dimensions. This study uses the CoI's multidimensional framework, drawing attention to the overlaps between the two theories, to explore faculty resilience during the COVID-19 pandemic.

METHODS

Sample

This research uses data from a broader interview study exploring how the online transition impacted faculty's approach to and thoughts about pedagogy. We used a non-random convenience sample to recruit participants from four universities in rural Northern New York. Two of the universities were public, two were private, and each has unique characteristics that differentiate it from the other three. Maple and Pine Universities (pseudonyms) were both private, with Maple being a technology-focused research institution and Pine, a predominantly undergraduate liberal arts institution. Walnut University is a public institution with a wide range of undergraduate degree offerings, well-known for performing arts and music education programs. Oak University, the other public institution, offers a range of degree and certificate programs, and has historically complemented its in-person classes with extensive online courses. All institutions are predominantly white, with student body sizes ranging from 2,300 to 3,300. The racial homogeneity of the institutions is largely attributable to the racial composition of the surrounding county, which is only 8 percent nonwhite.

Participants were recruited from the four universities via an email distributed by their respective dean or provost. Snowball sampling and referrals helped to maximize sample diversity. A total of 43 interviews were conducted in the summer and early fall of 2020. Table 1 provides basic profiles of the interviewees quoted in text. All names used are pseudonyms. The main ethnic minority group represented in our sample, Asian Americans, reflects the demographics of the broader institutions. Unfortunately, Black and Latinx faculty are not represented in the community or this study. Our results therefore are not presumed to apply to their own experiences of the pandemic, especially given the distinctly racialized effects of the pandemic.

Table 1: ***Key Characteristics of Quoted Interviewees***

PSEUDONYM	*PROFESSIONAL*	*DEMOGRAPHIC*
Chloe	Social Sciences Assistant Professor, teaching undergraduate lecture classes; highly active in service and advising, governance. Little research. Oak University.	50s, Asian woman, lives with spouse/partner
Winnie	Arts and Humanities Associate Professor, teaches upper-level undergraduates, has taught online classes, Hyflex in-person/online course flipped classroom w/ online videos and in-class case studies. Active in university diversity work, very research active. Oak University.	30s, White woman, lives with spouse/partner
Cassandra	Social Sciences Full Professor, teaching advanced undergraduate lectures. Department committee service; medium research active. Pine University.	40s, White woman, lives with spouse/partner, two children ages 12 and 18
Kelly	Arts and Humanities Assistant Professor, introductory and upper-level undergraduate discussion-based courses. Very research active. Maple University.	40s, White woman, lives alone
Karen	Arts and Humanities Associate Professor, Department Chair, Walnut University.	40s, White woman, lives with one teenage child

PSEUDONYM	PROFESSIONAL	DEMOGRAPHIC
John	Social Sciences Associate Professor. Very active in service; very research active. Maple University.	50s, White man, lives with spouse/partner, one child in 20s
Harry	Sciences Associate Professor. Low research active; very involved in service work outside the university. Oak University.	50s, White man, lives with spouse/partner, two teenage children
Jennifer	Social Sciences Full Professor, Department Chair. Very research active; tenure committee. Pine University.	50s, White woman, lives with spouse/partner, three children all under age 13
Janet	Clinical Health Sciences Lecturer for labs and clinics. Nursing Program Director and advisor. Oak University.	40s, White woman, lives with spouse/partner, three children ranging from age 2 to 17
Mary	Business Assistant Professor. Somewhat research active. Provides online/instructional support for faculty. Walnut University.	50s, White woman, spouse lives in another city, lives with her dog
Kristen	STEM Instructor, Teaches introductory courses. Maple University.	40s, White woman, lives with spouse/partner, three children under age 15
David	STEM Associate Professor, teaches introductory courses, active in campus activities.	40s, Asian man, lives with spouse, one child under 2yrs old
Mike	Associate Professor of Anthropology, teaches introductory and advanced courses to undergrads, somewhat active in research and also serves on IRB committee.	40s, White man, lives with spouse, two children, both under age 4

Data Collection

Individual semi-structured interviews, approximately 1.5 hours in length, were conducted by all four researchers over Zoom. The interview guide consisted of questions pertaining to the interviewee's transition online during the spring 2020 semester, including how they adapted their classes and evaluation plans, their work-life balance, their teaching philosophy, and their sense of purpose as an educator. Early interviews were conducted in pairs to establish a sense of respective styles and interests among the four researchers before switching to a mix of independent or paired interviews as schedules allowed. All components of the recruitment and interview process were approved by the Institutional Review Boards (IRBs) of each institution.

Analysis

Interviews were transcribed and imported into Quirkos (Quirkos, 2021) prior to the analysis process summarized in Figure 2.2. Initial codes were drawn from the literature, prior analyses, interview memos, and discussions. The coding frameworks were modified throughout the project as our understanding of the data evolved in a process similar to a "living codebook" (Reyes et al., 2021). Our initial code set evolved into a more fully developed framework that reflected the underlying themes of the CoI and resilience literature. Throughout the process, we actively sought to develop consensus and shared interpretations by discussing, clarifying, and reconciling disagreements in how codes were applied and interpreted across researchers—a strategy consistent with many recommendations for handling team qualitative analyses (Cornish et al., 2013; Richards & Hemphill, 2018). Codes were grouped into themes that aligned with the CoI's three elements (teaching, social, cognitive presence). Extensive analytic memos and summary tables further helped to identify aspects of the CoI and resilience uncovered in each interview (Miles et al., 2014).

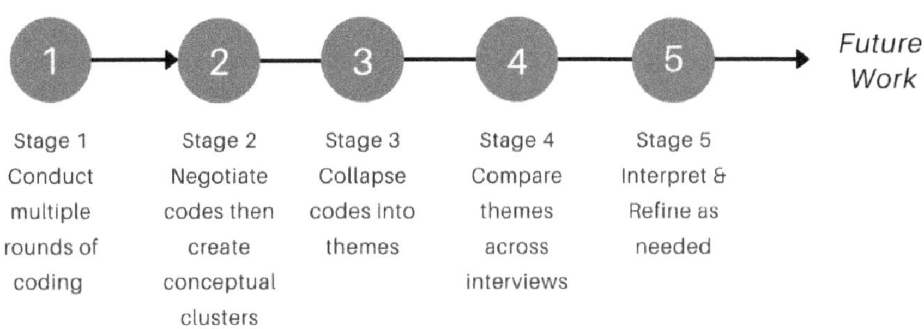

Figure 2.2 Overview of Analysis Process.
Created by authors.

FINDINGS

Our analysis exposed numerous examples of faculty problem-solving and adaptation in the context of the pandemic. Among our 43 interviews, we identified 24 faculty members who exhibited various forms of resilience in terms of at least one of the three dimensions of the CoI model. Notably, while the 43 interviewees had a balanced gender distribution, the resilience classifications were skewed toward women, with 8 men and 16 women represented. The results that follow highlight common themes that emerged among the various strategies faculty adapted in their transition to remote teaching. While many themes apply to multiple dimensions of the CoI, we have placed overlapping themes into their best-fitting dimension.

Teaching Presence

> I tried to do more . . . and at the same time, one of my messages to myself and to everybody else was this is the time of good enough. It's not . . . 'promote excellence' or 'be the best you can be.' This is: 'Okay, yeah, this is good enough . . . ' . . . you know, if you're always a 4–0 student . . . just relax, chill out, it's going to be fine.' (John)

The "Corona Curve"

Teaching presence refers to the ways that professors instruct their course, establish a curriculum, and focus day-to-day interactions. The first recurring theme that emerged in this context was described by Mike (quoted below) as a "Corona Curve," referring to relaxed grading standards and/or flexible deadlines. Cassandra describes her implementation of a Corona Curve:

> And so of course, I had all these [students] that . . . they're like, 'I can't concentrate.' And I'm like, 'I know . . . don't worry, we're gonna figure this out . . . We gotta be flexible.' I had zero late penalties whatsoever, even though normally there would have been like, 'Oh, that's a day late. That's 10% off.' . . . you can't hand it in after . . . But all of that went out the window.

The underlying motivations for implementing a corona curve seemed most often be traced to two factors—empathy and respite. A sense of empathy and uncertainty about how the pandemic was affecting students often led faculty to be more lenient than usual. Alternatively, or sometimes simultaneously, faculty expressed the need to establish the class as an escape from the chaos of the semester—a site for intellectual curiosity to flourish, not stress. For instance, Mike justified his implementation of a corona curve:

> I wanted my class to be a little bit of respite. So I cut the readings way back and I had them doing more observational writing. . . . I wanted them to be paying attention to how social distancing was changing social interaction. . . . I thought that would be beneficial to students to give them that structure.

Flexibility

A second theme that emerged was flexibility. Some faculty offered a range of formats for students to engage in course content, recognizing that many students faced barriers to class participation because of the pandemic. For example, Karen diversified the way she held class:

> . . . [I] continued synchronous classes, but I gave a number of different options because students had different levels of tech access or comfort or schedules. . . . I held them in two different formats because some students were better able to access [Microsoft Teams], which is supported by our campus. And some were better able to do Zoom. So they were able to participate in either or both. . . . And I also did asynchronous discussion boards . . . and put up all the recordings on Moodle and [placed students] in [groups] so that students could choose to sort of participate in any combination . . .

Karen's actions reflect an effort to preserve student engagement by designing the course to be more accessible.

Other faculty provided students with alternative content. Kelly selected an array of movie options for her post-apocalyptic film course on a new online streaming platform. Considering the depressing content of these films, she offered more optimistic alternatives for students who wanted a break from films that sometimes felt too close to reality as the pandemic unfolded. In this case, the redesign was motivated not just by accessibility, but also an explicit concern for students' mental health.

Reworked Assignments

A final theme involved faculty who rethought their assignments in light of both the pandemic and the new virtual setting. For example, to substitute for the use of mannequins in her clinical nursing class, Janet added role-playing exercises to a telehealth unit after the class migrated online. Here she describes portraying a pregnant domestic violence victim:

> I really tried to get creative. The one telehealth visit where the abuse was, I actually gave myself a black eye and [tied a] scarf around my neck. I put some fingerprints [on my neck] . . . I'm really doing that with makeup. . . . The students really had to use their health assessment skills because I wouldn't take my sunglasses off. Some of them got it and some of them did not get it at all until I finally pulled off my sunglasses . . . and they're all like, 'Oh my God, how'd we miss that?'

Leveraging online pedagogy and Zoom to provide a new and relevant experience was just one illustration of pandemic-fueled ingenuity. Other faculty tasked students with creating art assignments expressing pandemic anxieties, analyzing kinesthetics in YouTube videos, and considering the market ramifications of the global economic downturn. Also common was the addition of pandemic-related lecture topics ranging from the effects of unemployment on mental health to strategies for sterilizing biomaterials. Reframing the pandemic as an opportunity to try new ideas or increase the relevance of course content was a useful strategy for maintaining a strong teaching presence through the online transition.

Social Presence

> I would spend probably the first 10-15 minutes of a class just . . . checking in with my students . . . seeing how they're doing, what the challenges are. You know, are they keeping up? Are they able to access online? Those kinds of questions. (Kristen)

Social presence encompasses the ways instructors establish connections across the classroom—with and among their students. Resilience in this context entails overcoming the loss of human connection from transitioning online. Beyond straightforward adjustments (such as using conference software or online discussion forums), several examples emerged that shed light on the range of pedagogical adaptations.

Providing Expressive Space

The first theme we identified was the creation of additional space for emotional expression, support, and confiding, as Kristen's narrative (above) illustrates. Several faculty opened up to students, divulging their own pandemic-induced stress and exhaustion in an effort to create an empathetic connection. This empathy helped manage students' expectations for the professor's performance, while also signaling the professor's receptiveness to provide support. For example, Winnie notes:

> I . . . consciously tried to be a little more personal and a little more forthcoming, just as a way of saying, 'Hey, you know, we're all stressed and everybody's life is weird right now. And we'll figure it out. And I, as your professor, I'm not any more removed from that than you are. . . . I'm having just as tough a time figuring this out as you are.' And I do think . . . it helped in the sense that . . . they were able to see that I'm human too, right? . . . I'm still trying to figure it out just as much as they are.

The degree to which professors made room for emotional support varied greatly, and sometimes involved interventions that extended beyond the classroom. For instance, one professor offered his personal cell phone number to students that he sensed were having panic attacks. Other faculty, like Chloe, held in-class support sessions:

> I actually ran some virtual sessions where I taught them some basic meditation techniques, some basic breathing techniques . . . and some of the students thought it was funny because they were pooh-poohing it. . . . And during one session when we're doing one of these breathing exercises, one of them fell asleep on screen and started snoring, it was great. . . . He was convinced once we woke him up.

These examples reflect a dedication to providing students opportunities not only to learn, but also to develop coping strategies that enable them to be resilient in the face of adversity.

Reaching Out

A second recurring theme was an increased effort to communicate with students and to support their continued engagement with the course. For example, student feedback and surveys were used to guide course restructuring. Harry described using focus groups to test different adaptive learning software options in a pilot to select one for class, explaining: "It's their education. I don't know if you . . . get the students to buy in, and then it sucks, you're like, 'Yeah, you're partly to blame.'" He went on to say that he:

> . . . figured by sending out the updates and by keeping in touch with them . . . I could take some of their stress away and it took some of my stress away too. I had a lot of students say they appreciated it because there [were] a lot of professors that didn't get [ahold] of their students till after the spring break.

As Harry's experience highlights, seeking student feedback can create a sense of shared ownership over the course while also reducing stress by diffusing it across both faculty and students.

Other faculty increased communication efforts by reaching out directly to those who appeared to struggle or dropped off the map completely. This scenario was quite common, and most faculty we interviewed described having students suddenly cease attending. As John explains, he "lost probably three to four in [one class] and five to six in my [other] class. I bent over backwards to reach out . . . to connect to them. And just to make sure they were okay." Missing students often prompted emails, contacting university support services, and, less frequently, reaching out via text and phone calls. Although often fruitless, these efforts sometimes provided intervention through direct support or by way of referrals for access to campus services or equipment such as loaned computers.

Cognitive Presence

> It was the structure, it was connecting with one another . . . they did a lot of work together in breakout rooms and more hands-on learning. So I think it just gives [students] an escape mentally when [they] have to focus on something and complete a task. (Mary)

Cognitive presence happens when students are actively learning in a community of inquiry. It is facilitated by engaging students in critical thinking and problem-solving, listening to each other and the instructor, and describing/sharing their thoughts. Resilience in this case depends on the instructor's ability to convey a meaningful learning experience. Our interviews revealed a few instances where cognitive presence was bolstered during the pandemic, most notably among faculty with a firm foundation in pedagogical expertise and some, but not all, with online teaching experience.

The Intersection of Social and Teaching Presence

A common theme for cognitive presence was the importance of both structure and sense of community. While many interviewees expressed one or the other, those most resilient in this context notably emphasized both simultaneously. Although there were others, here we focus on two particularly obvious cases: Mary and Jennifer. Mary demonstrated resilience through several strategies that reflect her statement " . . . my mantra was structure and community or connection." She reorganized her course into two-week learning modules, carefully trimming assignments and content to retain key learning outcomes and scheduling periodic meetups to enable student interaction and communication. As part of her attention to structure, Mary required attendance regardless of whether or not students had done the readings. Her virtual café discussion board saw heavy student traffic, with students perhaps sharing more than they may have in person. "So I saw a lot of continued connection. And in some cases, deeper connection." These modifications reinforced cognitive presence by providing students' continued and consistent opportunities to interact with one another and with course content.

Jennifer, on the other hand, widely facilitated student initiatives even before the transition online:

> I give them the tools to learn the material . . . there's certain content that they do need delivered from me, but then there's a lot of it . . . we discover it together and apply it together. So I help them with the fundamental tools. But then I'd say about half of it is applying them to real world applications.

Like others, Jennifer saw the transition as an opportunity to enhance student learning. She enrolled students—and herself—in an online finance certification program through Bloomberg Terminals. "I took the modules with [the students], we talked about them together . . . and I think [that] gave us more chances in our breakout sessions than in our classroom to actually talk about what was going on in the world."

Also, like others but perhaps to an even greater extent, Jennifer revised her curriculum to directly connect to the pandemic, noting: "My [economics] class was the world situation . . . literally . . . I could show them CNN or CNBC . . . every single thing was on the front page of the *Wall Street Journal*, like every single thing was my class." To sustain the sense of connectivity and community throughout the semester, Jennifer's class routinely convened via discussion forums and virtual breakout rooms:

> I asked them all to put the camera on, and it was fine. And they were all okay with it and it would really help us engage in and we do a lot of breakout rooms and they all came to class and they all had their cameras on. And they did say that different professors and different classes didn't require cameras. . . . So by having the cameras on, they knew they were going to be actively engaging.

Although the use of cameras is a thorny issue and most faculty changed their approach as the online experience progressed, it appears that—like many—Jennifer's insistence on students turning their cameras on added value to their virtual classroom experience.

Efforts to provide consistent opportunities for communalization, expression of ideas, structure, and stability paid off with exceptional results in both of these cases. Mary reflected: " . . . the students got more confidence using technology for their purposes, and they connected with each other. And I felt like I connected even more so with them." Jennifer felt emergency teaching made her a better teacher and increased student engagement: "I had better attendance than when I taught in person." She felt she taught them some valuable tools for learning—different from what they normally would have learned in her course, but very important. However, establishing a community of inquiry did not come without tradeoffs:

> I've never gotten such good evaluations, but there were huge costs. Costs to my family, my life, you know, and to them, but I mean, I . . . conditioning on having to do that, I think it went okay. Would I do it that same way again? No, I'm going to try to do it so it's not quite as exhausting. And we'll see.

DISCUSSION

Garrison's CoI model has provided an effective lens for analyzing the ways that faculty adapted their courses as they transitioned to teaching online, and the themes that emerged align well with the three dimensions of the model. Faculty described a variety of strategies that exemplified resilience with respect to teaching presence—and even more so with respect to social presence. Ultimately, however, there were only a few examples—nine in all, two in particular—where faculty descriptions demonstrated resilience with respect to cognitive presence. These faculty were able to create deep and meaningful learning experiences for their students, thereby sustaining a Community of Inquiry in their online classrooms.

The CoI also sheds light more generally on emergency online teaching. The emergency transition was characterized by several competing challenges—limited time, limited energy, and limited skillsets of administrators, students, and faculty (Chow et al., 2020; Hodges et al., 2020). This frequently caused tension between different elements of the CoI—for example, devoting time and energy toward emotionally supporting students versus creating innovative assignments that leveraged online teaching tools and/or current events. Faculty were forced to triage among different dimensions of the CoI model, often sacrificing rigor and content mastery (cognitive presence) to maintain student motivation and well-being (social presence). Nevertheless, we identified 24 faculty who were indeed resilient in one dimension of the CoI or another. Incorporating the pandemic into the course can enhance student engagement by increasing content relevance, and democratizing decision-making builds student buy-in and motivation (Cavanagh et al., 2016). Similarly, an empathetic teaching presence has been shown to help students manage anxieties and fears about course material (Majeski et al., 2018; Meyers et al., 2019) and (we speculate) the pandemic as well. While fully balancing elements of the CoI was observed, it was rare and largely a function of prior pedagogical training and experience.

We observed examples of Quintana and DeVaney's preemptive resilience (2020)—for instance, when interviewees described pre-pandemic practices including recording and posting lectures online, incorporating current events, and using project-based strategies. Furthermore, some of our most successful faculty were, as previously mentioned, well-trained and experienced in online pedagogy and were likely more capable of pivoting online thanks to their existing skills. It was, however, challenging to identify these faculty cases in practice as their semesters often appeared calm and mundane because everything went smoothly. Understanding the preparation that went into making that transition smooth is valuable as it can inform future planning.

Furthermore, though these faculty's semesters appeared successful, they were also surrounded by stress and overwork. Though the classes went well, that does not necessarily mean the faculty themselves came out unscathed.

There were several strategies within the teaching presence dimension that aligned with the five dimensions of the CRP framework (Chow et al., 2020). For instance, refocusing assignments on the pandemic exemplifies the "creativity" dimension. Likewise, our description of a corona curve aligns with "adaptability." However, this framework fell short for describing resilience with respect to social presence. Many resilient strategies we documented (e.g., the creation of space for empathy, sharing, emotional support) were essential to the CoI but were not well encapsulated by the CRP framework. Future implementations of the CRP concepts might benefit from more explicitly considering the many ways that faculty retooled their social interactions with students alongside their teaching presence.

LIMITATIONS AND CONCLUSIONS

This study was limited by a number of factors. (1) As already mentioned, most of the participants were white and rurally based. A broader sample would quite possibly yield different results. (2) Our primary evidence was from faculty narratives, which are prone to desirability biases and memory lapses, especially given that a few of the interviews were conducted after the fall 2020 semester had started. (3) Cognitive presence was particularly hard to ascertain in this study, given that we were not able to observe classes and did not review teaching materials outside of shared syllabi. (4) Finally, we did not consider environmental and demographic factors that might have revealed potential disparities in adaptability. These include known correlates such as university policy, family pressures, and gender (McMurtie, 2020).

A final caveat is that these interviews are from the spring 2020 semester. Though this semester was unique, at the time of this writing crisis teaching has continued for over a year. Even our most resilient interviewees described being exhausted and stressed during the spring 2020 semester. Long-term exposure to this stress has undoubtedly had serious consequences: One recent survey found that half of faculty saw their enjoyment in teaching decrease since 2020, and a third considered leaving academia ("On the Verge of Burnout": COVID-19's Impact on Faculty Well-Being and Career Plans, 2021). Our results cannot inform discussions on the effects of long-term exposure on faculty, and it cannot be inferred that faculty who developed resilient pedagogy in one semester were personally or pedagogically resilient in the year that followed.

To conclude, this study found that faculty implemented a wide array of strategies to adapt to emergency remote teaching in the spring 2020 semester, and many exhibited signs of resilience in at least one dimension of the CoI model. Faculty adjusted their curricula and course designs, as well as the ways they interacted with students. These detailed findings can be helpful for faculty wishing to develop resilient strategies in the future.

There is a need to extend this work to include a more diverse sample group, as well as to consider contextual factors such as family and organizational pressures. Given the persistence of crisis teaching, it is also important to further investigate if resilience has persisted over time and if it has helped to mitigate the risk of burnout. The results of this study shed light on the fact that, even though the pandemic has been immensely challenging, some faculty have managed to adjust their courses successfully. Their reflections on personal and professional experiences during the spring 2020 semester lockdown offer a glimmer of positivity about what were otherwise dismal times.

REFERENCES

Barber, W., van Oostveen, R., Childs, E., & Harvey, J. (2019, June 12). *Situating Resilience, Grit and Growth Mindset as Constructs of Social Presence in the Fully Online Learning Community Model (FOLC)*. European Conference on E-Learning 2019.

Beck, D. (2015, September 9). Community of inquiry: Cognitive presence. *The EvoLLLution.* https://evolllution.com/programming/teaching-and-learning/community-of-inquiry-cognitive-presence/.

Broda, A. (2018, October 16). Communities of inquiry (CoI): Cognitive presence. *Model ELearning.* https://modelelearning.com/2018/10/16/communities-of-inquiry-coi-cognitive-presence/.

Cavanagh, A. J., Aragón, O. R., Chen, X., Couch, B. A., Durham, M. F., Bobrownicki, A., Hanauer, D. I., & Graham, M. J. (2016). Student buy-in to active learning in a college science course. *CBE—Life Sciences Education*, *15*(4), ar76. https://doi.org/10.1187/cbe.16-07-0212.

Chow, R. S., Lam, C. M., & King, I. (2020). Crisis resilience pedagogy (crp) for teaching and learning. *2020 IEEE International Conference on Teaching, Assessment, and Learning for Engineering (TALE)*, 384–391. https://doi.org/10.1109/TALE48869.2020.9368496.

Cornish, F., Gillespie, A., & Zittoun, T. (2013). Collaborative analysis of qualitative data. *The Sage Handbook of Qualitative Data Analysis*, *79*, 93.

Garrison, R. (2017). *E-Learning in the 21st Century: A Framework for Research and Practice* (3rd ed.). Taylor & Francis.

Garrison, R., Anderson, T., & Archer, W. (1999). Critical inquiry in a text-based environment: Computer conferencing in higher education. *The Internet and Higher Education*, *2*(2–3), 87–105. https://doi.org/10.1016/S1096-7516(00)00016-6.

Herrman, H., Stewart, D. E., Diaz-Granados, N., Berger, E. L., Jackson, B., & Yuen, T. (2011). What is resilience? *The Canadian Journal of Psychiatry*, *56*(5), 258–265. https://doi.org/10.1177/070674371105600504.

Hodges, C., Moore, S., Lockee, B., Trust, T., & Bond, A. (2020). The difference between emergency remote teaching and online learning. *Educause Review*. https://er.educause.edu/articles/2020/3/the-difference-between-emergency-remote-teaching-and-online-learning.

Irvin, M. J. (2012). Role of student engagement in the resilience of African American adolescents from low-income rural communities. *Psychology in the Schools*, *49*(2), 176–193. https://doi.org/10.1002/pits.20626.

Kurek, M., & Müller-Hartmann, A. (2019). The formative role of teaching presence in blended virtual exchange. *Language Learning & Technology*, 22.

Lazonder, A. W., & Harmsen, R. (2016). Meta-analysis of inquiry-based learning: Effects of guidance. *Review of Educational Research*, *86*(3), 681–718. https://doi.org/10.3102/0034654315627366.

Majeski, R. A., Stover, M., & Valais, T. (2018). The community of inquiry and emotional presence. *Adult Learning*, *29*(2), 53–61. https://doi.org/10.1177/1045159518758696.

McMurtie, B. (2020). The pandemic is dragging on. Professors are burning out. *The Chronicle of Higher Education*. https://www.chronicle.com/article/the-pandemic-is-dragging-on-professors-are-burning-out.

Meyers, S., Rowell, K., Wells, M., & Smith, B. C. (2019). Teacher empathy: A model of empathy for teaching for student success. *College Teaching*, *67*(3), 160–168. https://doi.org/10.1080/87567555.2019.1579699.

Miles, M., Huberman, M., & Saldaña, J. (2014). *Qualitative Data Analysis: A Methods Sourcebook and The Coding Manual for Qualitative Researchers*. SAGE.

Moore, A., & Mamiscishvili, K. (2012). Examining the relationship between emotional intelligence and group cohesion. *Journal of Education for Business*, *87*(5), 296–302. https://doi.org/10.1080/08832323.2011.623197.

"'On the Verge of Burnout': COVID-19's impact on faculty well-being and career plans" (pp. 1–23). (2021). [Research Brief]. *The Chronicle of Higher Education*.

Quintana, R., & DeVaney, J. (2020). Laying the foundation for a resilient teaching community. *Inside Higher Ed*. https://www.insidehighered.com/blogs/learning-innovation/laying-foundation-resilient-teaching-community.

Quirkos (2.4.1). (2021). [Computer software]. https://www.quirkos.com.

Reyes, V., Bogumil, E., & Welch, L. E. (2021). The living codebook: Documenting the process of qualitative data analysis. *Sociological Methods & Research*. https://doi.org/10.1177/0049124120986185.

Richards, K. A. R., & Hemphill, M. A. (2018). A practical guide to collaborative qualitative data analysis. *Journal of Teaching in Physical Education*, *37*(2), 225–31. https://doi.org/10.1123/jtpe.2017-0084.

Siegel, D. J. (2010). *The mindful therapist: A clinician's guide to mindsight and neural integration* (pp. xxvii, 288). W W Norton & Co.

Southwick, S. M., Bonanno, G. A., Masten, A. S., Panter-Brick, C., & Yehuda, R. (2014). Resilience definitions, theory, and challenges: Interdisciplinary perspectives. *European Journal of Psychotraumatology*, *5*. https://doi.org/10.3402/ejpt.v5.25338.

Chapter Three

COVID-19 Moments

The Photographic Narratives of Resilience and Productivity among MotherScholars

Sarah Symonds LeBlanc, Elizabeth Spradley, Heather Olson Beal, Lauren Burrow, and Chrissy Cross

The impact of COVID-19 sat front and center on the front page of the February 21, 2021 *New York Times*, filling the space with what appears to be a black-and-white image of nothing. It runs vertically from the masthead to nearly the bottom of the page. As your eyes focus on the image, you begin to see it is made up dots, a half of million dots. Making its way around social media, we see how people were moved by the imagery; the image was simple, yet powerful. It communicated what we already know: COVID-19 does not discriminate; each dot represented the same thing: one U.S. life lost to COVID.

The use of images, or in our case digital photos, is one way we communicated our narratives during the COVID-19 pandemic just as the February 21, 2021 image on the *New York Times* did. At the time of this writing, we are slowly emerging from 15 months of chaos caused by COVID-19. We documented the highs and the lows of what we experienced as we digitalized our memories, each captured moment reminding us of the upheaval, the new narrative we choose to write during COVID.

The authors began this process two months into the COVID-19 pandemic as part of a larger agenda focusing on MotherScholar. We use the term MotherScholar to designate ourselves as individuals and as a collective group.

Matias (2011) originally coined the term and Lapayese (2012) expanded upon the concept by writing that "Mother-scholars assert that when motherhood and intellect confront and inform each other, a new thinking emerges to capture the possibility of humanizing education beyond the private relationships between mothers and children" (p. xvi). Lapayese hyphenated the term, yet our group merges the two identities together (Spradley et al., 2021) reflecting how we constructed and negotiated our identities during the pandemic. MotherScholars are those who find ways to creatively blend their maternal identity into scholarly places and/or their scholarly identity into their mothering places (Burrow et al., 2021). The beginning of the pandemic forced us to cope and compose new family narratives (LeBlanc, et al., 2021) as we, along with other academic mothers, bore greater brunts of domestic duties as families locked down together (King & Frederickson, 2021). We moved our workstations around our homes as we baked, played, tutored, and provided entertainment all the while writing, emailing, Zooming, and grading (Spradley et al., 2021).

The purpose of this chapter is to discuss how five MotherScholars communicated support through the use of photographs and social media postings; in addition, we examine how that support contributed to our resilience during the COVID-19 pandemic. The bulk of our research from this project focuses on our narratives (LeBlanc, et al., 2021a; LeBlanc et al., 2021b; Spradley et al., 2020/2021; Spradley et al., 2021). This chapter unpacks narrative to examine digital memories and photos that communicate our journeys and build author-friend relationships. We begin by reviewing support and resilience literatures, especially in how they relate to MotherScholars navigating work/family (Clark, 2000). We then detail our method and analysis procedures before presenting results to speculate what all of this means.

PROLOGUE

Our story began before our first Zoom interaction. We use emails between Elizabeth and Sarah to capture the untold, undocumented beginning.

Somewhere in Nacogdoches, TX . . .

Elizabeth: I nervously opened my email. I currently had three co-authors, one of whom was an acquaintance and the other two who were strangers, and I had sent an email request to another stranger—friend of a friend type of thing—asking her to be a part of our MotherScholar writing team. Was I totally off base? After all, we were going to vulnerably disclose to one another about our COVID-19 experiences, share images from our lives, and share social media posts from our personal accounts. A part of me was nervous she would say no, but another part of me was nervous she would say yes.

Somewhere in Fort Wayne, IN . . .

Sarah: "So I just got this random email asking to be part of a research group talking about mothers as scholars," I told my husband as we passed each other during our "lunch periods." Despite both of us working from home, we rarely ate together. "Are you going to do it?" he countered. "I think so. A colleague from the last Hope conference recommended me. I'm a mother, a scholar, and well I have nothing to lose. So yeah." I hit reply and type my acceptance. "Elizabeth, thank you for the invitation. I would be honored to be part of the group." I hit send.

SUPPORT AND RESILIENCE

From the moment of our first Zoom (Spradley et al., 2020/2021), our work and family borders blended (Clark, 2000); Elizabeth's toddler burst into the closet she was working in to attempt an escape from her children during our session. The subject of our research as well as the identities that we accepted during our initial data gathering enabled us to cross the border between work and family consistently, bringing our family into our work and our work into our family (Clark, 2000). Organizational research (Fritz, 2014; McBride & Bergen, 2015) examines the various relationships present at work and opens the door to look at different and nuanced workplace relationships. We embody the virtual co-author relationship(s), which was both enabled and necessitated by COVID-19. To study this workplace relationship type, we examine support and resilience and how they impact the budding virtual co-author/friend relationship.

Social Support

Support is conceptualized as "expressions of care, concern, affection, and interest" (Burleson, 2003, p. 552). Demonstrating and showing support enhances relationships and well-being (Albrecht et al., 1992). Support is critical to the development and maintenance of friendships, romances, and families (Burleson, 2008). The impact of support among these various relationships is evident in areas such as postpartum depression (LeBlanc, 2021; Meluch & LeBlanc, 2021), cancer communities (Rising et al., 2017), handling contested illnesses (Russell, 2020), and organ transplants (Scott et al., 2011). Furthermore, we argue that the presence of support among working relationships is vital, especially in the field of academics. While underrepresented in the social support literature in comparison to health communication, organizational communication literature demonstrates the value of supportive workplaces, in which workers perceive they are valuable and have the help needed to fulfill their roles including relational, informational, and tangible support (Harris et al., 2011; Kossek et al., 2011).

The shift in teaching modalities at the beginning of COVID-19 impacted the lives of academics, especially academic mothers. MotherScholars were expected to take on the bulk of childcare while maintaining their academic workload (Lawless, 2021). Many MotherScholars found the lack of work and family boundaries challenging and unsupported (Hayden & O'Brien Hallstein, 2021; Lawless, 2021). The mothering in academia research focuses on the stress and pressure of MotherScholars, but little is mentioned in terms of supporting each other or mentoring. McDermott (2021) determined that the way many universities offered support did not consider faculty's diverse life situations. Our writing group defied the negative odds by supporting one another.

When exploring support within organizational communication, research focuses on compassionate communication (Gist-Mackey et al., 2021) or socialization or commitment to the organization (McGlynn & Richardson, 2014); our research extends this work to focus on the communicative behaviors we used to construct lines of support crossing academic disciplines and institutions. By examining our use of support, we are able to discern the impact these behaviors have on our professional and non-professional relationships.

Resilience

Buzzanell's (2010) work with Communication Theory of Resilience (CTR) contextualizes the concurrence of support and resilience in our MotherScholar professional and personal relationships. CTR "envisions resilience as a constitutive process through which people reintegrate and actively construct their new normal through language, interaction, networks, and attention to their identities and identifications, within their material environments and societal discourses" (Buzzanell, 2019, p. 69). The value of CTR to this chapter is the theory's aim to provide an explanation as to how humans communicate after a triggering event, like loss or hardships, to reframe, rebuild, and transform their lives in relation to others.

As MotherScholars, we experienced disruptions to our normal professional and personal lives as we worked and mothered from home. The pandemic was a *triggering event* that stimulated the five interrelated processes associated with CTR: crafting normalcy, foregrounding productive action,

Table 3.1 CTR Processes (Buzzanell, 2010)

Process	*Definition*	*Example*
Crafting Normalcy	Finding meaning and stability in the instability of the triggering event and its aftermath	Developing routines, deadlines, and discussion that offered stability and purpose to our MotherScholar disruptions
Foregrounding Productive Action	Not ignoring negative and difficult emotions, but working to foreground active progress toward a goal(s)	Acknowledging the COVID-19 threats to our maternal and professional ideals while focusing on MotherScholar projects that we had greater control over
Affirming Identity Anchors	Communicating identities embedded within collectivities that enable coping and resilience	Managing our MotherScholar identities together as we struggled to fulfill
Maintaining and Using Communication Networks	Supporting each other through social capital enmeshed in networks of relationships	Developing new collegial and friendly relationships with MotherScholars to communicate with and work with through the pandemic
Putting Alternative Logics to Work	Altering the organizing system through creative solutions	Labeling our COVID-19 work from home situation "disruptive" and move forward together with new research agendas

affirming identity anchors, maintaining and using communication networks, and putting alternative logics to work (Buzzanell, 2010/2017/2018/2019).

Of interest to us as we began this chapter was the way our task-oriented relationships as a writing team and our socially oriented relationships as five MotherScholars intermingled through our emergent communication network, which in turn became *resilient transformative action* narrated in the words and photos that follow.

Elizabeth's field notes:

At a Zoom mentoring meeting, Heather asks Elizabeth, "So, you and Sarah did not know each other before this project, right?" Elizabeth responds, "Right." "That's what I thought," replied Heather. Heather went on to explain why she asked the question. Lauren assumed that Elizabeth and Sarah were friends based on their shared academic discipline and their rapport throughout their MotherScholar communication. Lauren had made the comment to Heather, "It is so great that you, Chrissy, and I are so close and that Elizabeth and Sarah are so close that we could make this MotherScholar writing team work so well." Heather replied, "Actually, I am pretty sure that Sarah and Elizabeth were complete strangers prior to our first Zoom meeting."

METHOD

Friendship as Method

Methodologically, we blurred distinctions between outsider/insider, researcher/researched to embrace a friendship method that affords more intimate disclosures through data collection (Sassi & Thomas, 2012). Friendship as method is a relational approach to the qualitative research process touted by feminist researchers as a means of rich data collection, political action, and reflexive participation for consciousness-raising (Tillman-Healy, 2003). Tillmann-Healy (2003) describes "friendship as method" like ethnographic fieldwork; we must be in the world with others, gain entry, negotiate our roles, pass through stages, as well as navigate, participate, and observe. Mutual disclosures deepen the social support network and constitute data for our ongoing research agenda. Much like Jones's (2007) experience with a writing group, friendship emerged from a joint interest in scholarly writing and maternity. Our pre-existing identities granted us access to the MotherScholar culture, much like one does for ethnographic research. During the interviews beginning in May 2020, our friendships grew; our use of email and our Zoom conversations gave us access to the MotherScholar field site (Howlett, 2021). As a result, our friendship enabled us to engage in consciousness-raising and collective action in the research process by actively resisting socially constructed role limitations. We found that our similar dynamics endeared us to one another (Doherty, 2021): We are established in our respective fields, either tenured or on the tenure track with children of varying ages. We supported each other through our highs and lows during COVID-19. Despite the interview guides and/or prompts, these relationships grew out of natural contexts and showcased raw narratives resulting in personal benefits and professional opportunities that would not have existed before such a project (Burrow et al., 2020).

Data Collection

Arts-based research breaks the norms of traditional social scientific research. We draw upon three art-based genres: narratives, poetic inquiry, and autoethnography. Freeman (2019) suggests that the more creative the writing is "the more scientific it [narrative] would be" (p. 134). Poetic inquiry allows the poet to use personal narrative in a way that the audience can "relate, embody, and/or experience the work as if it is their own" (Faulkner, 2019, p. 210). Then, autoethnography bridges the creative arts with the social scientific (Adams & Holman Jones, 2019). Rather than presenting the data and applying it back to the existing research, we choose to present our story through our collective voices—our narrative, poetry, autoethnography, or visual representation.

To collect our photo-narratives in Fall of 2020, we conducted an additional Zoom session producing 51 pages of transcript. We decided on "participatory photography," meaning we agreed to take and share photographs representing MotherScholar support (Holm et al., 2018). During that meeting and through a subsequent email, Sarah clarified and asked for five to seven photographs and/or social media posts that captured each MotherScholar's social support and resilience experiences. A total of 36 photos, seven pages of single-space narratives, and 11 tweets comprise the photo-narrative data we drew on for this chapter.

Analysis

Analysis of our data began with Sarah surveying our data, identifying supportive relationships and their role in resilience, and noting how we communicated MotherScholar transformations during COVID-19. While assuming an open and iterative process of coding and categorizing data (Glaser & Strauss, 1967; Miles & Huberman, 1994), the social support and CTR literatures guided Sarah, with an attentiveness to the process of communicating support, resilience, and transformation and its temporal evolution through photo-narrative data. Consistent with qualitative methodology using member checks, Sarah organized the data into thematically segmented parts and shared the themes with the writing team for feedback, perception-checking, and reflection, resulting in the collaborative photo-narrative work in the next section (Chase, 2017; Lincoln & Guba, 1985).

THE PANDEMIC IN THREE PARTS

We tell our story in three parts starting with explanations of nervousness and emergence of new friendships (see above). After explaining the beginning of the friendships, we move into part one, which captures the initial minutes, hours, and weeks of COVID-19. Then, in part two we explore our use of social support; finally, part three emphasizes resilience and how the social support strengthened us and prompted creative expression. We close with an epilogue of Spring 2021, as we worked on this chapter.

Part 1: The Event

The impact of the COVID-19 pandemic was the catalyst that led to not only the development of our friendships but our use of social support and resilience. It is only fitting that our story begins with the various snapshots of how COVID-19 impacted us individually. Using pictures, narratives, and social media, we captured our emotional labor, isolation, worker bee, and struggle to balance mother and scholar.

From Elizabeth's fieldnotes entitled "Pre-MotherScholar Zoom Jitters":

> I remember being so nervous before our first Zoom session together. I had attended numerous Zoom meetings, but I had not set up a Zoom meeting prior to this one. Then, it all fell apart. I began the meeting, but no one was in my meeting room. They started emailing that they were waiting for the "host" to start the meeting. Zoom kept telling me that I could not start another meeting. Literally, I thought they would give up on me before we ever got started. But they didn't, and they even told me to stop apologizing when stuff like that happened. They reminded me that I was enough.

From Chrissy's fieldnotes entitled "A Million Questions":

> The blurring of roles . . . this is me in my office in a work meeting. I am communicating with my professional contacts in Zoom, while my 9-year-old watches TikToks on the floor in my office, out of sight. She has headphones on to minimize any noises from her device that keeps her entertained. It is almost like I am pretending she is not there. But she is always there, 24/7, day and night, my little mini-me, my shadow. During my workday her needs are an underlying current of my work. Did she do her schoolwork? How do I support her in math? . . . Does she need lunch? Does she get enough exercise? She probably watched too much TV today. All this running through my head like trickling background noise to my consciousness, as I participate in Zoom, teach class, write emails, present at conferences.

Our initial COVID-19 MotherScholar field notes reverberate with our anxieties, fears, questions, and uncertainties to which we answered, as best we could, with a façade of ordering, scheduling, and structure. Consider the following poetic narrative constructed by Lauren.

Lauren's "Noticeably Absent" poem:

> Could you organize and create a professional space of support,
> advocacy, achievement documentation, response for me like
> O.W.L.E. does?
> No, but make sure you send in your log of hours you've worked to
> prove to us that you have been working around the clock.
> Could you help me manage my mental health like a nature walk
> does?
> No, but make sure you are going above and beyond to be flexible
> for your students.
> Could you provide me space to escape and breathe and time to take
> joy and renew my heart like the Arts do?
> No, but you have 48-hours to complete this task.
> Could you send me a quick note acknowledging that I am doing a
> damn good job right now like my son does every day?
> ["You're on mute."]
> Could you show up and equip me with a few basic tools that I need
> to survive my job during a global pandemic, just like my Wolf Pack
> does?
> [Camera off]
> Could you literally just check on me during a historic, state-wide,
> blackout-causing winter storm like my Squad did when they brought
> gasoline to us from another city?
> No, but if you MUST bring your young children—who are shel-
> tering with you during a week with no heat, no power, and no
> water—to campus so you can access wifi to keep teaching you have
> *temporary* permission to do so.
> Could you light up my world like my husband did by not only
> upholding holiday traditions, but actually making them bigger and
> better?
> [Camera off]
> Could you offer me the simplest form of comfort like chicken fried
> steak and a glass of wine does?
> ["You're on mute."]

Lauren's poem points to the need for a semblance of organization. She and her social network fill that need through self-organization. In the absence of institutional resources for support, our reflections pointed to our communicative behaviors that supported the structures needed for our familial and professional roles.

Part 2: Support

Lauren: I love the support system . . . right here we created our own support systems.

As COVID-19 continued, we exhibited signs of support either directly or indirectly. For some, a simple email or text turned one's attitude from grumpy to happy. Not only did we turn to each other, but we turned to our social networks outside of our research team. We exhibited what Buzzanell (2010) refers to as affirming our identity anchors (each other and our networks) as well as maintaining and using our communication networks for support.

Visual Representation (social media)

From the Twitter Account of Sarah

Our immediate, face-to-face interactions with our families continually sought out support. Lauren's and Chrissy's narratives punctuate this section aptly illustrating both virtual and in-person support from friends, colleagues, and family.

Lauren's narrative entitled "Marco Polo Virtual Support":

> This year my friends have "virtually" lived in my house with me. Through *Marco Polo*, I have had a 24–7 lifeline to women who have watched me learn to cook, blown the wind at my back as I broke down in tears, hyped me up on the bad days, given me verbal hugs on the very bad days, clink! clinked! with me for professional accomplishments and personal achievements, and put into perspective the things that were making my life crumble to pieces. They've

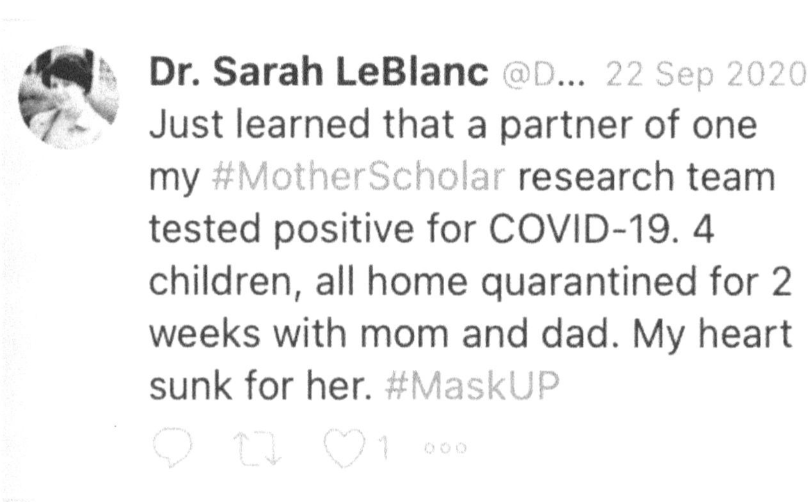

Figure 3.1 Sarah's Tweet.

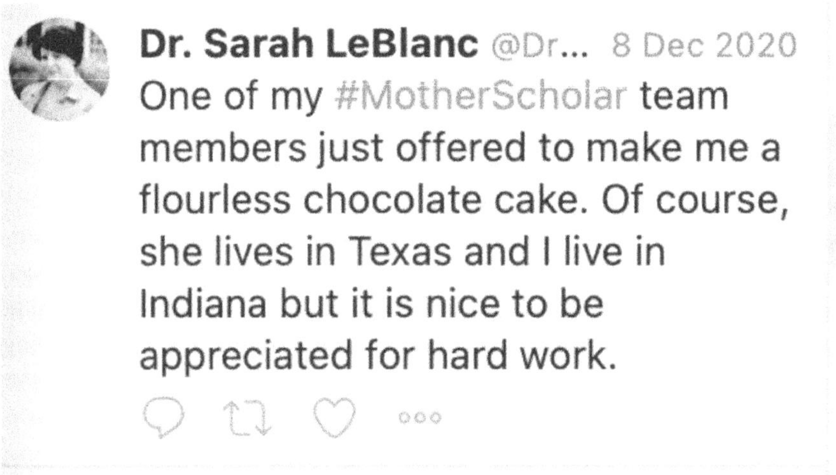
Dr. Sarah LeBlanc @Dr... 8 Dec 2020
One of my #MotherScholar team members just offered to make me a flourless chocolate cake. Of course, she lives in Texas and I live in Indiana but it is nice to be appreciated for hard work.

Figure 3.2 Sarah's Tweet.

> pushed me to talk about politics, police brutality, and the accurate pluralization of "octopus." They've listened to my kids tell jokes, they've warned me of family unfriendly policies coming down the pipe, they've advised me on email compositions . . . they've danced to entertain me, they've reminded me how special and valuable and smart and capable and strong I am.

From Chrissy's field notes entitled "(In)Visibly Safe":

> My 9-year-old daughter, my consistent shadow, my friends always know she is there, sometimes she peeks into a Zoom with them. She knows they are safe people, that they are happy to see her, that they know her name. She knows when to be seen and when to be invisible. Which meetings I give her the side eye to stay away, and which meetings I motion her to come over and talk to me. She knows and sees too much of my struggle. I worry about her mental health; I am not taking time to worry about my own. One night I was crying, and she looked at me and said, "Mama, it is always ok to cry." I had said that to her recently, and she knew she needed to say it back to me. COVID has been the worst year of my life, family members dying, extremely stressful work situations, a sick spouse, and a marriage separation, and moving myself and four kids into a rental house in the middle of work/school week. My child has seen me struggle, and she has seen my friends as my calm and constant source of support. . . . Some days I wonder if I am her shadow.

Part 3: Resilience

Our mutual use of support catalyzed professional and personal drives to foreground productive action during the rough times (Buzzanell, 2010).

Our challenges included being stuck at our home offices toiling away with diminished professional appreciation from the higher-ups and hitting metaphorical brick walls because of lack of communication or supplies required to be successful. In other words, our resiliency was threatened. Our shared social network functioned as a safe site to air these threats and a supportive site of active resistance to our limited resources. Because of each other's support, we practiced creative solutions to re-organize our MotherScholar lives (Buzzanell, 2010). Our visual and verbal narratives highlight our individual and collective accomplishments enabled by our supportive networks. Whether commemorating an organizational drive to give back to women in the community, artistically expressing a perceived frustration, or curating images of familial activity, these images and accompanying narratives demonstrate our MotherScholar resiliency.

Heather's image and narrative entitled "OWLE's Collective Action":

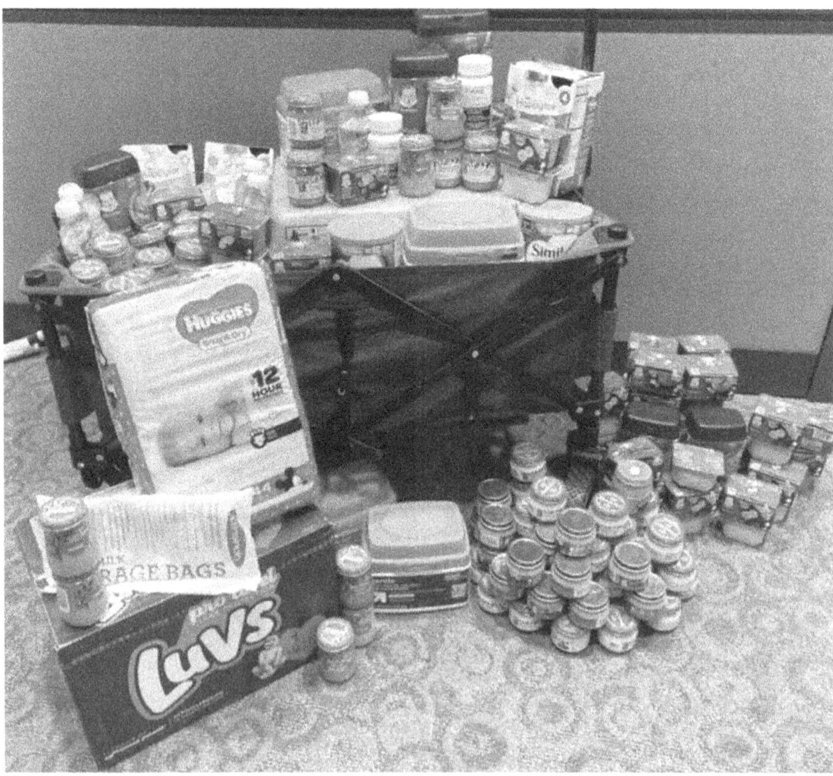

Figure 3.3 OWLE Pantry Drive.
Photo taken by Heather Olson Beale.

This picture is of a drive that the Organization for Women's Leadership and Equity (the new professional women's organization on campus that I started in September 2021) did for baby/toddler-related items for our campus pantry. They weren't collecting any such items. When we found that out, we worked hard and long to figure out a way to fill this need. This kind of work has also been very satisfying to me.

Lauren's Stationary Bike

This year there was no stopping; it was a constant go-go-go. . . . Some days it felt like I was on a stationary bike—pedaling at full speed, but still getting nowhere; no change of scenery; no end of the ride; no destination—and other days I was huffing and puffing my way up hills and down valleys, never knowing when I could stop for a water break, if I was on the right path, if the roads up ahead were smooth and gravel-free or steep and scary with loose pebbles ready to trip me up. My back tire kept me supported (spokes read: the names of my husband and children) and my front tire kept me steady (spokes read: the attitudes, practices, identities that kept me going; for example, MotherScholarhood grounded me, Teaching brought me joy, a glittery personality kept me positive, etc.) as I just kept pedaling and tried to enjoy the ride.

This is the creative, familial resiliency that resided with our immediate family's pandemic adaptations. We decided that our home would be a place to play, create, and grow—through structured and unstructured activities. We collaborated for special occasion desserts, gardening, outdoor play/projects, holiday activities, cardboard creations, and special snack time with mom.

In sum, Sarah tweeted on July 14, 2020, "4 women I have never met but am collaborating with are quickly becoming some of my favorite people. Their emails bring me smiles. #academicpartnerships #motherscholar." Similarly,

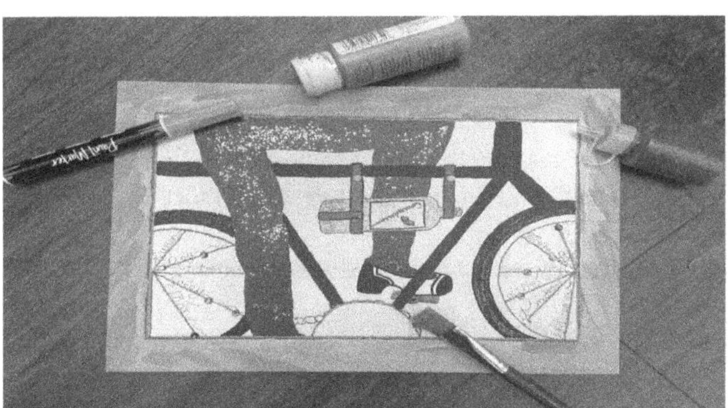

Figure 3.4 Lauren's Stationary Bike.
Artwork and Photo by Lauren Burrow.

Chrissy wrote, "this year has been one the best of my professional life, while one of the worst of my personal life. What a strange paradox." Yes, the negative and positives of pandemic life featured prominently in our photo-narrative work; but our MotherScholar networks provided support for productive action and affirmed our MotherScholar identity anchors.

EPILOGUE

A Group Zoom Call

> Chrissy: we should all submit to the International Congress on Qualitative Inquiry next year when it is in person. That way we could all finally meet in person and celebrate all of our work. No more raising our glasses at screens.

This chapter sheds light on the role of support to prompt resiliency through social networks, especially the MotherScholars authoring this piece. Despite the enormity of COVID-19, and perhaps because of it, we offered essential support. We acknowledge the hardships COVID-19 posed for women in academia, especially caregivers, as their personal and professional workloads and work-life boundaries were exacerbated by COVID-19. With each new shift in our personal narratives, we had a counterpart in our group we could reach out to who would understand the frustration, be able to empathize, and say the right thing to help us keep going.

Of concern to us is the lack of institutional support for other women academics to foreground productive action, enable support networks at work, or identify alternative logics that would constitute a new normal to affirm their maternal and scholarly identity anchors. As soon as colleges and universities made the modality switch to online education, women academics began to feel the impact (Almanssori & Hiller, 2021). Mothers handled more of the domestic responsibilities while trying to maintain a good academic face (Almanssori, 2021; Spradley et al., 2021). Our data demonstrates that we excelled both professionally (our MotherScholar research produced six chapters and articles) and in our mother roles (survived homeschooling, COVID-19 scares).

Gender disparities existed in higher education before COVID-19 (Moodley & Gouws, 2020); COVID-19 widened the disparity gap as many academics mothers took on a brunt of childcare and domestic responsibilities (King & Frederickson, 2021). None of this additional physical, mental, and/or emotional work women academics completed during the initial months of COVID-19 is factored into promotion and tenure procedures (Moodley &

Gouws, 2020). As a result of gender disparities in higher education, many academic mothers lack institutional support and mentoring. Lawless (2021) and Hicks Roof (2021) were told that they would have it easy on their maternity leave, only to have COVID-19 disprove that myth. Research projects fell apart, and they felt their newborns lacked the attention they deserved. When Lawless (2021) wrote about reaching out to colleagues, she heard echoes of earlier words that she was lucky to be on maternity leave.

We began this chapter by describing the picture on the front page of the February 21, 2021 *New York Times*; each dot represented a life lost to COVID-19. While we will mourn those we have lost, a representation of how the rest of us persevered is just as important. We may not have persevered in similar ways, using similar resources, or even developed new friendships; but many of us, especially MotherScholars, will emerge from this pandemic realizing that we could—and we will—survive anything.

REFERENCES

Adams, T.A. & Holman Jones, S. (2018). The art of autoethnography. In P. Leavy (Ed.), *Handbook of Arts-Based Research* (1st ed., pp. 141–64). Guilford Press.

Albrecht, T. L., Burleson, B. R., & Sarason, I. (1992). Meaning and method in the study of communication and social support. *Communication Research, 19*, 149–53.

Almanssori, S., & Hillier, K.M. (2020/2021). Frontline workers from home: A feminist duoethnographic inquiry of mothering, teaching, and academia during the initial stages of COVID-19 pandemic. *Journal of Motherhood Initiative, 11/12*, 171–88.

Burleson, B. R. (2003). Emotional support skills. In J. O. Green & B. R. Burleson (Eds.), *Handbook of communication and social interaction skills* (pp. 551–94). Lawrence Erlbaum Associates.

Burleson, B. R. (2008). What counts as effective emotional support? Explorations of individual and situational differences. In M. T. Motley (Ed.), *Studies in applied interpersonal communication* (pp. 207–27). Sage.

Burrow, L. E., Cross, C. J., Olson Beal, H. K., & Smith, S. (2020). The skits, sketches, and stories of motherscholars. *Qualitative Report, 25*, 4245–73.

Buzzanell, P. M. (2010). Resilience: Talking, resisting, and imagining new normalices into being. *Journal of Communication, 60*, 1–14.

Buzzanell, P. M. (2018a). Organizing resilience as adaptive-transformational tensions. *Journal of Applied Communication Research, 46*, 14–18. https://doi.org/10.1080/00909882.2018.1426711.

Buzzanell, P. M. (2018b). Communication theory of resilience: Enacting adaptive-transformative processes when families experience loss and disruption. In D. O. Braithwaite, E. Suter, & K. Floyd (Eds.), *Engaging theories in family communication: Multiple perspectives* (pp. 98–109). Routledge.

Buzzanell, P. M. (2019). Communication theory of resilience in everyday talk, interactions, and network structures. In S. R. Wilson & S. W. Smith (Eds.), *Reflections on interpersonal communication research* (pp. 65–88). Cognella.

Chase, E. (2017). Enhanced member check: Reflections and insights from a participant-researcher collaboration. *Qualitative Report, 22*, 2689–2703.

Clark, S. C. (2000). Work/family border theory: A new theory of work/family balance. *Human Relations, 52*, 747–70.

Doherty, E. (2021). "It's just like a break-up": A qualitative analysis of turning points in female friendships in early to middle adulthood. *Communication Quarterly, 69*, 43–66.

Ellingson, L. L. (2009). *Engaging crystallization in qualitative research: An introduction*. Sage.

Ellis, C., Kiesinger, C. E., & Tillman-Healy, L.M. (1997). Interactive interviewing: Talking about emotional experience. In R. Hertz (Ed.), *Reflexivity and voice* (pp. 119–49). Sage.

Faulkner, S L. (2018). Poetic inquiry: Poetry as/in/for social research. In P. Leavy (Ed.), *Handbook of Arts-Based Research*, (1st ed., pp. 208–31). Guilford Press.

Freeman, M. (2018). Narrative inquiry. In P. Leavy (Ed.), *Handbook of Arts-Based Research*, (1st ed., pp. 123–40). Guilford Press.

Fritz, J. H. (2015). Researching workplace relationships: What can we learn from qualitative organizational studies? *Journal of Social and Personal Relationships, 31*, 460–66.

Gist-Mackey, A. N., Kunkel, A., & Guthrie, J. A. (2021). Prioritizing ourselves and our values: Intersectionality, positionality, and dismantling the neoliberal university system, *Academic Labor: Research and Artistry, 5*, 20–48.

Glaser, B. G., & Strauss, A. L. (1967). *The discovery of grounded theory: Strategies for qualitative research*. Aldine Publishing.

Gonzales, L. & Griffin, K. (2020). *Supporting faculty during and after COVID-19: Don't let equity go.* ASPIRE: The National Alliance for Inclusive & Diverse STEM Faculty.

Harris, J. I., Winskowski, A. M., & Engdahl, B. E. (2011). Types of workplace social support in the prediction of job satisfaction. *The Career Development Quarterly, 56*(2), 150–56. http://doi.org/10.1002/j.2161-0045.2007.tb00027.x.

Hayden, S. & O'Brien Hallstein, L. (2021). An ode to academic mothers: Finding gratitude and grace in the midst of COVID-19. In A. O'Reilly & F.J. Green (Eds.), *Mothers, mothering, and COVID-19: Dispatches from a Pandemic* (pp. 169–80). Demeter Press.

Hicks-Roof, K. (2020/2021). The continuous clock: A working academic mother during COVID-19. *Journal of Mother Initiative, 11/12*, 265–76. https://jarm.journals.yorku.ca/index.php/jarm/article/view/40619.

Holm, G., Shalström, & Zilliacus, H. (2018). Arts-based visual research. In P. Leavy (Ed.), *Handbook of Arts-Based Research* (1st ed., pp. 311–35). Guilford Press.

Howlett, M. (2021). Looking at the 'field' through a Zoom lens: Methodologivcal reflections on conducting online research during a global pandemic. *Qualitative Research, 1–16. https://* 1468.794120985691.

Jones, R.G. (2007). Drag queens, drama queens, and friends: Drama and performance as solidarity-building function in gay male friendship circle. *Kaledioscope, 6,* 61–84.

King, M.M. & Frederickson, M.E. (2021). The pandemic penalty: The gendered effects of COVID-19 on scientific productivity. *Socius: Sociological Research for a Dynamic World, 7,* 1–24. https://10.1177/23780231211006977.

Kossek, E. E., Pchler, S., Bodner, T., & Hammer, L. B. (2011). Workplace social support and work-family conflict: A meta-analysis clarifying the influence of general work-family specific supervisor and organizational support. *Perspectives in Psychology, 64*(2), 289–313. https://doi.org/10.111/j1744-6570.2011.01211.x.

Lapayese, Y. V. (2012). *Mother-scholar: Reimagining K-12 education.* Springer Science & Business Media.

Lawless, B. (2021). Examining inequitable workload in a time of crisis: A COVID-19 "sabbatical." *Communication, Culture and Critique, 0,* 1–4. https://10.1093/ccc/tcab016.

LeBlanc, S. S. (2021). Portraying real feelings with comedy on top: Postpartum depression storylines and domestic sitcoms. In M. A. Johnson & C. J. Olson (Eds.), *Normalizing mental illness and neurodiversity in entertainment media: Quieting the madness* (134–49). Routledge.

LeBlanc, S. S., Spradley, E.L., Olson Beal, H., Burrow, L., & Cross, C. (2021a). Communication theory of identity, identity gap theory, and MotherScholaring during COVID-19. *Iowa Journal of Communication.*

LeBlanc, S. S., Spradley, E. L., Olson Beal, H. K., Burrow, L., & Cross, C. (2021b). Being Dr. Mom and/or Mom, Ph.D. [Manuscript submitted for publication]. Department of Communication Purdue University Fort Wayne.

Lincoln, Y. S., & Guba, E. G. (1985). *Naturalistic inquiry.* Thousand Oaks, CA: Sage.

Malisch, J.L., Harris, B.N., Sherrer, S.M., Lewis, K.A., Shepherd, S.L., McCarthy, P.C., Spott, J.L., Karam, E.P., Moustaid-Moussa, N., Calarco, J.M., Ramalingam, L., Talley, A.E., Canas-Carrell, J.E., Ardon-Bryer, K., Weister, D.A., Bernal, X.E., & Deitloff, J. (2020). In the wake of COVID-19, academia needs new solutions to ensure gender equity. *Proceedings of the National Academy of Sciences of the United States of America.* 15378–81. https://doi.org/10.1073/pnas.2010636117.

Matias, C. (2011, April). "Cheryl Matias, Ph.D. and mother of twins": Counter storytelling to critically analyze how I navigated the academic application, negotiation, and relocation process. [Paper presentation]. American Educational Research Association (AERA) Annual Meeting, New Orleans.

McBride, M. C., & Mason, K. M. (2015). Work spouses: Defining and understanding a "new" relationship. *Communication Studies, 66,* 487–508.

McDermott, M. (2020/2021). Learning from the experiences of mothers of school-aged children on tenure track during the COVID-19 global pandemic. *Journal of Motherhood Initiative, 11/12,* 247–64. https://jarm.journals.yorku.ca/index.php/jarm/article/view/40618.

McGlynn, J., III, & Richardson, B. (2014). Private support, public alienation: Whistle-blowers and the paradox of social support. *Western Journal of Communication, 78,* 213–37.

Meluch, A. L., & LeBlanc, S. S. (2021). Up all night with Facebook: A new mother's use of an online community to find social support. In C. Liberman & K. Wright (Eds.), *Casing mediated communication* (pp. 231–43). Kendall Hunt.

Miles, M. B., & Huberman, M. A. (1994). *Qualitative data analysis: An expanded sourcebook*. Sage.

Moodley, K. & Gouws, A. (2020). How women in academia are feeling the brunt of COVID-19. *The Conversation*, https://theconversation.com/how-women-in-academia-are-feeling-the-brunt-of-covid-19-144087.

O'Reilly, A. (2020/2021). Academic motherhood and COVID-19. [Special Issue]. *Journal of Motherhood Initiative, 11/12.* https://jarm.journals.yorku.ca/index.php/jarm/issue/view/2317.

O'Reilly, A., & Green, F. J. (2021). *Mothers, mothering, and COVID-19: Dispatches from a pandemic*. Demeter Press.

Pietrabissa, G., & Simpson, S. G. (2020). Psychological consequences of social isolation during COVID-19 outbreak. *Frontiers in Psychology, 11*, https://doi.org/10.3389/fpsyg.2020.02201.

Rising, C. J., Bol, N., Burke-Garcia, A., Rains, S., & Wright, K. B. (2017). Perceived stress in online prostate cancer community participants: Examining relationship with stigmatization, social support network preference, and social support seeking. *Journal of Health Communication, 22*, 469–76.

Russell, L. D. (2020). Making collective sense of uncertainty: How online social support communities negotiate meaning for contested illness. In N. Egbert & K. B. Wright (Eds.), *Social support and health in the digital age* (pp. 171–90). Lexington.

Sassi, K., & Thomas, E. E. (2012). "If you weren't researching me and a friend . . . ": The mobius of friendship and mentorship as methodological approaches to qualitative research. *Qualitative Inquiry, 18*(10), 830–42.

Scott, A. M., Martine, S. C., Stone, A. M., & Brashers, D. E. (2011). Managing multiple goals in supportive interactions: Using a normative theoretical approach to explain social support as uncertainty management for organ transplant patients. *Health Communication, 26*, 393–403.

Skinner, M., Betancourt, N., & Wolff-Eisenberg, C. (2021). The disproportionate impact of the pandemic on women and caregivers in academia. *Ithaka S+R*. https://doi.org/10.18665/sr/315147.

Spradley, E. L., LeBlanc, S. S., Olson Beal, H. K., Burrow, L., and Cross, C. (2020/2021). Proving our maternal and scholarly worth: A collaborative autoethnographic textual and visual storying of MotherScholar identity work in COVID-19. *Journal of Motherhood Initiative, 11/12*, https://jarm.journals.yorku.ca/index.php/jarm/article/view/40614.

Spradley, E. L., LeBlanc, S. S., Olson Beal, H. K., Burrow, L., and Cross, C. (2021). Crystalizing layered approaches to mother-scholar expressions in COVID-19: A photovoice and autoethnographic study. [Manuscript submitted for publication]. Department of Language, Culture, & Communication, Stephen F. Austin State University.

Thibaut, F. & van Wijngaarden-Cremers, P.J.M. (2020). Women's mental health in the time of COVID-19 pandemic. *Frontiers in Global Women's Health, 1, online.* https://10.3389/fgwh.2020.588372.

Tillman-Healy, L. (2003). Friendship as method. *Qualitative Inquiry, 9*, 729–49.

Wang, C. C. (1999). Photovoice: A participatory action research strategy applied to women's health. *Journal of Women's Health, 8*, 185–94.

Chapter Four

The Ritual of the Bering Sea

Commodity, Country, and Mortality in Deadliest Catch

Derek Moscato

The rise of streaming television services and a proliferation of "binge viewing" media consumption behaviors, particularly during the global COVID-19 pandemic, have paralleled the growth of reality entertainment genres that emphasize the contemporary material underpinnings of environmental and spatial communication. The state of Alaska has served as a popular backdrop for such media productions. Reality television programs focused on the exploits of northerly and Arctic adventure, and resources extraction industries provide a lens into the time and space dimensions of television production, distribution, and consumption. But they also provide insight into how geographic mediation transforms viewing audiences at home through a larger cognitive and social process of media ritual. In conjunction with a global crisis like the coronavirus pandemic, the mediation of social structures and ecological space shifts rapidly in the face of volatile markets, government health regulation, and a transformed supply chain.

The case of Discovery Channel's long-running flagship program *Deadliest Catch* provides a substantive case in point. The program's evolution over nearly two decades echoes the challenges facing not only the larger Alaska fishery, but also mirrors macroeconomic and social forces that configure contemporary life. While in its early years the program focused on the workplace dangers of crab fishing on the Bering Sea, it has expanded its scope to incorporate overriding themes of nationhood, ecology, global economics, and the larger human experience. This media dynamic aligns with existing scholarly perspectives. In his seminal text *Communication as Culture*, James

Carey (2002) established a divergence between an understanding of media as a transmitting medium, to one that established mediation as a sequence of rites. While this view pays some attention to the narratives embedded within the production of news and entertainment content, it is equally concerned with the social, behavioral, and cognitive outcomes arising from the systems of communication in which such content is embedded and subsumed. Such a perspective emphasizes the role of media technology and production, but it also situates media as a potential conduit in overcoming both space and time and as a facilitator of community and social organization.

This process takes on particular significance during a global health emergency like the coronavirus pandemic. In the weeks and months after the onset of the virus, audiences moved from traditional news and broadcast services to the kind of programming that offered both escapism and companionship (Johnson & Dempsey, 2021). Television programs became a generator of conversations both "within the household and on social media—allowing a sense of connection with others" (para. 5). Long-running dramatizations, soap operas, and reality productions therefore took on a heightened role not only in terms of individual- and group-level cognition but also as an unlikely catalyst for civic engagement. *Deadliest Catch,* like many of its reality entertainment counterparts, provided more than surface-level storylines. It offered symbolic renderings of the commercial workplace and the larger national context in which they are placed. It also positioned the industry of crab fishing as an arena in which one contemplates social connections, workplace traditions, and the longer-lasting implications of real-world tragedy. The program's sixteenth season, which captured the crab fishing season during a trade war between Russia and the United States, and the early impacts of COVID-19 on the Alaska fishery and global crab market, was broadcast by the Discovery Channel during the height of the pandemic. This was a time when home media consumption surged in the wake of government-imposed lockdowns and stay-at-home orders (Adgate, 2020). That same sixteenth season offered new and updated narratives of longstanding family dynamics interrupted by life-changing events both on and off the fishing boats, including the onset of the COVID-19 pandemic. And it provided the narrative of the all-too-real tragedy of the sinking of the F/V *Scandies Rose*, in which five lives were ultimately lost to the Bering Sea (Hollander & Wieber, 2020). All of these storylines provided a sequence in which viewers might consider their relationship to work, ecology, and economy through a repetitive process that emphasizes larger social organizing units, including family and nationhood. This mode of receiving content that both shapes and maintains an understanding of the larger world lies at the heart of the ritual model of communication (Anderson, 2011).

ON-SCREEN ALASKA: COMMODITY, CONFLICT, COMMUNITY

Since 2005, *Deadliest Catch* has aired on television screens across the United States and the globe, and has become one of the most popular and long-lasting programs of the contemporary era. Depicting the lives of crabbers working in Alaska's Bering Sea, the program is now shown in more than 200 countries and is one of the most successful shows of its kind since the advent of the reality genre. By its third season, the *New York Times* dubbed the program "a cult hit" (Hale, 2007) and after 10 seasons it was still pulling the highest ratings for any program ever on Discovery Channel (O'Carroll, 2010). At the same time, it is credited with having started a long-running boom for Alaska- and Arctic-reality themed shows, which also include *Ice Road Truckers* (launched in 2007), *Ice Pilots* (2009), *Bering Sea Gold* (2012), *Ultimate Survival Alaska* (2013), *Yukon Gold* (2013), and *Alaskan Bush People* (2014). Its popularity owes to a combination of stunning videography, high seas drama, ecological danger, and narratives that are carved out by the unique nature of the crab fishing workplace. As one scholarly observation describes it, "Unlike so much reality TV, it is a show for looking at, not looking through, and at times it's as though you are inside an epic contemporary adventure novel" (Blundell, 2017, para. 18).

Financial imperatives and the global marketplace drive many of the program's narratives. The featured boats, with names like the *Cornelia Marie*, *Time Bandit*, and *Northwestern*, regularly earn millions of dollars from king or opilio crab fishing. This translates into handsome paydays for both captains and deck hands. Within and outside of the program, the fishing boat captains are measured by the financial success of their vessels (Covey & Ewell, 2015); and such measurement is gamified by show producers to induce greater excitement within the program. At the same time, scholars have examined the program through lenses of "expropriation and proletarianization" (Wells, 2015) as well as class and gender (Blair, 2013; Kirby, 2013; Buchanan, 2014). Furthermore, the program's production is understood as the labor of both crab fishermen and television workers (Wells, 2015). This formula has allowed the program to "carve out a distinguished place in the history of U.S. maritime storytelling" while juxtaposing "extreme danger with cowboy-style free enterprise, bravado and macho sentimentality" (Blundell, 2017, paras. 2 and 4).

Yet it is the expression of labor and workplace ritual that drives a larger curiosity about the program's social legacy. For example, the mediation of logistics surrounding the crab fishery has shed new light on operations such as emergency medical response. As a case in point, Buttner (2020) points to the Iliuliuk Family and Health Services health center on Unalaska Island in the Aleutians. The facility is immersed in the larger Dutch Harbor maritime community, which sees an influx of over 6,000 seasonal workers during the fishing seasons and a workforce drawn from many countries and several continents. Yet it is the cycle of resources extraction and commodification that underpins the bulk of storylines. Primary sector reality television shows about fishing, logging, and mining make masculinity, competition, and bravery prominent, but they also showcase U.S. symbolism, with Americans represented as particularly skilled at navigating and exploiting natural resources (Clark et al., 2020). The staying power of programs devoted to raw materials presents a paradox, however. Even as jobs creation in these industries plateaus, particularly in hard-hit regions, the programs about them and by extension their audiences continue to grow (Clark et al., 2020). This paradox sheds light on the complex relationship between ecological-philosophical themes of idealism and materialism within this form of environmental media. Even in the face of diminished natural resources, the demand for programming about their extraction holds steady. Thus, even as on-screen Alaska serves up polar adventure and escapism, it also serves as a metaphor for the contemporary challenges of the global economy and the commodities workforce.

THE DISCURSIVE-MATERIAL CATCH

The confluence of communicative and material considerations within media processes comprises what Carpentier (2017) articulates as a discursive-material knot. This perspective highlights how discursively produced phenomena, such as language and symbols, interface with economic, spatial, and other geographic variables. A critique of the idealism emphasized by Laclau and Mouffe (1985) is that it reduced material forms to socially-constructed conceptions (Joseph, 2003). Yet communication formats within the arena of civic life, including community media, but also specific content such as documentary films, afford a perspective that intertwines the symbolic and material:

> The knotted interaction of the discursive and the material—in always particular and contingent ways—structures large-scale assemblages, such as state apparatuses, armies, or markets, but it also enters into the micro-processes of the everyday without these different levels ever becoming disconnected. (Carpentier, 2017, p. 4)

Here, the knot serves as a metaphor that underpins the complexity and necessity of the relationship between these two drivers in communication processes. Unlike views that emphasize how materiality receives its meaning through discursive output, thus situating it in a passive mode, Carpentier's knot points to the agency and dynamism of materialism while providing a platform for agency, participation, and engagement.

This speaks to the core catalysts of ecological media. The concepts of nature and environment as produced and consumed in media spheres are socially-constructed and therefore produce a recurring dialectic within traditional media texts but also the genre of reality television programs. Pointing to Prometheanism—a view of nature as serving human interests (Dryzek, 2013)—these media discourses reinforce invocations of extraction processes as historically grounded and socially desirable (Murphy, 2017). Integrated into this overarching dialogue is a robust debate about the limits of the planet's natural resources, and whether human action through innovation and technological advancement can expedite or hinder real solutions.

This ongoing deliberation—whether articulated through production techniques, the actions of program participants, or the interplay of immediate audience reception and longer-term cognition—comprises an important dimension of the discursive-material knot: the structure/agency dimension. Contrary to structural views, it emphasizes human agency and freedom: "the overdetermined and contingent logic of structure, which is both enabling and disabling, is combined with a plurality of subjectivations and identifications, invitations and dislocations" (Carpentier, 2017, p. 8).

DEVOTION AND REDEMPTION IN POLAR MEDIA

Because of the contingencies described above, the proliferation of Arctic and Alaska reality television programs presents a special challenge for the media scholar. Such artifacts are often understood through lenses of nostalgia (Kraszewski, 2017), representation (Fleras & Dixon, 2011), and political economy (Moscato, 2017). But to a surprising extent their impacts are felt beyond these realms and extend into civic life. The communication scholar James Carey revived the sometimes overlooked tradition of empirical approaches in communication, particularly by drawing from John Dewey and the notion of an engaged public sphere, as well as Durkheim's work on ritual (Carey, 2008; Blue, 2019). Further, Carey's work draws extensively from the Canadian geographer, historian, and international communication scholar Harold Innis, who understood media systems through their linkages to the material world and raw materials in particular (Carey, 1967).

The popularity of programs such as *Deadliest Catch* owes in great part to both tried-and-true narrative formulas and of a loyal audience that returns to the program every season for an assemblage of vivid nautical scenes, sequenced music and sound effects, and emotional soliloquys from victorious captains and exhausted deckhands. This devotion to a media artifact speaks to Carey's ritual view of communication. This rendering of communication processes connects media to the prayers, chants, and ceremonies that themselves drive the transmission of religious ideas and articulation. As opposed to views that uphold the relaying of information as the most important facet of communication, the ritual view "sees the original or highest manifestation of communication not in the transmission of intelligent information but in the construction and maintenance of an ordered, meaningful cultural world that can serve as a control and container for human action" (Carey, 2008, p. 15).

Here, Carey reconnected communication to the interdisciplinary nature of the Chicago School and situates mass communication as a form of social binding, moving it away from the previously dominant behavioral science model that once characterized mass media studies (Pooley, 2007). In doing so, he joined other social sciences of his time that were rebelling against the science-centric (or scientifism) approach that put blind faith in the combination of quantitative methodology and natural science. Like his fellow insurgents, Carey elevated "history and particularity" (Pooley, 2007). But this era of communication also saw Carey aligned with other scholars accounting for active audiences and the particulars of their engagement with media (Livingstone, 2002). In key ways Carey's ritual view shares objectives with Katz's (1979) uses and gratifications theory of mass media, in understanding specific audience engagements with media texts and also the nuances of transmission of content from producer to media consumer.

A material view of civic life informs this understanding of communication. Drawing from Durkheim's *The Elementary Forms of the Religious Life: A Study in Religious Sociology* (1915), Carey's ritual view points to a range of media artifacts that discursively organize social life and processes, including news stories and public speeches but also creative works such as architecture and the performing arts (Carey, 2008). More recent considerations of Carey's perspective have situated digital practices and customs as a contemporary form of information ritual, especially as they help to construct both individual and social reality (Sen, 2017). This presents a paradox of solitary and self-directed audiences who are simultaneously connected to the social world. In the case of reality television programs documenting social-ecological phenomena, the degree to which such a linkage is made might be contingent upon not only the descriptive action of production variables such as videography and narration, but also their "suggestive and elliptical nature." Thus, the documentary reality program might easily evolve from its traditional conventional boundaries to the loftier realm of art filmmaking (Grimes, 2002).

As a result of its malleability, ritualistic media therefore can serve the ends of institutions and other dominant structures, and is easily leveraged for ideological purposes. Through the ritual lens, Durham's (2008) analysis of news coverage of Hurricane Katrina establishes a disruption of the news media's rites of consensus with government, in contrast to a "sphere of consensus" that defined the media-government relationship after the September 11, 2001 attacks. A related view from Carlson (2001) argued that, in the spirit of Walter Cronkite and the popularity of his nightly newscasts for millions of Americans, journalists need to understand their professional role in both historical and contemporary contexts by recognizing the importance of ritual. A failure to do so has in part led to a decline in journalistic authority and a news industry that is increasingly unable to face the challenges of the current information environment.

Ultimately, this multi-layered process of transmission, reception, engagement, and action provides a foundation for shifting the larger understanding of community. Carey's ritual and culture-fused view of media draws from Dewey's articulation of the great community, itself comprised of transportation and mass media systems. Yet this notion of community is elastic, with its ebb and flow subject to the whims of the technological nature of its rituals. These rituals feature techniques and objects, but they can also include modes of hierarchy, control, and authority (Marvin, 1990). Thus, the rituals that comprise contemporary media serve to enrich communities even as they set the stage for their disintegration.

Building on this consideration of community dualism of technology-driven utopia versus dystopia, Anderson (2011) identified a digital media culture that would bring people together under a common culture and "facilitate dialogue in a ritualistic way that brings back some of the positive aspects of the oral tradition and transforms them, so that people across the globe can join the conversation" (p. 97).

THE RITES OF BERING SEA PASSAGE

Even as a populist form of entertainment within the mass media, reality television programs like *Deadliest Catch* make an impactful yet counter-intuitive contribution to the evolving literature dedicated to ecological discourses, particularly those centering the human experience in relation to nature. By extension, the Arctic's Bering Sea serves as an appropriate and compelling geographic site for analysis of this cultural artifact, given emergent global dialogue about themes of natural resources, environmental protection, climate change, and the ebb and flow of global commodities markets. The central topic of crab fishing serves as a microcosm for similar tensions playing out in numerous industries amid the globe's planetary ecological challenges, such as well-publicized battles over public lands, energy production, and resources extraction. The rites emergent from a discursive/material knot framework provide one means to contextualizing and identifying the meanings embedded in the program. A material/discursive lens identifies a cluster of discourses that give meaning to the natural world. In a context of extraction activities, these discourses can signify anthropocentrism and Prometheanism. But they also amalgamate discourses of ecological protection and the integration of humankind and nature. This approach helps bridge conceptual understanding of *Deadliest Catch* discourses as they relate to polar ecology and the Arctic's political economy, but it also helps explore the specific rites emergent from the program and their impacts on audiences.

During the sixteenth season, four overriding rites of passage were identified: 1) Commodity conflict between the U.S. and Russia; 2) The primacy of family connections; 3) The tragedy of the F/V *Scandies Rose* and the overarching theme of mortality it raised; and 4) The onset of COVID-19 at the conclusion of the season. The first rite invokes many of the narratives and tropes of the Cold War, as the program positioned the United States and Russia as arch-rivals in the quest to fish the Bering Sea, but also to patrol the fishery and bring crab to market. "It's USA versus Russia," declared the program narrator in the program's first episode, " . . . and everyone is vying for an edge" (Season 16, Episode 1). As the single-largest competitor to Alaska's fishing fleet, Russia presents an intriguing yet somewhat mysterious foil to the exploits of the American fishery. Russia's new fishing regulations were seen as aimed at cracking down on illegal fishing while restricting supply and raising prices, in turn intensifying the efforts of the Americans. Captain Sig Hansen articulated this Bering Sea economy in stark commodified terms: "This is looking to be one of the most profitable and competitive seasons in decades," he said from the bridge of the F/V *Northwestern*. "Because the Russians are now rationalizing their industry, there's going to be a race to get that crab to the market to get the highest price" (Season 16, Episode 1).

Thus, the urgency of U.S.-Russia conflict was an integral narrative driver in Season 16 as it rationalized the focus on American patriotism, but also the evolution of the crab fishery as a uniquely global enterprise. It even sent Captain "Wild" Bill Wichrowski onto Russian shores as a potential captain-for-hire in this evolving foreign market. The new regulations for the Russian crab fishery, which played a dramatic role in pushing American fishers to obtain their quota, were articulated by the show's own narration as it described the F/V *Saga*:

> New boat owner Jake Anderson and Captain Johnathan Hillstrand squeeze the gooseneck to catch a last-minute staggering 17,000 pounds of king crab. . . . Now facing a king crab price in free fall, Jake and Johnathan hunker down for a grind, eager to catch their crab before the Russians slash the American price to rubles on the dollar. (Season 16, Episode 7)

The rite of U.S.-Russia conflict drives a narrative of fluctuating commodity prices and regulatory environments. But it also emphasizes the tropes and metaphors that have defined the complicated and rhetorically exaggerated relationship between the two nations for nearly a century. Jake Anderson echoes some of these as he summarizes his boat's successes on the Bering Sea in the pursuit of king crab:

> Looking good, Johnny Boy. That's some good-looking crab. You keep fishing like this, the Russians don't stand a chance against you. Ruck you, fussia. Pow like "Rocky IV"! Pow! (laughs) After grinding through 28 exhausting days at sea. . . . Damn straight. I'm looking to make a statement with this crab I'm catching. (Season 16, Episode 6)

The Cold War mythology is furthermore integrated into labor relations on the boats. For example, the show conflates the nationality of deckhands with the global dynamics of the fishing markets. When Bill Wichrowski of the F/V *Summer Bay* is forced to fire a rookie employee from Russia for insubordination, the dispatching is presented to viewers as a contrast between respect for the fishery and a "problem" employee through the captain's parting words to his departing employee:

> . . . You know the least about anything in the fleet . . . you know what your position is? Your position as labor is, somebody says "go move" you go move. That is your job. And you have never done that from day one. . . . You know what, we're done talking. You are relieved of your duty. I want you off the boat now. (Season 16, Episode 6)

The captain's bridge serves as a stage for the performance of management, including authority, negotiation, and conflict. But it also puts a spotlight on the nautical families that comprise the fleet, including parent-child and sibling dynamics.

This second rite of family primacy is woven into every season of *Deadliest Catch*. Many of the boats on the program are family owned and operated. A case in points comes from the F/V *Northwestern* captained by Sig Hansen. In Season 16, Hansen's daughter Mandy joined the boat as a co-captain, which entails an array of responsibility for navigation, deckhand management, vessel safety, and the science of crab fishing itself. Despite earlier challenges, she and father, Sig, celebrated a substantial haul as the season approached the half-way point: "With Mandy helming the Northwestern for their last haul . . . And Captain Sig on the hook, father and daughter finish what they started. Yeah! . . . Reeling in the last of their 80,000 pounds—a $920,000 catch" (Season 16, Episode 7). The Hillstrand brothers presented a similar dynamic. Johnathan Hillstrand is introduced as being lured out of retirement to snag the "extra quota" with his friend Jake Anderson. Hillstrand, who helms the F/V *Time Bandit* in other seasons, brought along his brother Neil, nephew Philip, and wife Heather. Hillstrand declared triumphantly during the first episode that "I brought the whole damn family!" These immediate families serve as a microcosm of the Alaska fleet as a larger, cohesive social structure. And they underpin the connection of the program's participants to the extended community during good times but particularly in the aftermath of a real tragedy.

The deadly sinking of the F/V *Scandies Rose* in the Gulf of Alaska was one such event. The December 31, 2019 sinking, which occurred during the filming of Season 16, caused five deaths among the fishing vessel's crew of seven. The build-up of ice on the boat during especially cold and stormy weather, which can cause ice to form in the interior of the crab pots, was identified as a cause of the accident. This is an ongoing danger to boats, and more than 60 crab boats among the Alaska fleet regularly confront some of the most hazardous weather in North America in their pursuit of snow and king crab (Bernton, 2021).

While the F/V *Scandies Rose* was not one of the boats featured on the program, its captain and deckhands were friends and colleagues with crew members from across the show's fishing boats. Thus, the news of the fate of the F/V *Scandies Rose* presented a pivotal moment for a program like *Deadliest Catch*. Here, program participants were cognizant of their role in real-life events that are much larger than the boundaries of the tightly-packaged episodes in which their efforts are normally consumed. As *Northwest* co-captain Mandy Hansen declared, "I just can't believe that it went down. It wasn't supposed to happen"(Season 16, Episode 8). This shock was echoed by Captain Josh Harris: "You always gotta be on your toes out here. Tomorrow's never promised." Meanwhile, F/V *Lady Alaska* captain Scott Campbell Jr. articulated the notion of familial ties on the Bering Sea: "These are our brothers, and they're not coming home." These laments from crew members culminate with memorials at sea on the fishing vessels, including a symbolic tribute on the F/V *Summer Bay*, where a single rose represented each crew member lost to the ocean: "In these calm seas, we offer up these five roses so that our brothers may rest easy. . . . Farewell" (Season 16, Episode 8).

A perspective that resonated with many from the entire Bering Sea crab fishery, but also the viewers who have followed their exploits at home, was offered by F/V *Saga*'s Jake Anderson: "I've dealt with a lot of death in my life. It hurts. It doesn't feel good. I'm just worried about surviving and moving forward" (Season 16, Episode 8). These existential sentiments permeated the entire fishing fleet and provided a foreshadowing of the fishing challenges that would lie ahead, but also of a looming health pandemic about to rattle Alaska's fishery. Here, the ritual of mortality blurred the line between dramatization and reality and enveloped the audience into a larger community. It would also set the stage for the season's final act.

As *Deadliest Catch*'s sixteenthth season drew to a conclusion, a final rite crystallized the theme of mortality and civic loss. As the boats were closing out their season, word went out to the fishing fleet that a new pandemic was shutting down the country and putting the market for crab in peril. Governments from East Asia were threatening to shut down ports and the crab trade. In turn, the Alaskan fleet rushed to meet its quotas before all was lost. The narrative shifted from the U.S./Russia rivalry to the crab fishery's integration with the globe through an unprecedented international health crisis. Inside the boats, meanwhile, the news of the pandemic created confusion and panic, as the crabbers contemplated their own vulnerability and fears. As the fishing vessels arrived at Dutch Harbor, both captains and deckhands were aware of their integration with the larger world even in one of the most isolated geographies. A number of captains and crew members from the Pacific Northwest, including F/V *Northwestern*'s Sig Hansen, also recognized they were returning to the place where the coronavirus first took hold in the United States. "I'm scared," Hansen declared to the program's narrator, Mike Rowe. "I'm not the kind of guy that's afraid, and I'm telling you right now, I'm afraid" (Trock, 2020).

Here, there is a greater realization that fishing the Bering Sea does not provide immunity from the ravages of the disease, which had already caused havoc on supply chains and commodity markets. For the viewer at home, the mediated onset of a health pandemic that they, too, were experiencing added a different kind of reality to Alaska's best-known reality television program. The expected fishing crises—dangerous weather, mechanical failure, interpersonal conflict, financial loss—were replaced with a shocking tragedy in the sinking of F/V *Scandies Rose* and a new existential threat in the coronavirus. The rites and rituals of *Deadliest Catch* were not displaced but rather diverted. Yet the material underpinnings of the program's sixteenth season reminded viewers that the Bering Sea fishery is no longer a world apart. A nautical mythology exacerbated by a foreign nemesis was displaced by the narrative of an impending health crisis on the home front. The notion of ritual, solidified by conflict with an understood national rival, gave way to conflict with a fast-moving, unseen combatant. Even as a health pandemic shook up global supply chains and the Alaska fishery, it was easily woven into the civic narrative that drove this mediation of nature, labor, and polar adventure forward.

In its sixteenth season, Discovery Channel's *Deadliest Catch* produced discursive/material renderings of the Alaska crab fishing industry that embedded viewers in this otherwise unseen social world. These rites of Bering Sea passage included some of the foundational narratives of the long-running show, including those focused on labor, danger, interpersonal conflict, and climate change. Through engagement with the tragic sinking of the F/V *Scandies Rose*, it also included the rite of mortality and a documentary-like examination of the dangers of the Bering Sea workplace. Yet true to its linkages to the commodities marketplace and the global economy, the program also brought to viewers new insights about how a pandemic like COVID-19 might disrupt the market for crab and simultaneously shift the culture of commercial fishing. In other words, *Deadliest Catch* dramatized an economic cycle that featured not only micro-level depictions of the fishery, but also macro-level renderings of its place in the global economy. And true to Carey's model, it leveraged the technology of a particular spatial medium to reconfigure civic structures and expand the boundaries and possibilities of family and community in American public life.

REFERENCES

Adgate, B. (2020). Nielson: How the pandemic changed home media consumption like never before. Forbes. Retrieved from: https://tinyurl.com/2jcfxf4v.

Anderson, H. (2011). Siblings in Cyberspace: Carey's Ritual Model of Communication in the Digital Age. *Intersect: The Stanford Journal of Science, Technology, and Society*, *4*, 92–100.

Bernton, H. (2021). Expert testimony on deadly Scandies Rose sinking forces new look at safety rules for crab boats. *Seattle Times.* Retrieved from: https://www.seattletimes.com/seattle-news/expert-witnesses-in-scandies-rose-sinking-say-coast-guard-regulations-dont-account-for-ice-buildup-in-alaska-waters/.

Blair, N. (2013). The working-class heroes: Analysing hegemonic masculinity in occupational reality TV. *The Plymouth Student Scientist, 6*(1), pp. 137–160. http://hdl.handle.net/10026.1/14013.

Blue, G. (2019). Science communication is culture: Foregrounding ritual in the public communication of science. *Science Communication, 41*(2), 243–253.

Blundell, G. (2017). *Deadliest Catch*: Discovery Channel Alaskan adventure's 13th season. *The Australian.*

Buchanan, B. (2014). Portrayals of masculinity in the discovery channel's *Deadliest Catch*. *Reality Television: Oddities of Culture,* 1–20.

Buttner, M. (2020). Real rural: There's remote EM, and then there's Unalaska. *Emergency Medicine News*, *42*(9), 24–25.

Carey, J. W. (1967). Harold Adams Innis and Marshall McLuhan. *The Antioch Review*, *27*(1), 5–39.

Carey, J. (2002). A cultural approach to communication. *McQuail's reader in mass communication theory*, 36–45.

Carey, J. W. (2008). *Communication as culture, revised edition: Essays on media and society*. Routledge.

Carlson, M. (2012). Rethinking journalistic authority: Walter Cronkite and ritual in television news. *Journalism Studies*, *13*(4), 483–498.
Carpentier, N. (2017). *The discursive-material knot: Cyprus in conflict and community media participation*. Peter Lang.
Clark, K., Hawkins, R., & Silver, J. J. (2020). Gender, nature and nation: Resource nationalism on primary sector reality TV. *Environment and Planning E: Nature and Space*, *3*(4), 1196–1214.
Covey, S., & Ewell, P. L. (2015). The relationship between managerial orientation and productivity: An examination of captains from Discovery Channel's *Deadliest Catch*. *SAM Advanced Management Journal*, *80*(3), 57.
Dryzek, J.S. (2013). *The politics of the Earth. Environmental discourses* (3rd ed.). Oxford University Press.
Durham, F. (2008). Media ritual in catastrophic time: The populist turn in television coverage of Hurricane Katrina. *Journalism*, *9*(1), 95–116.
Durkheim, E. (1915). The elementary forms of the religious life. Joseph Ward Swain, trans. *New York*, *60*.
Grimes, R. L. (2002). Ritual and the media. In *Practicing Religion in the Age of the Media* (pp. 219–234). Columbia University Press.
Hale, M. A (2007, April 3). Third season at sea, preoccupied with danger. *New York Times*. https://www.nytimes.com/2007/04/03/arts/television/03hale.html.
Hollander, Z. & Wieber, A. (2020). 'From sleeping to swimming, it was about 10 minutes,' says survivor of fishing boat sinking. *Anchorage Daily News*. Retrieved from: https://www.adn.com/alaska-news/2020/01/02/crab-boat-that-sank-on-new-years-eve-leaving-5-presumed-dead-was-headed-into-area-under-gale-warning/.
Johnson, C. & Dempsey, L. (2020). How coronavirus changed TV viewing habits for good. *Conversation*. https://theconversation.com/how-coronavirus-might-have-changed-tvviewing-habits-for-good-new-research-146040.
Joseph, J. (2003). *Hegemony: A realist analysis*. Routledge.
Kirby, L. A. (2013). Cowboys of the high seas: Representations of working-class masculinity on *Deadliest Catch*. *Journal of Popular Culture*, *46*(1), 109–118.
Laclau, E., & Mouffe, C. (1985). *Hegemony and Socialist Strategy: Towards a Radical Democratic Politics* (1st ed.). London/New York: Verso.
Livingstone, S. (2002). Relationships between media and audiences. *Media, Ritual and Identity*, 237.
Marvin, C. (1990). Reconsidering James Carey: How many rituals does it take to make an artifact? *American Journalism*, *7*(4), 216–226.
Moscato, D. (2017). The political economy of Arctic reality television: The spatial communication of *Ice Road Truckers* & *Deadliest Catch*. *Arctic Yearbook*, *2017*.
Murphy, P. D. (2017). *The media commons: Globalization and environmental discourses*. University of Illinois Press.
O'Carroll, E. (2010). *Deadliest Catch* hauls in biggest audience ever. *Christian Science Monitor*. Retrieved from: https://www.csmonitor.com/From-the-news-wires/2010/0628/Deadliest-Catch-hauls-in-biggest-audience-ever.
Pooley, J. (2007). Daniel Czitrom, James W. Carey, and the Chicago School. *Critical Studies in Media Communication*, *24*(5), 469–472.

Sen, B. (2017). Information as ritual: James Carey in the digital age. *Cultural Studies Critical Methodologies*, *17*(6), 473–481.

Trock, G. (2020). *Deadliest Catch* Sig Hansen talks COVID-19: 'This is serious . . . I'm afraid!" Retrieved from: https://theblast.com/126179/deadliest-catch-sig-hansen-talks-covid-19-this-is-serious-im-afr/.

Wells, R. (2015). The labor of reality TV: The case of *The Deadliest Catch*. *Labor: Studies in Working-Class History of the Americas*, *12*(4), 33–49.

Chapter Five

Developing Voice Resilience

Building on Spiral of Silence Theory

Alana M. Nicastro and Shelly M. Valdez[1]

While turbulent and uncertain times are part of life, preparing in advance to navigate them is difficult and sometimes rare. It is often in hindsight that we reflect on what could or should have been done, not done, voiced, or left unsaid. Though we cannot predict the future, we can prepare ourselves for how we face it by developing a voice that stands amid turbulence. The COVID-19 pandemic offered an opportunity to understand and learn from its confusion, crisis, and conflict so we might develop a resilient voice that can hold us steady in ambiguous or tempestuous times.

One way to do so is by listening to and learning from those we consider expert voices around us. However, the voices we relied on to guide us in the pandemic were varied and contradictive of one another: "the virus is under control," "numbers are spiking," "don't buy masks," "wear a mask," "stay away from one another," "isolation is emotionally dangerous," "it's a hoax," "it's deadly," "it's just a flu," "it will go away by summer," "it will be here for years." Yet we needed to choose which voices to rely on as we tried to navigate the new pandemic world and persevere through the months of unknowns and changing facts and opinions.

One expert voice to whom America turned was Dr. Deborah Birx, a physician and diplomat who served as coordinator of the White House's Coronavirus Task Force and was a face of expertise among White House personnel. Dr. Birx drew both praise and criticism for her role. On one hand, she was able to manage the tension between what she knew was actual pandemic data from her team as opposed to the confidence of the president who purported to believe an entirely different set of facts and proposed solutions. On the other hand, many of us were stunned as we watched Dr. Birx sit in awkward silence during a White House press briefing when former President Trump publicly offered the idea of injecting disinfectant into the body as a potential coronavirus antidote on April 23, 2020. He stated,

> I see the disinfectant that knocks it out in a minute, one minute. And is there a way we can do something like that by injection inside, or almost a cleaning? Because you see it gets inside the lungs and it does a tremendous number on the lungs, so it would be interesting to check that.

Her decision to remain silent in the face of this altered, untrue, and even damaging data and conjecture evoked shock and disbelief in many, including the authors. To put it bluntly: We were angered and, for a time, shut down by what we read and heard, asking ourselves, "How and why does one lose (give up?) one's voice? How might one maintain one's voice and not be silenced, especially when so much is at stake? What are the personal and societal implications for silence?" Our reaction and response offered an opportunity to dig in and extrapolate new meaning from the incident that might illuminate a human condition and aid us in our own communication and decision-making about when and how we use our voice.

Shortly after leaving her position in the White House in January 2021, Dr. Birx addressed her role and explained her silence, thus allowing us to explore, analyze, and learn from her experience and aid us in the ability to project our own authentic voice into any situation. To accomplish this, the spiral of silence theory (described below) serves in this chapter as a foundation from which to study Dr. Birx's voice in her role as coordinator for the Coronavirus Task Force. In addition, to help explain the complexities and nuances of this case, the theory is expanded and modified. The chapter's critical edge, however, is a proposed voice resilience framework that adds power and moral conviction as components to enact a resilient voice, whether in-the-moment or over time. The notion of "voice resilience" was introduced by King et al. (2019) to describe willingness to voice following a negative response to prior voicing. This chapter expands on that definition.

THEORY AS FOUNDATION

Communication theories give us windows from which to view and make sense of our world. We use them to explain, predict, and understand phenomena (Abend, 2008), as well as to contest and widen existing knowledge (Swanson & Chermack, 2013). Communication theories also help us grow closer in relationship through interconnection and understanding of one another, especially helpful and necessary during the isolation and restricted communication in a pandemic. Finally, dissecting, magnifying, and when necessary, transmuting theory can help us analyze our own circumstances and make decisions based on those analyses.

Therefore, we turned our attention to Elisabeth Noelle-Neumann's spiral of silence theory—a mass communication theory—arguing that public opinion is a powerful force in contemporary society and a form of social control (Noelle-Neumann, 1974, 1979; Salmon & Glynn, 2009). The theory rests on the idea that to avoid isolation individuals either share or withhold their opinions based on perceived public opinion. And furthermore, once one view has been shared and accepted, those individuals enter into a spiral where some speak up while others are silent thereby stabilizing public opinion as conflicts are resolved through spirals of silence (May, 2009).

Public opinion, as defined by Noelle-Neumann (1979), is "in the sphere of controversy that one can express in public without isolating oneself" (p. 150). Her theory states that individuals risk possible social isolation or punishment due to going against the majority-held public opinion. It should be noted that, although Noelle-Neumann's theory is "among the most cited and replicated theories in social sciences" (Miller, 2005, p. 278), it is also controversial, in part, because it goes against the idea of individual autonomy. The spiral of silence theory has inspired a massive body of research that seeks to explain, confirm, disprove, or alter it. In fact, a search in our local university data base yielded 14,700 articles and books on the subject. For purposes of this chapter, we focus on the interplay of intersectional perspectives and entanglements within social media, culture and identity, and organizational structure.

In recent years, studies have included issues that were non-existent at the time Noelle-Neumann proposed her theory. For example, the onset and proliferation of online social media has led to research on its influence on public opinion and the concomitant effect on voice versus silence (Hampton et al., 2014). A meta-analysis of 66 studies involving 27,000 participants confirmed both online and offline opinion climate and opinion expression effects were similar but that participants were less likely to express opinions about "intrusive issues" within their social circle of friends, family, or neighbors (Matthes et al., 2017; Moy et al., 2001). This applies in general to the finding that consonance of one's opinion with family and friends, rather than society at large, both predicts willingness to speak out (Moy et al., 2001) and likelihood of the individual expressing an opinion (Ives et al., 2015). Contextual differences within an online environment such as one's perception of congruity with other commenters or perceived anonymity within the online environments (Wu, 2017) also serve as predictors of willingness to voice.

In addition to the influence of social media, there are multiple cultural/identity factors that can determine one's perception of public opinion, for example, individualistic versus collectivist culture, gender, race and identity, equal opportunities to influence, as well as personal characteristics including conflict styles and self-image (Scheufele & Moy, 2000). Any or all of these can have an influence on expression versus silence as does the nature of an issue itself, with more long-term public issues having a different effect than emerging issues (Brouard & Guinaudeau, 2015; Yeric & Todd, 1989). Yet silence enables the continued and unquestioned chemistry and sustenance of the spiral itself, encouraging hidden privileges (Niemistö et al., 2020) with those in positions of power or those who have more specialized knowledge or roles. This is especially true in highly hierarchical cultures where social identities may be regulated or constricted (Carmona & Ezzamel, 2016; Kärreman & Alvesson, 2004; Niemistö et al., 2020), such as government and military. Bowen and Blackmon (2003) further confirmed that relative privilege might also impair or conceal social exchange, therefore leading to silence.

In fact, employee voice in which there are differentials of power and authority within the work environment has sparked another area of research regarding spiral of silence, both within and across organizational hierarchies. Included in this research is the use of social media within an organization. Employees can use discursive tactics to speak up on internal social media to be heard and gain support for their cause (Madsen & Johansen, 2019) and avoidance strategies to explore forms of self-censorship (Hayes, 2007). Palekar et al. (2015) suggest that value proposition (deciding to be silent at present to express in future when they may have greater position or authority) makes the spiral of silence much more dynamic and changes the shape of the spiral itself. They proposed additional explanatory spirals to illustrate dynamism within the theory: "inverted" spiral of silence in which an individual progressively moves from passivity to participation (silence to voice), "cylindrical" spiral of silence in which passivity (silence) is consistent, and "hourglass" spiral of silence in which a passive individual may sporadically vacillate into active participation.

The nuance of spiral of silence along with its 50 years of critique and expansion often operates intersectionally. The authors believe integrating spiral of silence with Patricia Hill Collins (2019) intersectionality as critical social theory addresses multiple differences and intersecting identities that we may not see: the often-hidden inequities, disadvantages, and subordination residing in saturated belief systems. Various power structures interact in the public sphere, and we often need augmented explanatory power to assess "attitude certainty" and expression of politically minority opinions (Matthes et al., 2010).

We are all part of many social systems and unable to escape an inevitable silencing effect in some of those systems—we may be silenced, silence others, and use silence as strategies depending on our role in the system in which we are operating at the time. A theoretical lens is therefore helpful to make sense of this communicative phenomenon and apply it, not just in this specific case, but also in a larger context.

A CASE STUDY: DR. DEBORAH BIRX

Let's put theory into the context of Dr. Birx's role as coordinator of the Coronavirus Task Force. As noted above, after leaving her position in the administration, Dr. Birx admitted in her first public interview on CBS *Face the Nation* with Margaret Brennan (aired January 24, 2021) that the data she had given to the White House was being altered or replaced altogether and that she knew that certain "treatments" suggested by the administration were not just harmful but potentially lethal:

> I saw the president presenting graphs that I never made. So, I know that someone or someone out there or someone inside was creating a parallel set of data and graphics that were shown to the president. I don't know to this day who, but I know what I sent up and I know that what was in his hands was different from that. That worries me. . . . I've built my career on data transparency and accountability (Birx, 2021a).

With these personal convictions in mind, why withhold from the general public verifiable information that could save American lives? And further, why not publicly denounce verifiably false information that could cost American lives? There are certainly a number of possible answers to these questions, ranging from evil intentions to ignorance, neither of which we believed was the case and certainly Dr. Birx's own actions during her term as well as her statements in interviews after stepping down from the role negated either of these options as valid reasons for actions or lack thereof. Dr. Birx may have shared the majority opinion held by the American public that the virus was real and dangerous, but not the minority opinion voiced by Trump's closest allies that it was not. It is also possible that at least some of the White House's closest allies may have held different opinions but also felt silenced.

When asked during her CBS interview if she felt censored by the White House, Birx affirmed, "I was not able to do national press," and went on to explain her personal conviction: "I was not going to go outside of the chain of command." Chain of command refers to the hierarchy of authority and accountability within an organization, which is stringently adhered to in the military culture dependent on obedience to authority and hierarchy to save lives in battle. Dr. Birx's beliefs are rooted in our military system in which she spent the first 28 years of her career (U.S. Department of State, n.d.).

The obligation to uphold duty was further conveyed when asked if Joe Biden's presidential inaugural gathering in January 2021, which included numerous military personnel, was a massive super-spreader event, Dr. Birx (2021a) replied:

> It could be. When you bring 30,000 people together where you know that they're most likely to have asymptomatic infections and you haven't pre-screened, pre-tested, and serially tested all of these troops. These are dedicated troops. They're going to do their mission. I can promise you that they will sacrifice their own health to do their mission, because that's—that's where I came from. You sacrifice for others out of the military.

Paradoxically, although Dr. Birx believed that she acted ethically by following chain of command, it appeared her personal morale suffered. She noted in the same interview that although she felt it was her duty to remain silent in the face of presidential misinformation, her understanding of the suffering and deaths that the information caused has led her to regretfully, "think about it every day" (Birx, 2021a). In a subsequent interview on March 28, 2021 with Dr. Sanjay Gupta on CNN's *Pandemic Doctors Speak Out* she noted, " . . . there were about 100,000 deaths that came from that original surge," Birx said. "All of the rest of them, in my mind, could have been mitigated or decreased substantially" (Birx, 2021b). How do we find the coherency in this disconnect between one's moral and ethical beliefs and the decision to remain silent?

While serving in her White House role, Dr. Birx faced a series of disagreements and decision points that directly conflicted with her life of commitment to public service in a time of crisis. As a retired colonel with a 28-year military career, Dr. Birx was certainly familiar with and indoctrinated into a hierarchical command culture. While such a culture may be necessary when the flow of information must be controlled within an organization, it restricts free and independent thinking, decision making and flexibility, which is necessary when conditions are ambiguous or changing (Klein, 1999, 2003). And, more importantly, it restricts or altogether silences the voices of some who may have important information that could alter outcomes for the better. It is that lost voice that could have potentially saved lives.

Dr. Birx insisted that she is a scientist, not a politician, and as such she built her career on "data transparency and accountability" (Birx, 2021a). Surprisingly, this did not propel her to make that a public priority when confronted with what she believed was a higher moral obligation to adhere to chain of command. Rather, she chose an alternate route to circumvent direct chain of command by meeting individually with state governors where she could state her views and offer what she knew was correct data about

COVID. However, although she was in the position of expert authority while with the governors, her words and actions with them still went against chain of command, contradicting what had been put forth by the president in his public briefing.

Dr. Birx considered her role as coordinator of the Coronavirus Task Force a "terminal" event in that it was temporary and one from which she would retire, noting, "You can't go into something this polarized and not be tainted by the outcome" (Birx, 2021a). This could lead us to believe that with any potential loss of future position removed, one might feel freer to voice a minority opinion, in this case an opinion or belief in contrast to one's employer and/or colleagues. But potential loss of face and loss of respect remain.

She also mentioned the ongoing challenges female leaders face. Here we see intersectionality at play for Dr. Birx who, although holding a position of authority by virtue of her formal role, simultaneously held a position as an under-represented voice by virtue of her gender. A recent study of women's representation and voice in media coverage of the coronavirus (Jones, 2020) found "only a third of quotations in articles concerning the pandemic were attributable to women" and those varied by article category and topic with a clear divide "in female voice between traditionally feminine and masculine issues" (p. 1). Further, in coronavirus related articles in the U.S., Australia, and the UK, only four of the top 20 mentioned politicians in those countries were female. Therefore, the political responses the public saw in those countries "had a largely male face" (Jones, 2020, p. 1). According to the theory, majority opinion supports voice while minority opinion supports silence. Noelle-Neumann (1977) and many others have confirmed that if two groups differ significantly in their willingness to express views publicly, the group displaying more willingness is more likely to "have the future on its side" (p. 50), thus leading the conversation and subsequent actions.

Dr. Birx also shared what she deemed "an extraordinary moment" when she was publicly berated by the Speaker of the House, Nancy Pelosi. She acknowledged the gender biases she faced and framed this incident by explaining:

> I know what they've [women] had to go through to get to where they are. I also have now much more respect for women who are involved in journalism because when I was on the road, I could see that dynamic. It's also why I started calling on all the women first, because, you know, they would be out-shouted sometimes by their male colleagues. I mean it's difficult out there. Gender is still a very real and very difficult piece (Birx, 2021a).

Her response to these gender challenges was "focusing solely on the mission" and consciously thinking of ways to overcome them:

> The whole time I had to be serious to be taken seriously; and I could never let emotion come into this. That no matter how frustrated I got, no matter how beaten down I got—I had to keep pushing as hard as I could (Birx, 2021a).

But perhaps more significant given her professional history, experience, and accomplishments is that when finding herself in her new role, in a new situation in which she was unfamiliar with the culture, she found it hard to get a "footing" and did not know how far she could "push the envelope" (Birx, 2021a). Certainly, her training as a leader in both military and government service as well as within the scientific and medical communities must have prepared her to exercise voice in both chaotic and disturbing interactions. She did not appear to reveal how that training did not lend itself to her work within the pandemic, but the fields in which she garnered her professional experience would all have included training in dealing with new, changing, and chaotic situations.

Dr. Birx also mentioned there were several parallel and contradictory stories about the nature of the virus that were leaked to the press. It was her intention to stay clear of those stories that she considered not grounded in "truth" and avoid the "slippery slope" effect (Birx, 2021a, 2021b). Thus, her silence was a strategy she used to attempt to control the narrative in the moment, avoiding any planted story that was in direct opposition to hers. She also highlighted several tactics she felt were effective in informing the public about the impact of the coronavirus and to communicate health advisories, thus reclaiming the narrative. Through these tactics she mitigated potential loss of her position and reputation while finding alternative ways to use her voice to inform the public. These included:

- coordinating with allies for support,
- taking extensive notes (i.e., emails, reports, requests to expand testing, and how to improve therapeutics) in hopes they would one day come to light even if "not in [my] lifetime," which is telling of her belief this event would be studied as well as her mistrust of the public narrative and its purveyors,
- addressing the management of COVID as relating to the larger health infrastructure frailty (i.e., treating illness over prevention and racial/ethnic disparities and inequalities) as opposed to specific targeted responses of the day,
- avoiding contradicting or criticizing others in public,
- circumventing White House censorship by working directly with governors ("on-the-ground learning") to accomplish the work while keeping her "head down" (Birx, 2021a).

Communication scholars, leadership practitioners, and consultants are routinely asked by the organizations in which they work and consult how they can facilitate conversations to build confidence, trust, and skill. The answers are often framed in ethical training, i.e., using examples of ethical dilemmas to illuminate the decision-making process when there is no one right answer. For example, if a situation calls for a decision that would most certainly result in an ambiguous or even a negative consequence regardless of one's actions, examining how an option is chosen sheds light on the internal process that can then be applied to situations that are less ambiguous or negative.

When asked about her biggest mistake during her tenure with the task force, Dr. Birx said she always thinks she could have done more and said more (Birx, 2021a). This in itself is telling of the dilemmas she faced at the time. We have seen that in the case of the earlier "disinfectant" example at the White House briefing, Dr. Birx's two most obvious choices were to remain silent or to contradict her boss, i.e., contradicting her commander in chief in a public forum, both of which had potentially profound negative consequences. She chose public silence and therefore, what appeared to be complicity purportedly to keep her role in which she could meet privately with governors to relate her message, a role she believed would be of value to the American public: "You don't give up . . . you make it the least terrible it can be" (Birx, 2021a). That is, Dr. Birx appeared to believe that speaking and silence both had negative repercussions, the lesser of which might occur with her silence.

Yet, her actions, or lack thereof, caused emotionally reactive and negative judgment by many across the country, as witnessed by subsequent news stories and comments surrounding that briefing. Certainly, silence in the face of ethical and moral wrongdoing is not a new phenomenon. There is, for example, a massive body of literature about silence in the face of fascism during World War II (see Geoff, 2003; Tubach & Patterson-Tubach, 2011). During the Civil Rights movement in the U.S., many, including Dr. Martin Luther King, Jr., urged the public to speak up about injustice. He is often quoted as saying, "Our lives begin to end the day we become silent about things that matter" (King, 2003).

Dr. Birx's choice to speak about her own silence in interviews once she left her position was a present-day example of finding voice after having been silenced (or chosen to be silent) and after damage had been done. And it provided the fodder for studying the decision-making process involved in how, when, and why we choose to use or silence our voice.

BUILDING ON THEORY FOR FURTHER APPLICATION

Most of us are not faced with the very public and critical decisions Dr. Birx had to make, and when faced with even lesser decisions we often fall into self-judgment about what could have been done or said. These interior streaming monologues that play over and over in our minds are defeating and draining. Existing theories, including spiral of silence, do not explain the specific and nuanced combination of events and circumstances faced by Dr. Birx. While they do give us clues as to how to adjust expectations and preserve voice, they fall short and leave us wanting more. Having another analytical tool is important for the development of a resilient voice. We therefore propose four additions to Noelle-Neumann's theory:

1. Spiral of silence proposes that voicing opinions that go against the majority opinion leads to social isolation. Others have furthered this idea by including other repercussions. We take this one step further to propose that repercussions boil down to *fear of loss* and includes not just social isolation but other types of loss such as emotional isolation, physical isolation, loss of face, loss of love, loss of livelihood, and even loss of life. For example, Dr. Birx noted in the CNN interview that both she and her family received death threats, which would have had an impact on her decisions. Further, we propose that as the amount of perceived loss increases, so does fear. As fear increases, the willingness to voice decreases.
2. Noelle-Neumann (1974) proposed that the determining factor—the silencing effect—was dependent on where one stood with regard to the minority or majority opinions, i.e., how closely aligned one was with the opinion regardless of one's social, professional, or personal position. We propose that the determining factor is *perceived power differential.* While the (widest) top of Noelle-Neumann's spiral represented majority opinion, we propose that it is not identification with numbers of people who hold similar opinions but identification with where one stands with respect to the perceived position of opinion holders that determines voice or silence. So, the top of the spiral would represent those with greatest power as perceived by the observer who decides whether or not to voice, For example, if one holds a view that is in contrast to a view of one more powerful (by virtue of a professional position for example), even if surrounded by others who share your view, it may not be fear of social isolation but indeed fear of loss of livelihood that could keep one silent. In Dr. Birx's case, she held the view of medical and science experts who shared her knowledge of the facts at the time, but she was

in a position less powerful than the president for whom she worked. Voicing her views in direct contradiction with those perceived as having greater authority and power might easily have led to loss of her position. However, when she was speaking with the governors, she was in a position of power greater than those to whom she spoke, by virtue of her position in the federal as opposed to the state governments, and was, therefore, freer to speak.

3. We propose that we all exist and function in multiple spirals depending on the groups in which we live and work, our roles within those groups, and situations that can fluctuate at any given time. We move within and around a spiral or many spirals each oscillating and dynamic, context-dependent, and messy.
4. It is common knowledge that a moral component is inherent to the spiral of silence in that it would not necessarily apply to a situation such as whether to put ketchup or mustard on one's hamburger. What is missing from the original work, however, is the absence of the strength of one's moral conviction about an issue. We propose that the stronger one's moral conviction about any specific issue, the more that factor would interplay with fear of loss and the higher up on the spiral one might be, thus more likely to voice. Again, the example of Dr. Martin Luther King, Jr. and other civil rights workers both past and present come to mind in that moral conviction exceeded fear of loss—allowing them to act even in the face of death threats and ultimate assassination. Malala Yousafzai and Greta Thunberg are more recent public figure examples.

PRESENTING THE VOICE RESILIENCE FRAMEWORK

At this point, unfortunately, the idea of spirals become unwieldy and less helpful and less able to account for the nuances within systems and situations. We therefore propose a new framework with which one can assess not just the likelihood of silence versus voice but can also determine if and how one might choose to find the freedom to move from silence to voice—or not; as well as voice to silence.

In any group, role, or situation, two main factors come into play: perceived power and moral conviction about the specific situation or idea, both of which interact with the level of fear (not just of social isolation but of many other kinds of loss) that must be overcome to not remain silent. Let's be clear about what we mean here. We all have a set of moral convictions about situations and circumstances we face in our lives. These are the principles that guide decision-making and actions. Sometimes these moral convictions compete with one another. By saying one has low moral conviction about a situation, we do not imply that one has no morals or conviction, but that one's conviction at the time and in the moment is outweighed by a different, competing conviction about something that intersects at a particular point in time in one's life. In the case of Dr. Birx, it appears from her statements that disrupting chain of command held a higher sense of moral duty *at the time* and *in the moment* than the moral conviction to do no harm.

Our proposed framework is an analytical tool that acknowledges the tension between voice and the broader context to help us become more aware of how and when we use our voice versus remain silent.

Silence in the public face of the White House press briefings may also have been a function of Dr. Birx's perceived power differential between her and the president. Lower on the chain of command (and therefore with less formal authority), her belief was that her role was one of support—not contradiction—so she remained silent rather than risk loss of face, loss of position, and most importantly, loss of power to assist the American people in other contexts, such as meeting with state governors. In private meetings, however, her perceived power in that context may have been greater than those with whom she met and fear of loss decreased thus the ability and willingness to voice increased. In addition, her moral conviction to duty (chain of command) may have been greater than her moral conviction to do no harm (medical oath) in the context of the White House versus her meetings with governors.

Applying Noelle-Neumann's spiral of silence revealed the complexity of Dr. Birx's situation and the need for the theory, and its updated renditions, to be transformed even further to allow for voice to be understood as dynamic, nuanced, and at times, contradictive. We find this notion to be freeing and

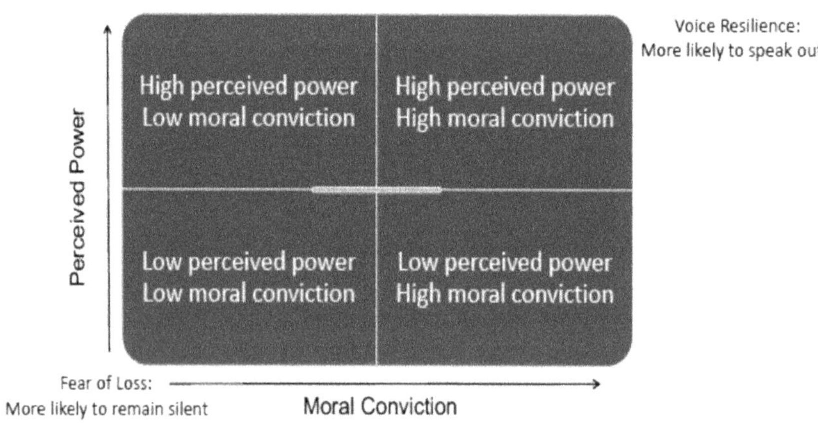

Figure 5.1 Voice Resilience Framework.
Created by Nicastro & Valdez.

uplifting, knowing that we might be silenced not by choice, but it is within our capacity to move on and between the spiral(s) while assessing the context that develops voice resilience. Theory has the potential to build bridges. Combining our four additions to the original spiral of silence theory with our Voice Resilience Framework reveals the rich takeaways from Dr. Birx's complex story. Voice should be measured and understood on the spiral continuum, allowing it to naturally oscillate given the complex world in which we live and behave. This work is a starting point—a place from which to persevere in a space of resilience, comfort, and productivity.

REFERENCES

Abend, G. (2008). The meaning of 'theory.' *Sociological Theory, 26*(2), 173–199. https://doi.org/10.1111/j.1467-9558.2008.00324.x.

Birx, D. (2021a, January 24). Interview by M. Brennan. *Face the Nation* [Television broadcast]. Washington DC: CBS Broadcast Center. https://www.cbsnews.com/news/transcript-deborah-birx-on-face-the-nation-january-24-2021/.

Birx, D. (2021b, March 28). Interview by Dr. Sanjay Gupta. *Pandemic Doctors Speak Out* [Television broadcast]. Atlanta: CNN Cable News Network. https://www.cnn.com/health/live-news/covid-pandemic-doctors-cnn-special/index.html.

Bowen, F., & Blackmon, K. (2003). Spirals of silence. The dynamic effects of diversity on organizational voice. *Journal of Management Studies, 40*(6), 1393–1417. https://onlinelibrary.wiley.com/doi/10.1111/1467-6486.00385.

Brouard, S., & Guinaudeau, I. (2015). Policy beyond politics? Public opinion, party politics and the French pro-nuclear energy policy. *Journal of Public Policy, 35*(1), 137–170. https://doi.org/10.1017/S0143814X14000221.

Carmona, S., & Ezzamel, M. (2016). Accounting and lived experience in the gendered workplace. *Accounting, Organizations and Society, 49,* pp. 1–8. https://doi.org/10.1016/j.aos.2015.11.004.

Geoff, E. (2003). Hitler's silent majority? Conformity and resistance under the Third Reich (Part Two). *Michigan Quarterly Review 42*(3). http://hdl.handle.net/2027/spo.act2080.0042.319.

Hampton, K., Rainie, L., Lu, W., Dwyer, M., Shin, I., & Purcell, K. (2014). *Social media and the 'spiral of silence.'* Pew Research Center, Washington, DC. http://www.pewinternet.org/2014/08/26/social-media-and-the-spiral-of-silence/.

Hill Collins, P. (2019). *Intersectionality as critical social theory.* Duke University Press. https://doi.org/10.2307/j.ctv11hpkdj.

Ives, A., Kennedy, J., & Sylvester, C. (2015). *Spiral of Silence and Fear of Social Isolation in Faith-Based Campus Organizations* [Poster presentation]. University of Wisconsin. https://minds.wisconsin.edu/handle/1793/74488.

Kärreman, D., & Alvesson, M. (2004). Cages in tandem: Management control, social identity, and identification in a knowledge-intensive firm. *Organization, 11*(1), pp. 149–175. https://doi.org/10.1177/1350508404039662.

King, D. D., Ryan, A. M., & Van Dyne, L. (2019). Voice resilience: Fostering future voice after non-endorsement of suggestions. *Journal of Occupational and Organizational Psychology, 92*(3), 535–565. https://doi.org/10.1111/joop.12275.

King, M. L., Jr. (2003). *I have a dream: Writings and speeches that changed the world.* (J. M. Washington, Ed.). HarperSanFrancisco.

Klein, G. (1999). *Sources of power: How people make decisions*. The MIT Press.

Klein, G. (2013). *Seeing what others don't: The remarkable ways we gain insights.* Public Affairs Publishers.

Madsen, V. T., & Johansen, W. (2019). A spiral of voice? When employees speak up on internal social media. *Journal of Communication Management, 23*(4), pp. 331–347. https://doi.org/10.1108/JCOM-03-2019-0050.

Matthes, J., Morrison, K., & Schemer, C. (2010). A spiral of silence for some: Attitude certainty and the expression of political minority opinions. *Communication Research, 37*(6), 774–800. https://doi.org/10.1177/0093650210362685.

Miller, K. (2005). Communication theories: Perspectives, processes, and contexts (2nd ed.). McGraw-Hill.

Neill, S. (2009). *The alternate channel: How social media is challenging the spiral of silence theory in GLBT communities of color [Master's thesis, American University].* Wayback Machine Archive. https://web.archive.org/web/20110629083241/http:/www.american.edu/soc/communication/upload/09-Neill.pdf.

Niemistö, C., Hearn, J., Karjalainen, M., & Tuori, A. (2020). Interrogating silent privileges across the work-life boundaries and careers of high-intensity knowledge professionals. *Qualitative Research in Organizations and Management, 15*(4), pp. 503–522. https://doi.org/10.1108/QROM-06-2019-1775.

Noelle-Neumann, E. (1974). The spiral of silence a theory of public opinion. *Journal of Communication, 24*(2), 43–51. https://doi.org/10.1111/j.1460-2466.1974.tb00367.x.

Noelle-Neumann, E. (1979). Public opinion and the classical tradition: A re-evaluation. *Public Opinion Quarterly, 43*(2), 143–156. https://doi.org/10.1086/268507.

Palekar, S., Atapattu, M., Sedera, D., & Lokuge, S. (2015, December 13–16). *Exploring spiral of silence in digital social networking spaces* [Paper presentation]. 36th International Conference on Information Systems (ICIS). Fort Worth, TX, United States. https://core.ac.uk/download/pdf/301367551.pdf.

Salmon, C. T., & Glynn, C. J. (2009). The spiral of silence: Communication and public opinion as social control. In D. W. Stacks, & M. B. Salwen (Eds). *An integrated approach to communication theory and research* (2nd ed., pp. 325–359). Routledge.

Scheufele, D. A., & Moy, P. (2000). Twenty-five years of the spiral of silence: A conceptual review and empirical outlook. *International Journal of Public Research, 12*(1), 3–28. https://doi.org/10.1093/ijpor/12.1.3.

Swanson, R. A., & Chermack, T. J. (2013). *Theory building in applied disciplines.* Berrett- Koehler Publishers. Accessed May 2, 2021. ProQuest Ebook Central.

The Spiral of Silence Theory. (n.d.). *Elisabeth Noelle-Neumann: Her life and scientific work.* Retrieved March 5, 2021, from https://noelle-neumann.de/scientific-work/spiral-of-silence/.

Tubach, F. C., & Patterson-Tubach, S. (2011). *German Voices: Memories of life during Hitler's Third Reich.* University of California Press. https://www.ucpress.edu/book/9780520269644/german-voices.

U.S. Department of State. (n.d.). *Deborah L. Birx, M.D.* U.S. Department of State Diplomacy in Action. https://2009-2017.state.gov/r/pa/ei/biog/224406.htm.

Wu, T. (2017). *Exploring the predictors of the spiral of silence in online news discussions* [Doctoral dissertation, University of Connecticut]. https://opencommons.uconn.edu/dissertations/1396.

Yeric, J. L., & Todd, J. R. (1989). *Public opinion: The visible politics* (2nd ed.). F. E. Peacock Publishers.

NOTES

1. This paper reflects the opinions of the authors and not those of the United States Marine Corps, Department of Defense, or federal government.

Chapter Six

What Reassurances? What Reality?

Governor Cuomo, COVID-19, and the Politics of Masculine Protection

Laurie E. Naranch

It has been a remarkable rise and fall for the now former New York State Governor Andrew Cuomo, who became a hero, an unexpected comfort, and even a sex symbol to many when he began daily COVID-19 briefings on March 2, 2020. Livestreamed around lunchtime on the state's website, the briefings were widely available on social media such as Facebook, Twitter's Periscope, YouTube, and carried on cable television (CNN, Fox News, MSNBC) and broadcast on the Albany National Public Radio station WAMC. Many found his approach and the content of the briefings to be a salve in a challenging time. By the end of March 2020, viewers were nearly one million a day (Weiner, 2020) with the governor's office reporting 59 million viewers overall when the briefings ended in June 2020 (Vienneuve & Hill 2020). Cuomo received the Founder's Award Emmy in November 2020, given to an individual or organization who "crosses cultural boundaries to touch our common humanity" (International Emmy Awards 2020), an award that was rescinded the day after he resigned as governor on August 24, 2021, due to sexual harassment and assault allegations as detailed in New York Attorney General Letitia James's report (2021). The *Report of Investigation into Allegations of Sexual Harassment by Governor Andrew M. Cuomo*, published and released on August 3, 2021, found credible evidence of sexual harassment and abuse of eleven women in a toxic workplace environment in its 165-page report.

Even before the charges of sexual harassment and assault were in the public's eye and the subject of the attorney general's investigation, there were questions about just how effective and transparent Cuomo and his administration were in regard to pandemic death rates. Attorney General James issued a report in January 28, 2021 showing that nursing home deaths were undercounted by the state by as much as 50 percent in June; the numbers purposely underreported by Cuomo's top staff to keep up the image of a more effective state response as measured by death rates (Goodman et al., 2021). In February 2021, Queens Assemblyman Democrat Ron Kim publicly questioned the effectiveness of Cuomo's pandemic response in relation to nursing home deaths; Kim reported on the harassing phone call Cuomo made to him reporting that Cuomo said "he would destroy me" (Lee & Morales, 2021). In taking this exchange public, Kim exposed the toxic and often bullying environment of the Cuomo administration (McKinley 2021). In a February 24 essay in *Medium*, former Cuomo aide Lindsay Boylan (2021) accused Cuomo of experiences of sexual harassment and other improper behaviors naming Cuomo. Moreover, many journalists and health professionals have argued that New York State, rather than being a leader in addressing the COVID-19 pandemic, delayed an initial response to shutdowns and mitigation leading to a disproportionately higher number of deaths in Black and Latinx communities (Barkan 2021a, 2021b; Paumgarten 2020; Lasch & Paumgarten 2021).

Despite these accusations of abusive, negligent, or criminal behavior, the three-term governor first elected in 2010 enjoyed favorable public opinion as shown in a Siena College Research Institute poll from July 2021. Voters said they approved of Cuomo's handling of the pandemic 51 percent favorable to 32 percent not favorable, his managing of the vaccinations 66 percent favorable to 20 percent not favorable, keeping New Yorkers informed at 60 percent to 27 percent, and reopening the state at 54 percent to 33 percent. Voters gave Cuomo a negative assessment on the issue of reporting nursing home deaths, 60 percent reported he did not handle this well to 22 percent thought otherwise. When asked about what Cuomo should do in the then context of the revelations about failures of pandemic management and charges of sexual harassment and assault, one third of voters said he should run for re-election, 39 percent said he should finish the term but not run again, and 23 percent said he should resign immediately (Siena College Research Institute 2021). That is, even after evidence of the underreporting of nursing home deaths, charges of harassing behavior and sexual assault, Cuomo continued to have favorable ratings in terms of his handling of the pandemic. Now Cuomo has resigned and the appeal of his pandemic response can be put into this context. Rather than a simple story of leadership strength and salvation in a public health crisis, we need a more complicated and complete story about the comfort the pandemic briefings provided for so many along with the crush of workplace toxicity, abuse, and lack of disclosing important health information to the public.

Even as the charges of sexual harassment and abuse became public, former aide and Cuomo critic, State Senator Alessandra Biaggi, noted that many voters were struggling to reconcile the heroic pandemic image of the governor with the abusive leader since he was “a man many turned to during one of the scariest periods of their lives.” Biaggi said, “What’s hard for people to hold in their mind is a discordant belief that at the same time that this person made you feel safe, he was doing things and making decisions that were not only bad, but riddled with misconduct” (cited in Lerer, 2021a). To experience a “discordant belief” when someone you think is protecting you is also engaged in deception and abuse is familiar to critics of abusive, intimate power in the private sphere (RAINN 2021), but it is also a recognizable public phenomenon. Iris Marion Young (2007) suggests using a feminist lens attuned to gendered dynamics of power to help explain how the George W. Bush administration’s war on terror puts citizens in a position of dependents—like women and children in traditional patriarchal relations—setting the stage for a trade-off between security and obedience to growing antidemocratic actions. While the trade-off between security and liberty is an old one in democratic politics, what Young (2007) points to is how this may not be noticed when it takes a seemingly benign form to protect others, and specifically women and children. Taking inspiration from Young’s analysis, but turning to the novel experience of the COVID-19 pandemic, this chapter seeks to understand the discordant meanings of Cuomo’s leadership in terms of his performance of both care and dominance and what that reveals about our collective desire for leadership in a health crisis, even leadership that can undermine public knowledge, effective policy responses, and equity in the workplace.

I suggest that what was reassuring is that Cuomo offered a seeming contrast to the toxic masculinity of then President Donald Trump and his administration’s chaotic pandemic response. This toxicity appeared in the form of Trumps’s aggressive rhetoric, demonizing groups such as the Chinese, and by association all Asians and Asian-Americans, the denigration of scientific experts or those questioning the federal government’s response to a public health and economic crisis, and his politicization of pandemic health mandates such as masks as a liberal ploy threatening freedom (Viglione 2020; Diamond 2021; Dugyala & Jin 2021). Hegemonic or dominant expressions of masculinity, however, can take many forms (Connell & Messerschmidt, 2005; Aboim et al., 2016). Cuomo offered a seemingly more benign executive masculine leadership role of protector, one who cares for his family and the citizens of his state and nation. In an unprecedented health and economic crisis, Cuomo validated our anxiety and fear of the virus. He calmed our concerns about how government will respond to its duty to protect through the actions he took at the state level and how he conveyed that information. Moreover, Cuomo’s ability to speak in science-based, policy, commonsense, and familial terms resonated with people as he made the personal political by blending love and toughness in his pandemic briefings. Yet, Cuomo, too played on our acceptance of male dominance in leadership roles to keep his control in the workplace and secure his national media image.

The command Cuomo performed rhetorically in words and visuals (the PowerPoint slides accompanying the briefings, the staging of the briefings, his appearance as an executive), coupled with the emergency powers granted to him by the state legislature in March 2020, revoked March 5, 2021 (Chapel, 2021), helps to explain the comfort he could offer as the one leading the charge to address this health and economic crisis (see also Schacht, 2020). What was hidden in plain sight though was the danger of the white male protector who exercises a patriarchal or paternal style of power not through overt domination, but through the rhetoric of protective care, that he alone has the knowledge, love, and toughness to make things better. This form of hierarchy positions the father figure as the one in control—of messaging, of resources, of care. While no response to a crisis is without controversy, and the responsibility to protect is a part of leadership, an accounting of what deceptions and abuses occurred is essential to public health, workplace equity, and democracy, which relies on trust, protecting life, and ensuring fairness.

THE POLITICS OF MASCULINE LEADERSHIP

American political life has been dominated by the values of toughness and machismo associated with male leaders (Jeffords, 1994; Kimmel, 1996; Katz, 2016). Assumptions of strong leadership privilege stereotypical masculine characteristics regardless of the gender of the candidate—valuing toughness over deference, hardness over softness—which makes it more challenging for other forms of leadership, or women in general, to be taken seriously. Political science scholars Susan J. Carroll and Richard Fox (2018) have traced the pitfalls for women candidates and office holders in negotiating gendered expectations of leadership even in light of differences of party, geography, opposition candidates, and other contextual factors. Women candidates and leaders, more so than their male counterparts, negotiate expectations of both masculine and feminine stereotypes since displaying toughness is especially challenging for women given the macho presumptions of who looks and acts like a leader and the still male-dominated institutions of government (Dittmar, 2015, pp. 88–89; Carpinella & Bauer, 2021). Despite the fact that some find stereotype expectations between male and female candidates not so stark in campaigning (Sapiro et al., 2011), stereotype expectations still shape the world of political expectations when it comes to leadership. We still operate in a world where political actions are viewed favorable when they appear as stereotypically masculine (active, assertive, honorable) versus being stereotypically feminine (passive, diplomatic, cooperative). This poses a challenge for other ways of acting in political life and for broader gender equality in leadership. It also explains why it can be so hard to root out bullying and harassing behavior especially when targeting women or anyone else who is in a subordinate role since this behavior is seen as normal or a typical behavior among politicians (Kimmel 1996; Katz 2016).

The logic of masculine protection allows us to see how male leaders even when blending gender stereotypes of masculinity and femininity—assertiveness and care—still do so within a framework of male dominance even if they seem to counter the worst effects of macho aggression and abuse. This is one reason Young's (2007) work is valuable to trace the interplay of gender expectations of leadership which may blind us to the costs of male protection. This form of protection has its attractions. Young writes that the "good man" in a protector role "keeps vigilant watch over the safety of his family" and that the logic of masculinist protection includes the figure of the "selfish aggressor," the "bad man" against whom the good protector acts (2007, p. 119). In return for this protection those in a subordinate relationship, such as the feminine woman, are not submitting to a violent bully, but rather happily deferring to this protection. "She looks up to him with gratitude for his manliness and admiration for his willingness to face the dangers of the world for her sake" (p. 119). Analogizing this logic of masculinist protection from the personal to the public sphere, Young (2007) builds a case that Bush utilized the rhetoric of protection, of the nation and of saving women and girls, as justification for the war in Afghanistan and Iraq. Bush was not known as a defender of women's rights in the United States, nor for democratic protections against unnecessary surveillance threatening privacy rights. By positioning himself as a defender of women and girls elsewhere, he made the actions of his administration and the move to war more palatable to many who otherwise would not think so. While the pandemic is not the same as justifying war to a population for national security, there are analogies to be made in terms of the logic of masculinist protection that help explain the favorable ratings of Cuomo's pandemic leadership. Cuomo performs the position of the "good man" in his pandemic briefings. In this case there is not an external enemy. Instead, we have juxtaposed to the protector the internal threat of the Trump administration and Trump himself, who threatens public health through inaction or denial of the science of the disease. Of course, for many Republicans and Trump supporters, Cuomo was never their protector but a hindrance to the president and economic recovery. However, to explain Cuomo's broad appeal as a pandemic leader means acknowledging the protector role he embodied in this global health crisis.

To call attention to the discordant experience of Cuomo's actions as protector and abuser, it is useful to notice how he positioned himself as a defender of women even before the pandemic. Cuomo had many senior women working for him and he promoted women's rights in legislation, such as his 2012 Women's Equality Agenda and the Reproductive Health Act he signed in 2019; however, many saw this as motivated to solidify his own power (Lerer, 2021b). Likewise, Cuomo also formed the Women's Equality Party (WEP), which did little to support women candidates or anyone opposed to Cuomo's administration. The origin of WEP in 2014 was to hold off an unexpectedly robust primary challenge from Zephyr Teachout and position Cuomo as a leader for women rights (Grim, 2021). Women, usually white women, have benefited from working with patriarchal male leaders seeing themselves as exceptions to the rule with how other women are treated. Rebecca Traister (2021) reinforces this, "Powerful white women have often benefited from, and thus worked to uphold abusive patriarchal power systems" (p. 18). One such beneficiary is Secretary to the Governor Melissa DeRosa, who served as Cuomo's enforcer "under the guise of girl power" (Traister 2021, p. 18). It is an old tactic of white patriarchal power to allow some white women, and some women of color, to have important roles to play but always in deference to the male leader, positioned in dependent roles as an aide, daughter, wife, supporter, or the public writ large.

Thinking about how Cuomo could effectively be both a protector to the public and also abusive to others and the public trust, I suggest Cuomo performs leadership through a "comforting crush" of masculinist protection. "Comfort crush" has two meanings to note—on the one hand, the meaning in popular culture refers to a character you desire who makes you feel safe (Urban Dictionary 2021). On the other hand, the downside to this "crush" is evident when that comfort turns intimidating and abusive.

Living in New York and working from home when my college went fully online, I watched or listened to Cuomo's briefings several times a week starting in March 2020 until they ended in June. At the time I was listening not as a scholar, but as a college professor and concerned citizen. In returning to the briefings more critically to understand their appeal, I bring together an archive of media reports and popular culture sources. I also sample pandemic briefings to test the claim about masculine protection as both comforting and crushing to equity and democratic health. I chose six pandemic briefings to read inductively paying attention to the presentation of scientific data, the rhetoric of comfort, and policy actions taken to protect our health and well-being. I include the first briefing, every fifth Monday briefing from March 2, 2020 to June 8, 2020, which happened to be day 100 after the first coronavirus case, and the last briefing on June 19. I relied on the archived briefings on the New York State Department of Health page

"Past Coronavirus Briefings" which brings you to the YouTube site. I also procured the official transcript from the governor's website when available or from transcriptions available via YouTube. For depth and contextualization, I added popular press sources that describe Cuomo's comforting crush, his briefings, and PowerPoint slides. I examined both words and visual forms of communication to explore the power of the briefings. Dan Schill (2012) argues that it is important for scholars of political communication to study the power of visual symbols. The staging, dress and appearance, tone, and PowerPoint slides we see are powerful forms of nonverbal communication.

CUOMO AND THE COMFORT CRUSH

New York Governor Andrew Cuomo offered his first COVID-19 pandemic briefing on March 2, 2020. He would offer 111 briefings, his last on June 19, 2020. Even those not historically favorable to Cuomo's moderate brand of liberalism, or those who were critical of his transactional, often vindictive, and controlling leadership style, had praise for Cuomo as the pandemic started to tear through New York City and the state. Ben Smith (2020) writes in the *New York Times* that "Andrew Cuomo Is the Control Freak We Need Right Now" saying that those bullying, micromanaging traits have a benefit in a crisis. Rebecca Fishbein (2020) writes in the feminist cultural venue *Jezebel* of her worries about being alone in her apartment, if her father would survive, if she will hug anyone again. She reports that it's Cuomo who offers an edgy comfort. She writes,

> Andrew Cuomo, Dear Leader, will take care of me. He loves me. He is the only one who is here for me. He will help me get through this. And when I finally do, I will need an endless amount of anti-brainwash therapy so I can rightfully yell at him for using prison labor to make hand sanitizer.

In a conversation with journalist Kara Swisher, the comedian Chelsea Handler also expressed a love for Cuomo, and then a deep disappointment after the abuse allegations saying that during the pandemic, "I was very turned on by his morning news conferences, as many of us were." (cited in Swisher, 2021). Handler continues, "And then I found out all the stuff we found out about him . . . so my crush with him is, yes, O-V-E-R" (cited in Swisher 2021). The term "Cuomosexual" was first popularized by comedian Randy Rainbow, who said that he identified as #Cuomosexual (Chapin, 2021), a hashtag printed on many t-shirts. Even the well-known New York actor Robert De Niro praised Cuomo on *The Late Show with Stephen Colbert* (2020). De Niro speculated that when the movie is written about this era we will see that Cuomo is "doing what any president should do" and that he could see a President Cuomo in the future.

At least part of Cuomo's appeal was that he often demonstrated empathy and performed care by talking about his family. This is not unusual given that (white) men have often presented themselves as the ones who are responsible for others and the household in the liberal social contract tradition (Pateman, 1988). Cuomo made reference to his then 88-year-old mother, Matilda, his three adult daughters (Cara, Michaela, and Mariah), and "the boyfriend" as well as to his brother, the CNN host Chris Cuomo, on whose show he appeared during the pandemic (in pre-pandemic times he did not do this given the familial relationship and crossing of journalistic lines). Positioning himself in a traditional masculine role, Cuomo could be father, son, brother, executive, and simultaneously always in charge. Cuomo embodied recognizable expressions of male leadership in speech, dress, and posture, speaking with authoritative, declarative statements, strong voice projection, wearing a traditional white-collar suit or casual golf shirt while sitting at the center of a table. Drawing on the specificity of his Italian-American background and New York identity also allowed him to use cultural expectations of "toughness" that tracks with stereotypical masculine expressions of hardness, aggression, and control. This is also an identity he referenced in his book *American Crisis: Leadership Lessons from the COVID-19 Pandemic* (2020).

Using the now famous PowerPoint slides, which were often humorous, frank, serious, and/or data driven, Cuomo took a more academic style of presentation with the PowerPoint slides and made them an organizing tool to inform and speak to the public. Indeed, the PowerPoint slides were a hit on their own, showing how Cuomo transformed a wonkish and academic way to organize information visually and succinctly into a distinct part of his pandemic briefing genre. News outlets made lists of the best of Cuomo's pandemic slides. *Business Insider* (2020) listed the 27 best PowerPoint memes such as "This will be over." and "It's not 'you' or 'me' it's 'we'" demonstrating the humorous way Cuomo suggests that we are all in this together. Other lists from *Yello Substack*, a digital newsletter about visual politics; *Vulture,* an online magazine that tracks the U.S. cultural landscape*;* *Mother Jones,* the progressive news outlet; and even *Art in America* illustrate the power of the aesthetic and rhetorical innovation of the PowerPoint slides with the combination of data, policy, empathy, and irreverent or commonsensical concerns. Shannon Mattern (2020) writes in *Art in America,* "His slides mix impersonal factual delivery with second-person exhortations, first-person declarations, and philosophical introspection. One slide reminds us: 'Today is Saturday,' with 'Saturday' emblazoned in gold. This statement of truth is accidentally hilarious in its self-evidence." This content and the visual presentation resonated with viewers and helps explain the comfort Cuomo offered and what made those briefings "must see TV." In tapping into all of these performative roles, Cuomo embodied the protector in ways that made him and his message attractive to the public.

Looking at a sample of Cuomo's pandemic briefings, we see a pattern of his blend of confidence and control with humor and care that offered comfort in repetition of facts, coupled with the performance of empathy. March 2, 2020, the first pandemic briefing. Cuomo sits in the center of a draped table. Sitting near—not in our social distancing mode yet—are New York City Mayor Bill de Blasio and health care professionals. Behind Cuomo are the flags of the United States and New York State. Cuomo wears a dark suit, white shirt, and red tie. He speaks in the manner for which he will be nationally recognized (McKinley & Goldmacher 2021) as measured, calm, decisive, and reasonable as he presents content with the appearance of candor and scientific insights. Cuomo mentions that the first infected person documented in New York is a health care worker who did not take any public transportation, though she recently traveled. The state will contact people who were on her flight "out of an abundance of caution." Cuomo says it's a matter of not if, but when there will be more cases. He recognizes the anxiety the public has. To illustrate this, he describes a call he had with his daughter after she saw news of the positive test case.

> And I could hear in her voice she was nervous. And my daughter said, 'don't tell me to relax. Tell me why I should be relaxed.' Which is a very big difference there. So, I want to make sure I tell the people of New York what I told my daughter. In this situation, the facts defeat fear. Because the reality is reassuring. It is deep breath time.

After giving some explanation about the mortality rate, he notes that children do not appear as vulnerable. Moving to a conclusion he says look at the facts and the facts will dictate reality. He says, "I get the emotion, I understand it, I understand the anxiety. I'm a native-born New Yorker, we live with anxiety. But, the facts don't back it up here." I mention these aspects of the briefing to illustrate the form and content of the briefings that will recur. The setting out of facts, the care in how to speak of the anxiety out there, and the example of his own family experience as a source of connection and comfort. He is in charge and the state is taking action to help. The protector role is in play, the comforter is here.

April 6, 2020, socially distanced on the panel are Cuomo and four others, including Secretary to the Governor Melissa DeRosa, who will regularly be at the briefings. "Good morning, the start of another workweek, or not," he begins in recognition of what has changed. The setting is the Red Room of the New York State Capital with its impressive architecture and wood wainscoting which will often be the site of future briefings. The tagline on the bottom of the slides—which will be readily recognizable as the briefings continue—states in capital letters: "STAY HOME. STOP THE SPREAD. SAVE LIVES." There are concerns about hospital capacity in New York City. Cuomo also thanks first responders and health care workers whose photos appear on the slide show with their first names and job title.

At the 18:47 mark Cuomo reports that he had good conversations with his daughters Cara and Michaela about the difficulties unfolding in the pandemic. He says it's hard to hear number of deaths, and he sees his job to prevent this loss, "we like to think we can control everything, we can't." On the slide labeled "Perspective" he reiterates, "We will lose people—the virus takes the most vulnerable." The last slide says "New York Tough = compassionate, unified, loving, smart." These themes of compassion, unity, intelligence, and love are ones that he returns to again and again in these briefings.

May 11, 2020, pandemic briefing. He jokes, "Scattered applause, scattered people, scattered applause" as he enters the room. The coverage of the briefings has reached national outlets (O'Kane, 2020). Cuomo has issued an Executive Order mandating mask wearing as of April 17, 2020. We see reporters in the audience, socially distanced, and they appear to be wearing or adjusting masks. At this stage Cuomo is optimistic that "we are on the other side of the mountain" and he says reopening plans are for May 15, the upcoming Friday. This leads into his "Personal Opinion" slide and riff on how now people do not see competence in government today. But that is what he wants to show. Cuomo analogizing himself to Lincoln, saying an informed public will keep the country safe. Putting himself in the company of Lincoln as a great unifier and protector of the nation is clearly how he wants to be seen.

June 8, 2020 pandemic briefing include remarks on the murder of George Floyd. Reporters in the audience are wearing masks. On the slide we see the word "Day" in white, "100" in yellow font on a blue-sky background. The sign interpreter, which was ordered by a federal judge (Campbell, 2020), is in the corner of the screen revealing that inclusion was not always the case in the briefings for the deaf or hard of hearing community. Cuomo is optimistic about New York reopening. This is a briefing on the longer side at over 45 minutes. He says we went from the one of the worst situations in the nation, and on the globe, to one that is better than the rest of the United States (6:28). Soon after this he mentions the death of George Floyd, noting that now we have dual crises. The slide says, "Opportunity for NYS to lead nation in wake of George Floyd murder." This is Cuomo taking on a more national profile, and clearly wanting to do so as a broader protector of the nation from the harms of the pandemic and racism. Cuomo was not generally seen as a leader on police reforms and antiracism, but he had been consistent in his work with African American community leaders in New York whose support he relied on in elections (Durkin, 2021). At the end of the briefing Cuomo takes a number of questions from reporters. Cuomo wears a dark suit, white shirt, and purple tie; he is not masked in the briefings when he is speaking. Here we see Cuomo following the format of previous briefings and wanting to be more nationally relevant in speaking about the murder of George Floyd. Both his role to comfort and lead, and a national audience, are in mind.

June 19, 2020, the last briefing. Cuomo is sitting at his office desk, a sign interpreter is on the lower right of the screen. Cuomo says, "Good morning, today is Friday, Juneteenth" (the day emancipation was delivered to slaves in Texas 1865). There is a photo with his three daughters on the table behind him. Cuomo says New York will recognize Juneteenth as a holiday. There are no PowerPoint slides. He says the numbers are showing the lowest weekly infection rate, lowest death, despite 25 souls lost each day to "remember in prayers." While COVID isn't over, he says in the past three months we have "done the impossible," New York went from "worst to first" in handling the pandemic. He thanks people for their support, including his daughters and people who sent letters and tweets. He continues, to the 59 million viewers who shared in these daily briefings, thank you for the support and "don't worry I'm not going anywhere," he concludes. The briefing takes just over nine minutes. The conclusion is an uplifting slide show of where we have been since the first briefing and it sets the stage for Cuomo as a conquering hero, even the redeemer of health and good government. That hero myth, however, has not been borne out. The comforter had crushed the very things he claimed to value: transparency, public health, equity, and cooperation in governing, and it was hidden behind the protector role in a time of crisis.

THE ONGOING AFTERMATH

The New York State Attorney General's report was released on August 3, 2021. The investigation found that Governor Andrew Cuomo had sexually harassed 11 women, several of whom were aides, unlawfully retaliated against one woman, and created a toxic work environment. Cuomo announced he would resign effective 14 days later. Cuomo resigned on August 24, 2021. Lieutenant Governor Kathy Hochul was sworn in as New York's first woman governor, promising a new era of transparency in government with "a dramatic change in culture" and no tolerance for individuals who cross the line (Hochul, 2021).

Lessons from the pandemic are still to be learned. One thing that we have learned, however, is how easily we the public accept what I have referred to as the logic of masculine protection, especially when we are in a crisis. We crave, rightly so, direction and effective government. Protection is, after all, an essential element of the social contract. Yet if this protection follows the logic of masculinist protection, this form of stereotypical male power can hide uncomfortable truths about failures to act to protect our health and the inability to call to account abuses of power. This happens precisely because it is so familiar as a hierarchical political style of behavior that depends on dependents. All too commonly those dependents are women in general, people of color, and those without resources. This isn't the power of an authoritarian-leaning macho man, but a more benign but no less potentially abusive leadership style when unchecked. It is, as Traister (2021) writes, a kind of power that

> could be petty, corrupt, threatening, skeezy; it could be handsy at weddings and harassing at the office; it could lie and cover up and be sent to jail and still it would be our norm and all we had to turn to in a storm, through a pandemic. We had to pin our hopes on it as a refuge from other, worse brutal white patriarchs. And so we learned to love it, to tune in to its daily briefings and allow its self-assuredness to wash over us.

This is different from the shock doctrine and incompetence of President Trump, which is inflammatory, violent, overly brutal and macho, and often insulting in its rhetoric (Honig, 2021). While Trump has a "shock doctrine" effect in the polity, Cuomo I suggest offered a "comfort crush" in pulling the polity in close, but too close for workplace and democratic health. Cuomo's pandemic briefings were powerful because it was familiar in its logic of masculine protection offering a broad rhetoric of care: caring for the science, caring for others, caring for family, and performing a series of relevant affects such as grief, frustration, and love. The downsides, however, are to limit our democratic health and the value of professionalism, civic service, and fair treatment in the workplace. This poses challenges to the trust and collaboration we need to meet the next crisis together.

REFERENCES

Aboim, S., Hearn, J., & and Howson, R. (2016). Hegemonic masculinity. In G. Ritzer (Ed.). *The Blackwell encyclopedia of sociology online* (2nd ed.). Wiley-Blackwell. doi:10.1002/9781405165518.wbeosh022.pub2 (pp.1–4).

Alter, R. (2020, March 23). 7 great moments in Cuomo's coronavirus PowerPoint slides. *Vulture: New York Magazine.* https://www.vulture.com/2020/03/governor-cuomo-press-conference-7-greatest-moments.html.

Barkan, R. (2021a, March 5). Andrew Cuomo was never a hero. Karma is coming for him, with a vengeance. *The Guardian.* https://www.theguardian.com

/commentisfree/2021/mar/05/andrew-cuomo-sexual-harassment-nursing-home-deaths-accused.

Barkan, R. (2021b). *The prince: Andrew Cuomo, coronavirus and the fall of New York.* OR Books.

Boylan, L. (2021, Feb. 24). My story of working with Governor Cuomo. https://lindseyboylan4ny.medium.com/my-story-of-working-with-governor-cuomo-e664d4814b4e.

Campbell, J. (2020, May, 12). Judge orders Andrew Cuomo to add sign-language interpreter to coronavirus briefings. *Democrat & Chronicle.* https://www.democratandchronicle.com/story/news/politics/albany/2020/05/11/judge-orders-andrew-cuomo-add-asl-interpreter-covid-19-briefings/3112892001/.

Carpinella, C. & Bauer, N. M. (2021). A visual analysis of gender stereotypes in campaign advertising. *Politics, Groups, and Identities, 9*(2), 369–386.

Carroll, S. J. & Fox, R. L. (Eds.). (2018). *Gender and elections: Shaping the future of American elections (4th ed).* Cambridge University Press. https://doi.org/10.1017/9781108277792.

Chapel, B. (2021, March 5). New York legislature strips Cuomo of extraordinary emergency powers, with a caveat. *NPR.* https://www.npr.org/2021/03/05/974083354/new-york-legislature-strips-cuomo-of-extraordinary-emergency-powers-with-a-caveat.

Chapin, A. (2021, March 22). What do Andrew Cuomo's former 'cuomosexual' fans think now? *New York Magazine.* https://www.thecut.com/2021/03/andrew-cuomo-cuomosexual-fans.html.

Colbert, S. (2020, May 7). The Late Show with Stephen Colbert. https://www.youtube.com/watch?v=B7H41OYIWrU.

Connell, R.W. & Messerschmidt, J. W. (2005). Hegemonic masculinity: Rethinking the concept. *Gender and Society, 19*(6), 829–859.

Cuomo, A. (2020). *American crisis: Leadership lessons from the COVID-19 pandemic*. Crown.

Diamond, D. (2021, March 29). Feuds, fibs and finger-pointing: Trump officials say coronavirus response was worse than known. *Washington Post.* https://www.washingtonpost.com/health/2021/03/29/trump-officials-tell-all-coronavirus-response/.

Dittmar, K. (2015). *Navigating gendered terrain: Stereotypes and strategy in political campaigns.* Temple University Press.

Dugyala, R. & Jin, B. (2021, October 3). Trauma and Trump make Asian American voters a more cohesive bloc, new poll reveals. *Politico.* https://www.politico.com/interactives/2021/asian-american-community-voting-trends-polling/.

Durkin, R. (2021, March 3). 'Go to your friends': Black leaders rally around Cuomo. *Politico.* https://www.politico.com/states/new-york/albany/story/2021/03/17/go-to-your-friends-black-leaders-and-voters-rally-around-cuomo-1368623.

Fishbein, R. (2020, March 19). Help, I think I'm in love with Andrew Cuomo??? *Jezebel.* https://jezebel.com/help-i-think-im-in-love-with-andrew-cuomo-1842396411.

Goodman, J.D., Hong, N., & Ferré-Sadurní, L. (2021, April 29). F.B.I. investigating whether Cuomo aides gave false data on nursing homes. https://www.nytimes.com/2021/03/19/nyregion/cuomo-nursing-homes-covid.html.

Governor New York State (2020–2021). https://www.governor.ny.gov; https://coronavirus.health.ny.gov/past-coronavirus-briefings.

Grim, R. (2021. March 15). Cuomo's 'women's equality party' might just be the most cynical political move of his career. *The Intercept*. https://theintercept.com/2021/03/15/andrew-cuomo-womens-equality-party/.

Hochul, K. (2021, August 24). Inauguration speech. *YouTube*. https://www.youtube.com/watch?v =J9BTZHZrgbw.

Hoffower, H. (2020, March 18). 'No bailout boondoggles': 27 of NY Gov. Andrew Cuomo's best PowerPoint slides. *Business Insider*. https://www.businessinsider.com/andrew-cuomo-best-powerpoint-slides-memes-nys-governor-coronavirus-briefings-2020-5#what-type-of-bread-shall-we-bake-in-quarantine-day-2451-22.

Honig, B. (2021). *Shell shocked: Feminist criticism after Trump*. Fordham University Press.

Jeffords, S. (2004). *Hard bodies: Hollywood masculinity in the Reagan era*. Rutgers University Press.

Katz, J. (2016). *Man enough? Donald Trump, Hillary Clinton, and the politics of presidential masculinity*. Interlink Pub Group.

Kimmel, M. (1996). *Manhood in America: A cultural history*. The Free Press.

Lee, M.J., & Morales, M. (2021, February 17). Cuomo said 'he can destroy me': NY assemblyman alleges governor threatened him over nursing homes scandal. *CNN*. https://www.cnn.com/2021/02/17/politics/cuomo-ron-kim-nursing-home/index.html.

Lerer, L. (2021a, March 15). Why Al Franken hovers over the debate about Cuomo's future. *New York Times*. https://www.nytimes.com/2021/03/12/us/politics/al-franken-cuomo-me-too.html.

Lerer, L. (2021b, August 11). Cuomo advanced a feminist agenda. Was that just politics? *New York Times*. https://www.nytimes.com/2021/08/11/us/politics/andrew-cuomo-feminism-womens-rights.html.

Mattern, S. (2020, April 13). Andrew Cuomo's COVID-19 briefings draw on the persuasive authority of PowerPoint. *Art in America*. https://www.artnews.com/art-in-america/features/andrew-cuomo-covid-briefings-powerpoint-slideshow-authority-1202683735/.

McKinley, J. (2021, March 5). As outcry over nursing homes grows, Cuomo lashes out at critics. *New York Times*. https://www.nytimes.com/2021/02/19/nyregion/cuomo-nursing-homes.html?searchResultPosition=1.

McKinley, J. & Goldmacher, S. (2021, February 22). How Cuomo, once on sidelines, became the politician of the moment. *New York Times*. https://www.nytimes.com/2020/03/24/nyregion/governor-andrew-cuomo-coronavirus.html.

New York State Attorney General. (2021, January 28). Nursing home response to COVID-19. https://ag.ny.gov/press-release/2021/attorney-general-james-releases-report-nursing-homes-response-COVID-19.

New York State Attorney General (2021, August 3) *Report of Investigation into Allegations of Sexual Harassment by New York Governor Andrew M. Cuomo.* https://ag.ny.gov/sites/default/files/2021.08.03_nyag_-_investigative_report.pdf.

O'Kane, C. (2020, March 24). New York Governor Andrew Cuomo takes national spotlight during coronavirus pandemic. *CBS News*. https://www.cbsnews.com/news/coronavirus-updates-new-york-governor-andrew-cuomo-takes-national-spotlight-during-coronavirus-pandemic-2020-03-24.

Pateman, C. (1998). *The sexual contract*. Stanford University Press.

Paumgarten, N. (2020, October 12). Andrew Cuomo, the king of New York. *The New Yorker*. https://www.newyorker.com/magazine/2020/10/19/andrew-cuomo-the-king-of-new-york.

Paumgarten, N. with Host Lach, E. (2021, March 11). "Politics and more" podcast from *The New Yorker* and WNYC. https://www.wnyc.org/story/andrew-cuomo-pandemic-hero-political-pariah/.

RAINN (Rape, Abuse & Incest National Network) (2021). https://www.rainn.org/?_ga=2.50622241.960972865.1626106044-997684343.1626106044.

Santiago, A. L. H., Sharpe, S., Dolby, N., & Williams, Z. (2021, April 8). All the allegations against Cuomo. *City and State*. https://www.cityandstateny.com/articles/politics/new-york-state/all-allegations-against-cuomo.html.

Sapiro, V., Cramer Walsh, C., Strach, P., & Hennings, V. (2011). Gender, context, and television advertising: A comprehensive analysis of 2000 and 2002 house races. *Political Research Quarterly, 64(*1), 107–119.

Schacht, L.P. (2020, April 8). Cuomo and Trump's sailing briefings in a propaganda world. *Brookings.* https://www.brookings.edu/blog/fixgov/2020/04/08/cuomo-and-trumps-daily-briefings-in-a-propaganda-world/.

Schill, D. (2012). The visual image and the political image: A review of visual communication research in the field of political communication. *The Review of Communication, 12*(2), 118–142.

Schwarz, D. H. (2020, April 27). The 31 best Andrew Cuomo slides. *Yello Substack.* https://yello.substack.com/p/the-31-best-andrew-cuomo-slides.

Smith, B. (2020, March 16). Andrew Cuomo is the control freak we need right now. *The New York Times.* https://www.nytimes.com/2020/03/16/business/media/cuomo-new-york-coronavirus.html.

Swisher, K. (2021, July 8). Chelsea Handler has a message for straight men. *Sway* [Podcast]. https://www.nytimes.com/2021/07/08/opinion/sway-kara-swisher-chelsea-handler.html.

Thompson, L. (2020, March 24). A series of reassuring and oddly endearing PowerPoints from New York Governor Andrew Cuomo. *Mother Jones.* https://www.motherjones.com/coronavirus-updates/2020/03/a-series-of-reassuring-and-oddly-endearing-powerpoints-from-new-york-governor-andrew-cuomo/.

Traister, R. (2021, March 15–28). The cruelty and the casualties: Inside Andrew Cuomo's toxic workplace. *New York Magazine*. https://nymag.com/intelligencer/article/andrew-cuomo-misconduct-allegations.html.

Viglione, G. (2021, November 3). Four ways Trump meddled in pandemic science—and why it matters. *Nature.* https://www.nature.com/articles/d41586-020-03035-4.

Villeneuve, M. & Hill, M. (2020, June 19). 100 days of Cuomo: Governor ends daily COVID-19 briefings. *AP News.* https://apnews.com/article/us-news-andrew-cuomo-new-york-virus-outbreak-ny-state-wire-5a63c14d5684e995f6827057f895efd6.

Williams, Z. (2021, March 18). Melissa DeRosa was on the rise, then the last two months happened. *City and State New York,* March 18, 2021. https://www.cityandstateny.com/articles/politics/new-york-state/melissa-derosa-was-rise-then-last-two-months-happened.html.

Young, I. M. (2007). The logic of masculinist protection: Reflections on the current security state. In Michaele L. Ferguson and Lori Jo Marso (Eds.), *W Stands for Women: How the George W. Bush Presidency Shaped a New Politics of Gender.* Duke University Press (pp. 115–139).

Zimmerman, J. F. (2008). *The government and politics of New York State.* (2nd ed.). State University of New York Press.

PART 2

Creativity and Productivity

Chapter Seven

Being There and Not

Slippery Simulacrums of Song

David Staton

Graduation. Travel. Weddings. Being there. It's something, many things really, we've missed out on during the pandemic. For some, there are no substitutes, no solutions, no quick fixes. If part of your DNA is tethered to a church, you've had to, at varying times, limit your attendance, which cuts into the community and the communal ideas and ideals of a congregation. And no singing, as harmonic vocalizing may spread the virus, and no sacred communion (too close). One clergyman, when asked about the viability of virtual church, expressed the absence this way in a *New York Times* article: "You can't program the body and blood of Christ in 1s and 0s of digital code" (Hansen, 2021). For him, there is no sacred simulacrum. But, we still persist, we persevere, and, one way or another, prayer prevails. From ministerial YouTube videos to a host of live streaming applications (Dacast, streamingchurch.TV, TruthCasting, etc.), we've expanded opportunity. "Come as you are in your car" was the slogan adopted by one church in New Jersey (Chow, 2020). One might consider sports another kind of religion. It, too, has similarly been impacted as for many months fans were prohibited from attending live competition. However, as we adapt and adopt, we accommodate: a case of stagecraft (writ large) and spectacle meeting wishful thinking underscore any number of simulated participatory acts. Rather than in-person attendees at stadiums and arenas, many televised collegiate and professional sporting events were filled with life-sized cardboard cutout fan photographs and engineered crowd sounds developed by digital gaming giant Electronic Arts echoed through the empty spaces. For $299 you could get a cutout image of yourself (or your dog, for $149) in a very good seat at Dodger

Stadium. We've also Zoomed, Skyped, and Teamsed our way into countless classes and conferences all for the sake of being there.

Being There is also the name of a film in the National Film Registry. Oh yes, going to the movies, that's something else we've missed, not that we've been without any number of theatrical releases—thank you, Disney+, HBO Max, Apple TV+, Amazon Prime Video, and the host of other all-star streaming services. That 1979 movie concerns Chance, a middle-aged man who has lived and learned all worth knowing from watching television. Baudrillard (1981) would say Chance is guided by the map, not the territory; however, his naiveté is interpreted by those in his orbit as a sort of genius-level wisdom in a world in which life is a state of mind. *Being There* also provides the title for one of my deserted island playlist must-haves, the sophomore effort by Wilco, the longtime Chicago-based rock band. That double-album recording contains twisted tales of intimacy and anxiety and disasters large and small. It's a group I've experienced (not simply seen or heard or went to, *experienced*) many, many times. But not recently. Recently I've not been there. And I not only miss the thing itself, but all the things that went with the thing itself; and the attendant and certain lovely feeling of presence. I've been almost there.

ALMOST THERE

Benjamin (1935) understood reality and presence surrounding art as being reliant on experiencing the original—mechanical reproduction eliminates the art object's aura. The genuine article was "an instrument of magic" a space of contemplation; its reproduction requires no attention and results in an absent-minded consumer (241). That sort of interaction and experience only grew with the proliferation of broadcast media, and along with it came McLuhan's edict, "the medium is the message" (1964). This idea was later quoted in admonitions by Debord in *The Society of the Spectacle* (1967): "The spectacle's social function is the concrete manufacture of alienation (11). Later still, Baudrillard asserted that sometimes the map, not the thing itself, was useful in understanding the territory in that we gain a distance and different perspective. He deftly describes this moment, suggesting it becomes a new experience: "When the real is no longer what it used to be, nostalgia assumes its full meaning. There is a plethora of myths of origin and signs of reality; of secondary objectivity and authenticity" (7). Hence, a new "old" reality we are yearning for may become synthetic, the simulacrum redirecting the focus to what we have, not what we have not, "it masks the absence of a basic reality" (6), Baudrillard notes. This is the third of four orders of simulacrum described in the French scholar's *Simulacra and Simulation* (1981). It's likely the most eyebrow raising of his reality iterations as it suggests we live in an utterly constructed world that is grounded in the hyperreal; there is no prototype to mimic by reproduction as the "real" has ceded to an imitation of appearance, "it is of the order of sorcery" (6). If that sounds daunting consider the digital products we knowingly and sometimes unknowingly interact with each day in a host of spaces: artificial intelligence, virtual reality, "fake news," audio tracks created by algorithm, and deep fakes. We live in the hyperreal, which does sort of conjure sorcery.

Perhaps you're a wizard, but for the rest of us we've all had to back a number of things out of our personal equations during the pandemic; adapt, adopt, *and* transition. Mostly, we've had to change our expectations, then recalibrate whilst anticipating more change, more instability. If your day-to-day belief system has remained the same throughout, carry on! But, if you're anything like myself, you've questioned the quotidian and reexamined, reimagined, and repurposed whatever "normal" once was. Of all of those things that were backed out of my routine, I felt the pangs of absence the most; my loss of health: I endured COVID-19 twice and had a major, reconstructive spinal surgery, the lack of energy and ability to exercise, an utter void of spontaneity, and a limiting of habitat. Of such deprivations, one that left a large space, and the one I tried to fill, was experiencing live music. I'm cognizant this is a non-consequential, blind passion, and I'm equally (self) aware that it's necessary to my well-being. It's been an and/both, more-is-better part of my life for many years now, opening doors and dialogues with utter strangers and shared experiences with longtime friends—everyone remembers their first and their worst, and they're happy to talk about it.

In a former career, I was paid to attend music spectacles. For me, the role of critic was (and remains) fulfilling on a number of levels, not the least of which is to act as an intermediary for those who can't attend, to bear witness to a live performance on their behalf. I continued to frequently attend live music events well after my reporting days were distant, from an acoustic performance at a local craft beer-tasting room near my northern Colorado home to a bewildered Beck playing Prince covers at an amusement park in Stockholm. No matter the venue, concert-going has been a core element of my existence. Giving voice to missing this, admittedly, seems trite in the throes of a pandemic. But it's extraordinarily, selfishly true—I felt the absence of the entirety of the live music experience, which had been delimited by a global scourge. These new boundaries were exhaustingly frustrating because they excluded such a rich local and regional music scene, including the concert mecca venue, Red Rocks Amphitheater, where the dozen or so tickets I'd purchased early on for five summer 2020 performances became objects of suspended imagination. As music venues shut down—among them the wonderfully creaky Gothic Theatre, the elegant Ellie Caulkins

Opera House, and the intimate Ophelia's Electric Soapbox—the presence of absence became manifest in myriad ways. The *Denver Post* headlined one story "Loss of concerts makes Denver question its cultural identity" (Wenzel, 2020) and noted the nearly $1.5 billion impact the live-concert industry has on the state's economy. I take such warm comfort from live music, because it is an engrained, embodied performative act. I looked to locate a portion of my identity amid the loss of livelihoods and leisure.

LIKE BEING THERE

In a turn of phrase, I believe necessity nurtures innovation. For those whom the music must play on, different delivery avenues surfaced; people were not going to the music, the music was coming to them via digital access. A bevy of providers and producers surfaced to ensure live performance continued and were viewed but, for me, *not* experienced. I became familiar with the varying degree of quality in live streaming and staged productions presented by Mandolin (generally superb!), Bandsintown Plus (a regrettable Q&A format with a forgettable host), and nugs.net (cinematic in scope and intention) to name a few. I will not deny there exists a rich history of recorded live music performance, and here I think of the cinematic biggies like *Monterey Pop*, *Woodstock,* and *The Last Waltz* or the indelible TV performances on *The Ed Sullivan Show*, *Top of the Pops*, and *Soul Train*. However, viewing performance via a live stream is a more contemporary performance iteration, and it is performed differently. It seems inconceivable to me, as I was waiting for countless hours on an America On Line dial-up connection during this bygone era, but the first concert was streamed on the net in 1993 by the trivia-question-worthy band, Severe Tire Damage. This other band, the Rolling Stones, would venture into that digital space the following year (Alfred, 2009).

Traditionally, during live performance a musician or singer is being watched by a viewer from a fixed perspective. That fundamentally changed with the exclusion of audiences the pandemic brought with it. The cameras are the onlookers. This may fundamentally alter the dynamic of music performance; ball players are still looking to put points on the board, but musicians may be looking for their closeup (they play from a score, not keep one). Whether you're watching on a mobile device or a wall-filling flat screen, the glaring asymmetry of giver and receiver is upended. Depending on the platform and provider, agency is generally ceded to the viewers; they receive the best seat in the house. And in an era of televised wish fulfillment for spectators, always closer and ever nearer shape the visual experience even more so in a time of social distancing. It is a highly mediated experience to the extent that applied technologies, e.g., Skycam video or micro closeups, inform a way of viewing that is at once visually immersive and emotionally disengaging. The action is always in your lap. Benjamin writes of this spatial and temporal arrangement that it "reactivates the object produced" (44). Perhaps my longing could be filled by this reactivation, this replacement in which the copy has no original.

During my most recent from-home concert experience, a pairing of Wilco and Sleater-Kinney at Red Rocks Amphitheater (August, 2021), I was seated in a super comfy red leather armchair, my wife on a *Titanic*-sized love seat and our two dogs nestled by our feet. I was drinking one of my favorite IPAs and had a gas fire insert with dancing flames available at our behest resting just behind our heads. As we settled in for our viewing of the performance, blankets and pillows tucked just so, the weather at the fully-exposed outdoor venue looked pleasant, though I have been there when it is not . . . very not. I also didn't have to worry about tipping over the drink of the person next to me or that overly-served patron who offers vile smells and cheap comments ("Play 'Free Bird,' dude!!!") as the performance is unfolding. And when nature calls, there's not a 20-minute slog to a washroom with floors coated in sticky concoctions nor the miasma of the skunky, sweet nectar of weed, alcohol, and high desert air. Rather, at the push of a pause button, I enter the world of time shifting and, moving carefully between dozing dogs, pad my way off in socked feet to take a wee break, simultaneously altering and navigating the temporality and distance between songs.

This is the transmuted message, a shift in aura, Debord's spectacle through a kaleidoscopic lens, that sort of new media process that redefines narrative and experience as Manovich (2000) explained in his exegesis on the subject. But what about new media is new? Is it a revolution, an evolution, or, as Silverstone (1999) argues, a "relationship between continuity and change" (10)? That topic has been tackled by many for a long time, and perhaps it's time not to once again unpack the idea, but to retire the expression; we all engage in contemporary media practice. A better frame for talking of this mediated experience might be to ask what's *different* about this media product? This is that which hides the absence of truth, Baudrillard notes (32); this distant digital delivery constitutes a secondhand truth. If I'd attended the Wilco/Sleater-Kinney show as planned, that analog experience would be different, perhaps something closer to a version of a truth, nearer to the aura. But, I've never seen Sleater-Kinney live, never participated in that particular listener-performer exchange; my sole understanding of the band is mediated.

Here is what mediated "truths" and a global pandemic does: it creates an affective space in which nostalgia is activated. I recall the fidelity of my mother playing hymns on her piano. It was my first in-person interaction with melodies. I had absolutely no question she was the finest musician to ever address the instrument. She was not. Near my childhood home there was a low-watt radio station, which you had to pass in order to trace the most direct path from "downtown" to our house. Four-year-old me would marvel at how that little building with the big lattice-work towers could house all those musicians, all those instruments, all that gear, and get their sound from the low-slung green "music hall" on Redwood Highway to our place on Redwood Avenue. I wondered how they could switch out all those people and equipment every three or four minutes. They did not. I was most assured in this fragile innocence; I believed my eyes and ears and that sets a pretty high bar.

Now I hunger for such wisdom, some sort of nourishment of in-person experience, the awareness that comes from realizing the ineffable quality and capacity of being human and of having a part of myself belong to something if only for the length of a song. Concert going has always provided that space. But pandemic time is largely predicated on screened encounters. It predisposes everyone to organize and restructure lives and information differently and adjust our vocabularies to include alternative facts, varying schemes of temporality, and abiding fear of missing something (anything). By unknowing compromise or willing acceptance, the simulacrum becomes the lived-in present. If everything is spectacle, nothing is. Does being there matter?

HERE WE ARE

Through the course of recovery (I have long COVID, there really isn't a recovery), I watched numerous streamed musical performances and, where the provider allowed, repeats. They were great. They were horrible. They made me wish for the genuine article, but this is the hyperreal thing Baudrillard addresses: he knew we were already there. "It is always the aim of ideological analysis to restore the objective process; it is always a false problem to want to restore the truth beneath the simulacrum." Because, the simulacrum is its own truth; "it bears no relation to any reality whatever" (6). It stands alone. Possessed of what Gillian Rose (2016) calls a good eye (I was involved for many years in the fine arts world after earning an Art History master's) and a pretty good ear (again, my music critic gig) I engaged in a sort of formal, hybridized textual analysis of a number of these performances: look and listen. My informal methodology relies on the strictly subjective personal, my "truth meter" which peaks into the red when I sense auto tune or vocal guide tracks or see/hear lip synching or detect voice-cloning software. I cannot accurately rely on aural evidence. And, too, images no longer bear the burden of proof because we live amid an era of PhotoShop and deep fake videos (it is impossible to unsee the mashup of Steve Buscemi as Jennifer Lawrence). We also have avatar-led virtual bands like Damon Albarn and

Jamie Hewlitt's long-running Gorrilaz. Both s(t)imulations have led us to a place very near the uncanny valley; a simulacrum in which you can't quite believe your eyes or ears becomes a necessary compromise. It's not misdirection, rather a new one. It's this, or very near it, that Baudrillard describes in *Simulacra and Simulation.* That text underscores my experience of and thus my critique of three live-streamed musical performances I interrogate in the following pages.

Phoebe Bridgers

Before she raised eyebrows and misplaced chat room furor by smashing a guitar during her debut *Saturday Night Live* performance (2/21), Phoebe Bridgers, one month prior, took the stage for a live performance with pianist Ethan Gruska that streamed on the subscription service Bandsintown Plus. There was some awkward banter between the two met by silence from the ghost audience; both musicians seemed keenly aware of the artificiality or genuineness of the concert, making dry puns about a Las Vegas audience as though they were dueting at a Glitter Gulch casino instead of an audience-free, sparse Los Angeles studio. The nervous energy was persistent throughout the hourlong set and I distinctly remember thinking how incredibly different Bridgers's singing voice, at once soothing and plaintive with an effective two-octave range, is than her speaking voice. That register is a husky bravado more akin to a heavy smoker who mistakes volume for value. This set came on the heels of Bridgers, with full band, holding forth in an empty Red Rocks Amphitheater for an hourlong immersive set streamed on the concert sponsor's website as well as its Twitter account. At capacity, the legendary amphitheater holds about 9,500 attendees. The Bridgers's performance was part of a three-day event and enjoyed a virtual audience of 8.5 million people. Repackaging the video for YouTube, nearly 650 thousand additional people have viewed her performance. One commenter on YouTube noted: "Watching a girl sing ethereal pop in a skeleton outfit she's been wearing for 3 years straight, playing a BC Rich Warlock (guitar) to an empty stadium. Well, ya don't see that routinely."

Therein, with vocabulary choice describing the commenter's experience of the performance, e.g., "watching" and "see," is revealed the passive privilege of ocularcentrism that underscores, occasionally undermines, the digital delivery of live music events. A concert, like a track and field meet, is a three-ring circus; the eye dances across a field of activity. But, if you're doing an insistent closeup on Phoebe's fret work, digital audiences can't see what the rest of the band is up to or scan the horizon or isolate the drummer's intense energy. It's all a bit prescriptive and reductive. Audio qualities such as tone and pitch and a decent mix ought to receive at least equal attention.

Another disorienting factor was that for this performance, Bridgers did not use the stage's traditional orientation, rather she set up the band facing the back of the stage with the majestic red cliffs (bearing digital projected viewer tweets and feedback) flanking the group, upward and behind their backs where an audience would normally be seated. It engendered a sort of sense of unease that didn't feel quite natural and yet made me wish for the real (being there).

> Nostalgia, in other words, weaves an optimistic thread of continuity throughout the experiential disruptions of identity. It allows us to interrogate the past, not as a repository of veridical events, but as memorial planes of certain affectual transcendence: an assurance that I was "thereness" on the "beach-ness." (Shields et al. 2011, 86)

The nostalgia I felt (for being outdoors at a concert in a "sacred" setting) was, Baudrillard would say, a "nostalgia for a lost referential" (47). And though I've never seen her perform in the flesh, I did feel a pronounced gulf between this performance and that lost referent. I felt a psychic ache, the pain of absence. What I wish was absent, as it turns out, was the special Q&A format that followed her set on the Bandsintown Plus televised gig. Bridgers fans, known as Pharbz, were able to submit some questions to the moderator, most concerning her dog; they were as vapid as the comments from the live chat viewers could participate in on their screens (you could also, mercifully, hide the chat box during the performance). The fanboy moderator leaned heavily into bro-speak and didn't do much to guide the brief chat with the artist toward any meaningful purpose. In my estimation, this augmented material brought nothing to the performance, further instilling a sense of distance and falsity.

Jeff Tweedy

A few days following the January 2021 Bridgers/Gruska show, I watched Jeff Tweedy perform a solo show on the Bandsintown Plus platform. The prolific Wilco frontman was playing songs from the full-length recording he made, *Love Is the King*, during the pandemic. During Tweedy's ongoing pandemic time, he's also written a book, his second, *How to Write One Song* (2020), and performed 200 live Instagram shows from his living room. This was a tight, short set played, once again, to a ghost audience. Tweedy is a craftsman and this was evident in his playing of a time-tattered Taylor guitar from which he burnished great sound; a natural complement to his well-weathered voice. But, again, an absence.

A great part of the thrill of experiencing Jeff Tweedy (whether solo as "Jeff Tweedy," with his son as "Tweedy," or as the leader of "Wilco") is stage banter. I know of no one quite so good as Tweedy at such wickedly sharp repartee. And, typically, he's admonishing the crowd for not policing itself very well; at a solo show about 16 years ago, when someone offered him drugs, his rejoinder was "No thank you sir, you may have heard I just got out of rehab." The grumpy guy shtick is real and really absent in this performance; Tweedy's natural foil is not there to parry with. I miss the familiar, discomforting back and forth. So does Tweedy. At a concert months earlier, on a chilly September evening in 2020, he'd performed at a drive-in movie theater in rural Illinois. There was a crowd albeit confined to their vehicles. Near the end of the show, Tweedy addressed the cars and concertgoers. "It's not the same. This just isn't the same," he said, his voice choking and eyes beginning to well with tears. A few car horns sounded and a few head lights blinked. The equation was imbalanced, the aesthetic differed; the traditional circuit was not complete. I have seen Tweedy choke up once before during a song he wrote and performed for his wife. For all of the feigned grief he conveys to audiences, he also loves the fans. He is a generous performer, prone to inviting audience members into swelling choruses of singalongs and at once jabbing at and celebrating those rituals so engrained in the concert form. But not tonight. This is a different day, a different deal, a different delivery, and that, writes Baudrillard, is the point:

> When the whole system becomes weightless, it is no longer anything but a gigantic simulacrum—not unreal, but simulacrum, that is to say never exchanged for the real, but exchanged for itself, in an uninterrupted circuit without reference or circumference (5).

It is this sense of dislocation and questioning simple precepts that has us evaluating relationships and reality. Affective stimuli lead us repeatedly to a newly designed space of reality; we find nostalgia almost visceral, but for naught because things change, systems diverge, viruses mutate. Melancholia is the regrettable outcome for some whilst others engage with the hyperreal as a condition, not just of the pandemic, but of postmodernism writ large, which liquidates all known referents, or, at least, renames and repackages them. I am, at least in spirit, like that closed-off husk of a person depicted in Dürer's engraving, *Melencolia I* (1514) And, regrettably, both inwardly and outwardly, I take measure of Baudrillard's words, "Melancholia is the inherent quality of the mode of the disappearance of meaning," (156) and find they are an apt description of self.

Norwegian Digital Jazz Festival

The Norwegian Digital Jazz Festival boasted 15 different sets over eight days and runs through the Christmas holidays season in 2020. At this festive time of year, I'm really looking for a connection, that humanness, to try to move beyond that feeling of melancholy, which you may know is black bile and the least desirable of the four humors Hippocrates tethered to health. This tele-concert series with some of Scandinavias's finest is a foray into a largely unknown musical area for me; I'm more comfortable in the traditional jazz vein, Bird, Miles, Monk. First up in the series was the pianist Bugge Wesseltoft performing from Oslo's Sentralen Performing Arts Center. Sparse, elegant, and *everything* I didn't know I needed. His playing captured a rare mastery of technique and poetry, and he brought it to the fore beginning with an interpretation of Paul Simon's "Bridge Over Troubled Water" that, initially, I couldn't quite place, so inventive was his interpretation. Next, he changed up with a Bach-inspired piece that, magically, seems to quote hauntingly from another Simon song, "American Tune." Such deft subtlety was mirrored in the visuals—sleek moves with delicate intention. Bob Dylan, Henry Mancini, and Yusuf Islam (the former Cat Stevens) were also given Wesseltoft interpretations. And for an hour, nostalgia and awe were reactivated within myself as I soaked in the transcendent union of the spectacle of images and sounds. This was its own impossibly, unique simulacrum; an authentic re-experiencing of all of those late night and early morning gigs I'd covered as an arts writer and, later, taken in purely on the basis of fandom and fun. There was something genuine about this instrumental performance; the simplicity, almost sacred, of one person fulfilling the promise of what an instrument is capable of arousing, or soothing, in us. I felt a psychic hug.

I did not find such comfort and solace in the additional festival offerings: one was plagued by technical problems, disrupting any sense of flow, rhythm or pace; another was an acid jazz combo, which I appreciate on its merits, but not for its musicality; another vocalist offered Joni Mitchell-esque phrasings, that fell short and felt long. And, as the lighting schemes appeared to become more garish and insistent, the rhythms more jagged, the worst of feelings overcame me: boredom. I have been, seen, and felt many things across many years of live music performance; I do not believe I would say I was ever bored. It was easy not to continue to watch. Really easy. My investment (the entire festival cost $50 to view and would take many hours of commitment) and a certain sense of risk aversion (things are rough enough without opening the door to possible disappointment) prompted me to shut it down. With the click of a button.

WHAT IS THERE?

For me, navigating the simulacrum is pretty straightforward; I'm a savvy media consumer/producer by training and by experience. The delivery of the spectacle becomes the mechanism we use to interact with the outside world and, before long, the idea of participating by simply witnessing through a televised image is grounded in its own unreality. The simulacrum has become, in the instance of streaming live music performances, just another mediated experience involving a screen. Tune in and turn on . . . or turn off as I did with several of the Norwegian Digital Jazz Festival offerings. That is not to say this simulacrum does not have its rewards; again, in view-on-a-screen-being-there there are generally, no liquid-courage inspired shout-outs for the band to play a third encore and, of course, the convenience of logistics. I return to the idea of and/both in my knowing embrace of the simulacrum. I can move between multiple realities. Clones and CGI, simulacrum and science fiction, green screens and uncanny valleys are constituted by implicating bodies, just as other real-world experiences rely on such calculus. And, too, nostalgia can exist within the hyperreal.

> Because music can relay the historical instance without the burden of its consequence, and because music circumvents the world of objects through its technology of signification, it has been generally taken as pure memory and an expressive tool for the becoming of pastness (Shields, et al., 87).

I'd certainly love to revisit Bugge's transcendent "Bridge Over Troubled Water" on screen with hope that I might locate that energy and release I encountered on my first visit to the space. But, given the opportunity to see him do so live at this current moment in a climate of anti-vaxxing and anti-masking, generates little nostalgia for the current live music experience. But, my informed hesitation really hinges upon this: the simulacrum cannot land at that rare, liminal moment that live music does in which, simultaneously, I am soothed and energized. That transcendent space where seeing and being becomes knowing. That previously mentioned and/both possibility is not fully available; mediation demands of me an either/or proposition. I'm open to the possibility that concerts as we remember them will return someday and all the parking hassles, pre-concert preparations, and warm, overpriced beer will be welcomed by many as an old friend. Venues and festivals are reopening, but I see what others see as promise right now as mostly a threat. When/if I return to my passion, it will present and re-present something quite different. Being there has changed because an integral part of the idea and ideal in practice is not just being there in spirit, but being there for one another. We are not there anymore.

REFERENCES

Alfred. R. (2009). June 24, 1993: Concert goes live on net June 24, 2000: President goes live on net. *Wired.* Retrieved from https://www.wired.com/2009/06/dayintech-0624/.

Baudrillard, J. (1994). *Simulacra and simulation* (S. Glaser, Trans.). University of Michigan Press.

Benjamin, W., Arendt, H., & Zohn, H. (1968). *Illuminations*. Harcourt, Brace & World.

Chow, A. (2020) "Come as you are in the family car. Drive-in church services are taking off during the coronavirus pandemic" *TIME Magazine*. Retrieved from https://time.com/5811387/drive-in-church-coronavirus/.

Debord, G. (1967). *The society of the spectacle*. Zone Books.

Hansen, C. (2021). What we lose when we livestream church. *New York Times*. Retrieved from: https://www.nytimes.com/2021/08/08/opinion/covid-church-livestream.html.

Manovich, L. (2001) *The Language of New Media*, MIT Press.

McLuhan, M. (1964) *Understanding Media: The Extensions of Man*. Signet Books.

Rose. G. (2016) *Visual methodologies: An introduction to researching with visual materials*, (4th ed.). SAGE.

Shields, R., Park, O., & Davidson, T. K. (2011). *Ecologies of affect: Placing nostalgia, desire, and hope*. Wilfrid Laurier University Press.

Silverstone, R. (1999). What's New about New Media?: Introduction. *New Media & Society*. *1*(1):10–12.

Chapter Eight

Theater Doesn't Work

(Co-)Creation in Pandemic Theater-Making

Izabela Derda

It is 7:00 pm on December 01, 2020, in Wrocław, the fourth biggest city in Poland. One of the Capitol Musical Theater actors enters the theater's big street-facing window, sits down on a black chair set on the white background and—does nothing. People pass by the window. Some stop and watch; others rush by unnoticing. Some theater fans stand in front of the window, watching. The actor does not try to engage with his "audience" nor react to their actions. He does not do anything to bring attention to himself, neither does he pretend he is unaware of their presence. He does not play with his phone nor read a book. He does not mean to perform; he just spends an hour and a half in stillness and then leaves. The next day another actor comes at 7:00 pm, sits for 90 minutes, and leaves. The routine is repeated for 23 days. Each day a different actor comes, sits still, and leaves.

Theater Doesn't Work, created by the assembly of the Capitol Theater is a "happening," an artistic endeavor to bring art to life and break down the barrier between artist and audience. It follows Berleant's and Kaprow's idea, inspired by abstract expressionists, that art does not have to be static and isolated from the audiences, but has the potential to be integrated into everyday life and offer a unique encounter for each person partaking in the experience (Berleant & Kaprow, 1967). But above all, it is an act of waiting. The actors wait to go back on stage and do their job. They wait for the theater to re-open. The performance neither violates COVID-19 regulations, nor denies the pandemic's existence, but rather comments artistically on the surrounding reality and highlights the irony of the situation:

> Our situation is quite absurd (. . .) Today, shopping malls are filled with customers in large glass windows; we can see what they have to offer. The churches gather the faithful who are experiencing Advent—the time of waiting. In the big glass window of the theater, the idle artist is also waiting, because THEATER DOESN'T WORK. (Imiela, personal communication, February 26, 2021).

The COVID-19 pandemic has forced theaters around the world into limbo, not knowing when and how they would be able to reopen their doors again. Performing arts' dependency on physical audiences placed theaters in a highly vulnerable place. Many artists and cultural institutions faced financial

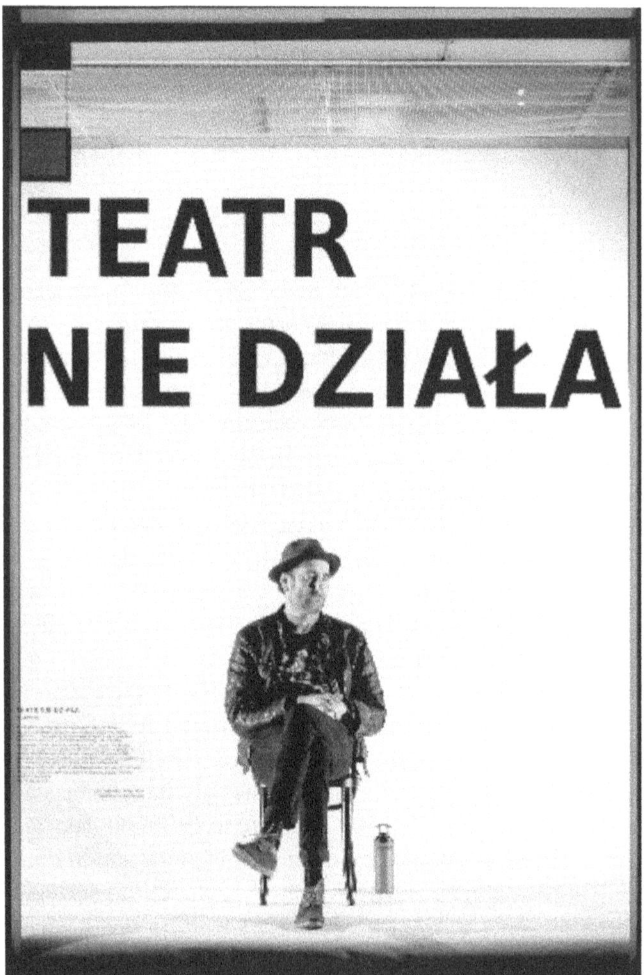

Figure 8.1 *Theater Doesn't Work.*
Source: BTWPhotographers for Capitol Musical Theater.

devastation (Betzler et al., 2020) as the absence of box office revenues were followed by the missing incomes from sponsorships, donations, and commercial services like catering, advertising, workshops, and finally the loss of government subsidies (IDEA Consult et al., 2021). The situation put numerous companies on the verge of extinction with just a few months' worth of cash on hand (Brown, 2020). Between March and September 2020, on Broadway alone, 1100 actors and managers lost their jobs (Whitten, 2020), and 52 percent of US-based actors and 55 percent of dancers stayed unemployed in the third quarter of 2020 (Guibert & Hyde, 2021). The fragility of the sector was exposed. In Europe, at least 32 percent of the cultural workforce is self-employed and lacked any kind of social protection during the crisis (IDEA Consult et al., 2021).

The dramatic financial situation pushed theaters to search for new ways of operating. With a series of restrictive regulations forbidding not only performances but also rehearsals and in-person meetings, the theatre, along with many other sectors, experienced an accelerated digital transformation in order to continue offering their art and services (Ponte, 2020), which placed many creators in unknown territory. The pandemic challenged them to reconsider their ways of working in creative teams, generating income, and finding and engaging audiences. The shift modified the very physical interaction of artists, the audience, and space, for hybrid productions, mixing offline and online realities.

DECENTRISM, THE "ART OF WITH," AND BRICOLEUR AUDIENCES

The Capitol's happening, *Theater doesn't work*, can be considered an example of *decentrism*, coined in 1987 by Adam Wiśniewski Snerg to describe fine arts. As much as 'centrist' art desires to fully expose the presented object or content, regardless of the chosen form, decentrism, in contrast, is interested in art where the center of the object depicted therein is located somewhere outside the framework of the work, but dominates the present surroundings. This principle of composition—by creating a tension between the hidden object and the visible background—strengthens the meaning of the object or its surroundings, depending on the role assigned to them (Wiśniewski-Snerg, 1987). Decentrism intentionally hides what is most significant and creates an imaginary (intuitive or philosophical) space in which it places the essential sense of artistic creation. Therefore, it is based on evoking appropriate associations, inviting the audiences to decode the hidden message. This is exemplified in the use of shadow as a popular carrier of meaning in the decentric art. The shadow emphasizes the physical existence of characters or objects not present by awakening recipients' imagination and inviting to them to see what the author has not presented (Andre & Baranowski, 2009).

Even though the concept of decentrism has been developed relatively recently, the idea that a piece of art remains incomplete until it is consumed by its end-user is rooted in the classical theories of aesthetics and semiotics. For example, Umberto Eco (1986) claimed that works of art were subject to numerous interpretations and that the reader, like the writer, was equally involved in generating meaning, making art consumption a "collaborative journey" (Govier, 2009, p. 3). Walter Benjamin supported participatory art in the 1930s, writing that art was greater the more it drove people to abandon their passive status as spectators (Benjamin & Underwood, 2008). In the performing arts, happenings need to be considered as manifesting "the art of with" idea (Leadbeater, 2009, p. 5) as they were conceptualized to "break down the barriers between the artist and the audience, art and the everyday" (Leadbeater, 2009, p. 7). In the twenty-first Century, the "participatory avant-garde" came to refer to art that was inter-subjective and dialogic in its construction as well (Leadbeater, 2009, p. 9). Today, the internet facilitates artwork that motivates audiences to participate through constant feedback and interaction, and encourages creative acts of those involved (Leadbeater, 2009).

Although the digital world allows for new encounters, the loss of materiality has an impact on the audience's experience and meaning co-creation. As Grundström (2018) lays out, while place and space should not limit the development of experiences, when audiences feel distant, the experience's perception can become impersonal (Walmsley, 2016) and less inviting of interaction (Lim et al., 2012). Therefore, the audiences' expectations are to receive the environment with a series of acts that can support their connection with the experience (Casetti, 2015) or perceive the gratification from attending (Bakshi & Throsby, 2014). Casetti (2015) labels this new form of spectators *bricoleur*-the audience assembles various elements into a comprehensive and personalized experience and, as with hybrid experiences, audience participation is becoming more bidirectional, with people actively co-creating or even reinventing the events (Casetti, 2015).

This chapter explores approaches to mediated theater performance co-creation. It investigates how the interference of technology changes the connection within artistic teams and with their audiences. The study takes a qualitative approach using digital ethnography, including participant observation and four case studies of theaters that shifted their processes. Interviews and observation offer an extensive overview of organizations' methods of dealing with the lockdown and of the rationale behind their choices, and highlights some of the patterns visible in the theater sector between March and December 2020.

BEYOND THE FRAME

While theater performance as an expression of resistance to the surrounding reality or political power cannot, by any means, be considered a novel idea, the case of Capitol Theater offers an example of a company that decided not to move the core of their activity online. For Capitol, the first COVID-19-related lockdown came a week before the *Stage Songs Review*, an annual festival held in Wrocław since 1976. The review could not take place nor be moved online. Instead, the team decided to offer *Viral Festival Television* during the original duration of the review; this was a series of daily online videos providing a humorous commentary about the events that did not happen and "things that do not exist" (Imiela, personal communication, February 26, 2021).

Capitol's activations can be seen as the execution of decentristic ideals. Both performances are built around actions outside the "frame" of the performance, and the meaning of "not happening" is incomplete without the audience's involvement. The audience participates in making meaning of "inexistent" events and contributes to co-creation by decoding the messages and building their own interpretations, similar to Eco's understanding of the art piece's completeness or Wiśniewski Snerg's (1987) vision of focusing on periphery and exterior. As Imiela expressed:

> Is this idle actor or actress actually performing or not? It turns out that viewers sitting on the other side of the glass had a very strong experience of participating in this happening. We seem to show the performer's passivity, but it affects people who watch it very strongly. And this inscription above the artist's head became very provocative - the theater does not work, but it has a strong impact. (Personal communication, February 26, 2021)

SEARCHING FOR CIRCULATION OF SOCIAL ENERGY

As the weeks of lockdown passed, individual artists and organizations began to search for ways of reestablishing connection with their audiences through digital means. The creators tried to lure theater lovers with performances shared straight from their digital archives, interactive tours, live-streamed performances, behind-the-curtain materials, and experimental forms (like WhatsApp-based storytelling) across all digital channels. Even though digital performances gained some attention before (Cerratto-Pargman et al., 2014), the pandemic has accelerated the adoption of digital means in the performing arts, which has also led to reshaping their relations with their audiences (Rae, 2020).

In the first reaction to lockdown, the digital environment became a natural space for showcasing performances, reconnecting with audiences, and alternative financing. Many theater companies reached into their institutional archives and offered online screenings of their on-stage productions captured live before the pandemic. Some of them enabled interaction in the form of liking and commenting during or after the show, and often added discussions with actors or the director to the content.

Mint Theater is an off-Broadway theater company focused on producing "lost or neglected" plays. Due to the "fragile" nature of the material with which they work, Jonathan Banks, the artistic director, started building an archive many years ago, so the plays and performances would not be lost again. Banks was not sure if or when he would be able to make use of those videos due to the union's regulations, and doubted people would be interested in watching pre-recorded theater. However, in March 2020, in the early weeks of the shutdown of the theaters in New York, Banks decided to share some of those recordings online with a core group of the theater's supporters. He put the videos into the packages containing the show, pre- and post-show talks, and discussions with the cast. Even though he considered the selected audience especially predisposed towards the Mint, the number of views was disappointing. He concluded that the audience was not interested in seeing the Mint's Productions Online.

Banks gave the online environment another try when the paycheck protection program provided a low-interest business loan from the federal government of the United States in June 2020, to support wages for continued work (CARES Act, 2020). In summer 2020, he organized the online Summer Stock Streaming Festival, making three shows available simultaneously for two weeks. He expected that people would not be interested in watching more than a few minutes of each show, but he hoped it could give people a sense of who they are as a theater, and increase interest after the pandemic.

> It turns out, I completely misjudged. We gathered a large and very enthusiastic audience who watched from start to finish or watched in two parts (. . .) and in retrospect, I can see that my first test was kind of exactly wrong, because 75% of the people who are watching our streams are people who have never seen one of our productions. (Banks, personal communication, February 25, 2021)

The outcome exceeded his expectations as the theater has tripled the number of individual contributors from the previous year. Even though it was still struggling financially, the Mint has increased its visibility and reached new audiences.

The practice of streaming pre-recorded performances, however, does not shift far from televised theater, which has been common since the 1920s

(Pszczołowski & Kougan, 1959). Examples include BBC broadcasts of Shakespeare's plays (Willis, 1991) and Disney+ streaming the hit Broadway musical *Hamilton* (DMED Media, 2020). However, streaming reached a new scale in the new online environment. Archives, usually serving a secondary role in theatrical practice (Morawski, 2020), now held a central position and allowed performances to have a dual existence for primary and secondary audiences (Auslander, 2006). If we consider theater "a mindset that allows for a free exchange of creative energy between an arts organization and its public" (as cited in Brown et al., 2011, p. 18), then, similar to TV theater, the experience of streamed theater can hardly be seen as a complete *circulation of social energy* between a stage and audience (Greenblatt, 1992). The experience is likely to lack the feeling of collectiveness (for some), as Imiela discussed based on his experiences with Capitol's audiences:

> the feeling of being somehow (a part of) a larger community, one organism. The feeling of receiving live experience of art; perception in the *real* world, this is what we need to *experience theater*, and this is something the screen cannot transmit. (Personal communication, February 26, 2021)

Audiences of streaming material need to "fill in the blanks" to build an understanding of the play and the *feeling of experience* from an incomplete set of information (Morawski, 2020).

The Mint's experience is not exclusive to their situation but rather something observed often in the dynamics between the theater organizations and online audiences. The audiences may complain about the unreality of the experience, the lack of a "wow" effect, its lower prestige, egalitarian character, and difficulties in engaging with and focusing on the performance (Buchner et al., 2021). Yet, they also compliment the better accessibility and convenience, the new ways of experiencing theater, and, above all, meeting the need for culture despite the pandemic (Buchner et al., 2021). Therefore, while exploring audience co-creation and the dynamics of the exchange occurring between audiences and creators, it is important to consider the pure relationship between a performance and its documentation (in this case in the form of a streamed recording), to understand the essence of the experience in online representations. But even more importantly, the relationship between the documentation and its audiences needs to be considered (Brown, 2005) including how the audiences "bricoleur" their experience (Casetti, 2015).

CO-CREATING (FOR) ONLINE

Theater performance is an aesthetic collaborative endeavor that is co-created through the interaction of multiple creators with diverse skills and a common goal (Walmsley, 2013). The pandemic did not leave those collaborative efforts untouched. From video-call brainstorm meetings, table reads and rehearsals, the utilization of digital tools for thought-exchange and delivery of online content, to greater freedom and responsibility for team members, the experience of lockdown and government restrictions pushed for new ways of co-creation.

Maciej Sobociński is a theater and live TV director who, every year, introduces a new performance based on Boguslaw Schaeffer's work during the Schaeffer's Era Festival. Schaeffer's world of creative imagination is full of vibrant performance and improvisation, music, dance, and artistic expression, "not limited by the frames of art, medium, scene or theme." The team behind the project did not want to resign their 2020 plans nor compromise the project or its scale by delivering Zoom readings or mini-performances but rather searched for ways to deliver an experience as close to the original vision as the situation allowed.

The project ended with two spectacles. The first one, *Schaeffer Puzzle Play 2020,* was a live online event based on improvisation inspired by Bogusław Schaeffer's scores. They consisted of a combination of scenes performed live in multiple locations, along with pre-recorded videos. As Sobocinski explained: "you will find everything that is characteristic of Schaeffer: music, theater, graphics, dance. Unpredictable, scattered like Schaeffer's scores, like puzzles from which a complete picture is assembled." The second project—*Schaeffer in L.A.*—was a live-streamed event happening in two cities simultaneously—in Warsaw, Poland, and Los Angeles, California. The event, strongly inspired by Schaeffer's dramas, raises issues of loneliness in a technologized world and questions the meaning of art and the artist's life, especially in the post-pandemic reality.

The fragmentation and fluidity of both performances pushed a search for new means of artistic expression and delivery. In both cases, the performance was designed to be streamed online live, yet artists could not meet in person or had to follow strict social distancing regulations. In LA, the actors and crews were also spread geographically, which led to scheduling and technical complications due to differences in time zones and issues with image and sound synchronization. It became important to ensure that the need for technological reliability did not dominate the desire for artistic excellence.

Sobocinski was meeting on Zoom with each actor to rehearse individually, as he would in person. This was followed by Zoom meetings of the entire cast for "table" readings. "In a sense, you are able to work with actors online, set the structure, even set certain pauses very precisely, as well as the emotional side," Sobocinski explains. However, more changes were visible as the team moved to the phase of physical rehearsals as Sobocinski directed the show from his house, looking at every camera-filled location in which actors were rehearsing (and later performing live). The vision was mixed live and sent to his computer, so he could see how the audience would experience the show, but he could also see and control every camera from his laptop, much like a live TV control room. Moreover, at the same time, he was connected with the crew through video calls on iPad to be present at the rehearsal more "physically" and be able to talk to actors "face-to-face," making the process truly hybrid and requiring all involved to adapt to the new workflow.

He believes that even if the process requires more preparation and precision, working with cameras gives him more freedom than in offline theater. He can guide the viewer more precisely and has a bigger impact on their perception. In this sense, he sees working online as liberating, despite missing the live energy exchange between actors and audiences. The audience's absence allows actors to focus better. "There is a different energy when we do not let the audience in, which always introduces a certain nervousness. Here we could have a certain intimacy, despite the technological bliss" (Sobociński, personal communication, February 19, 2021).

As film and TV techniques have been broadly applied to on-screen theatrical performances, they have influenced the framing and overall experience of theater consumption. Traditional stage-crafting practices were affected by cinematic thinking (though as discussed before, not for the first time), guiding spectators more directly through the story and its nuances, leaving less space for the audience's self-exploration of the stage and related happenings.

KEEPING IT REAL, KEEPING IT ALIVE

The nature of the performances being created for the personal screens, the ubiquitous presence of cameras, and hybrid way of working were influencing not only the traditional workflows and relations between stakeholders, but also the casting choices and requirements for actors. As the actors had to perform wearing face masks throughout (in the case of the LA-based cast) and could not be in any physical contact, Sobocinski searched for actors comfortable having only their body, eyes, and text at their disposal. As he explains: "Not every actor can play physical theater focusing on a body movement; it can be a struggle for 'traditional' dramatic actor. I had to have certain actors who were also acting and thinking that way" (Sobociński, personal communication, February 19, 2021).

Also, acting for the small screens of audiences' laptops and mobile phones, and working with cameras on stage required a cinematic rethinking of the means of expression. The traditional staging approach was challenged by the requirements of the screen-mediated experience and pushed for revised approaches to staging, acting and voice modulation:

> Actors need to hold back the emotions and be very intense at the same time. The means of expression must be slightly scaled-down and reduced. Every scream, every overexpression, every falsehood the camera easily unmasks, and online does as well. If you are watching something on your phone and something is 'too big', you will immediately see where it hits you; it is unnatural and artificial. You cannot play with simple tricks. (Sobociński, personal communication, February 19, 2021)

As Sobocinski explains, in his view, a camera requires more discipline, not only from the director (who now directs more elements than in traditional theater), but also from the actors. If the play is not translated into the cameras' language, emotions cannot transfer, and an audience stays bored and unsatisfied. The dramaturgy must be built so that the actor plays the most important scenes to the "viewer," that is, to the camera, and at the same time, they need to be able to play with a partner. These make stage situations denser. For this reason, while casting the Schaeffer-based performance, Sobocinski was looking for versatile actors who like to take risks and are open to experimenting.

> It takes a lot more teamwork; there is less self-focus. Actors have to re-learn to propose elements of their role for specific solutions. Conceptually, the world (in which they operate on stage) grew. They had to start thinking with the cameras. (Sobociński, personal communication, February 19, 2021)

Numerous directors share this notion of the need for flexibility and openness from all involved in online theater production. Among them, there are Andressa Furletti and Debora Balardini, artistic and executive directors of BR Group, a Brazilian theater in New York. Furletti and Balardini developed an immersive show based on a pre-recorded play and a series of smaller Zoom-based performances with their actors. They require "hybrid actors" to improvise, be unafraid to offer their own ideas, and to have freedom and responsibility. Even before the pandemic, Furletti and Balardini worked with "composition and improvisation"—through offering actors "some kind of skeleton of the show" (Furletti & Balardini, personal communication, February 26, 2021), but at the same time, expecting actors to bring their own ideas and interpretations to the work.

The idea of keeping actors present during online spectacles seems to be one of the leading challenges for directors in the pandemic. Sobociński was also searching for tools to keep his actors alert even if they could not see each other. He did not want the actors simply to deliver the pre-rehearsed structure and scenes; he wanted them to stay genuinely reactive. He mentioned that even though the experience was streamed for the audiences, the actors were performing live so that everyone involved felt that something might go wrong. It was giving them energy, resulting in an enlivened experience. Also, in the case of *Schaeffer's Puzzle*, each of the actors had one scene prepared about which other actors did not know, which they were allowed to use in their preferred moment. These surprises kept the spectacle structure fluid. Neither the actors nor the director knew the final shape of the performance, which was born in front of the viewers, a technique borrowed from the improvised theater.

None of these practices is genuinely new or unique within the online environment. Improvisation is a long-known technique of practicing presence, finding its roots in many cultural traditions—from Buddhists' meditation and awareness training, Hindi musicians' tuning instruments to the vibrations of the room, to shadow plays of political satire in Indonesia and Bali (Zaporah, 1995). It has also been noted that viewers are drawn to artistic improvisation since there is a dance between predictable structures and creation in the inevitable moments that arise when humans share in imaginative, collaborative activities (Spolin & Sills, 1999), which might be called a *hybridized improvisational attentiveness*.

FROM A SAFE DISTANCE, OR IT'S HARD TO SURPRISE US IN THE VIRTUAL WORLD

The uneasiness and lack of control for actors became an essential tool for directors to keep shows more 'alive' in the online setting. But experiencing the performance through the screens also placed the audiences at a "too safe" distance. For Imiela, this distance is an argument for not moving the theater performances to an online environment:

> The art should take risks. Art should examine our limits of comfort; when it knocks us out of everyday life, out of our comfort zone, then it provokes our emotions and thoughts, which is one of the obligations of art. And we have a much greater chance of taking a risk in the real world. We would rather be in a safe; we look through the screen, we are at a safe distance, nothing is required of us. It is psychologically easier. Moving to the web is convenient for the viewer, but it is not, what art is about. (Personal communication, February 26, 2021)

Many are looking for ways to throw the audiences off balance. Furletti and Balardini offered the example of their production *Inside the Wild Heart*. The show moved online by creating an immersive environment of an interactive multi-story house. Each room represented part of a play and part of a pre-recorded performance, which audiences could navigate as they wished, replicating the self-exploratory experience of the original performance. The audience was able to "travel" through the house in a nonlinear way, making their own decisions on what, when, and how to consume the performance environment and, therefore, partaking in bricoleur spectatorship as introduced by Casetti (2015). Furletti and Balardini observed that some people expected a "click, sit, and watch" kind of experience, but this was not what the play was designed for:

> It was really that we wanted to give the audience the feeling of disorientation when they enter the world of the play. This performance should give you this feeling like you don't know what to think or what to do, and sometimes you want to take a rest because the actress said something that made you question a lot of things in your life or another was like, Oh my god, I didn't know someone else thought about that as well or something that you go like. So sometimes we hear that it is not something people look for in the online theater. (Personal communication, February 26, 2021)

Sobociński also echoed the notion:

> I'm always trying to break 'the fourth wall; I don't like having this comfortably seated spectator, who just watches something through this 'window' (of the screen) from the safe distance. In a physical theater, I always try to surround the spectator, so the action is around him so that he can be in the middle of the events. So, in the case of online, this is even more important. If the audience can just see some actors walking and doing things from a distance, then it does not have a chance to work. (Personal communication, February 19, 2021)

In their view, the online stage needs to be created in a way that the viewer can be 'inside' of the happenings and close to the actors, aiming for eye contact and intimacy to keep audiences involved in the story.

The interviewees also highlight the difficulty controlling the broader environment in which the performance is consumed, including the construction of mood and feeling through the use of stage tools like lighting, music, sounds effects, or scents. Watching from the comfort of their homes, audiences feel 'too far' from the actors and action. In fact, at-home audiences have full control of the environment in which the play is consumed—their personal choices related to the environment setup may affect their perception and understanding of the play—and this can be seen as co-creation. At any point of the play, the audience can pause, rewind, or fast-forward the experience when it becomes uncomfortable or inconvenient, interrupting the flow of the show and, therefore, influencing how the experience is shaped.

> We want an increasingly predictable world. We can check everything exactly to the second. Everything becomes very predictable. In which we have a very limited possibility of surprises. Art likes to make surprises. It's hard to surprise us in the virtual world. (Imiela, personal communication, February 26, 2021)

MINIMUM THEATER, SO IT CAN EXIST IN ANY FORM

The theater is an art of co-creation. The design and production processes behind the theater performance need to be seen as creative processes and, as such, cannot easily be formalized into a well-defined sequence of tasks (Davies, 2010; Macdonald, 2007) but rather need to be seen as explorative journeys (Leadbeater, 2009). The traditional journeys of the theater experience have been highly disrupted by the pandemic, changing their nature, and exposing the fragility of the "theater performance." Joining the Zoom-craze (Loewenstern, 2020), many offered what we could call "minimum theater"—offering some snippets of the theater experience in the place of forbidden in-person immersion, while others pushed for the maximum, learning from social media and film how to fit the audiences' expectations and engage them in the process of co-creation. Both approaches are challenging common practices and require reinvention of the ways creators develop and deliver performances.

In the first place, the digital environment pushed a new dimension to the hybrid bricoleur spectatorship (Casetti, 2015), making audiences responsible not only for making sense of the meanings present in and outside the frame of the spectacle but also for the broader context in which the performances are consumed. Secondly, physical and online theater experiences need to be considered very differently (Mueser & Vlachos, 2018). Loses in the "energy circulation" (Greenblatt, 1992) have been reported by both creators and audiences (Buchner et al., 2021), and there is a risk of disconnection (Walmsley, 2016). As "arts attendance seems to be driven by some concept of identity" (Bunting et al., p. 64), there is a need to overcome the barrier of the screen and expand opportunities for social interaction.

If the pandemic has formed more longer-term shifts in artist-audience relations, the change in theater operations and financing needs to be seen as influencing these dynamics. The pandemic pushed theater companies to reinvent the way they operate. The turn to a digital environment opened opportunities to expand means of artistic expression and invited the application of audiovisual techniques to enhance and control the online content. At the same time, it demanded new approaches to drive the casts' and audience's attentiveness. Streaming theater opened a path for better accessibility, however, theater companies that lacked the necessary resources for such a pivot were left behind. Many theater companies had to invest in equipment and swiftly develop the required skills to become video content producers. Suddenly in the same market as film and TV platforms, theaters experienced new challenges of supersaturation and choice fatigue (Newell et al., 2008). It will be interesting to observe whether theater companies will continue extending their online presence after the pandemic situation normalizes. If so, the question is whether the assembly of compositions will evolve, what new roles theatrical companies will develop, and whether it will affect financing models.

Finally, it needs to be noted that in many cases, theater companies and artists engaged in online performances outside of their regular institutional program or mission. Some aimed at fulfilling the need of actors to engage with their audiences and to keeping a sense of belonging among their teams. Others used them as marketing efforts, or eligibility to access national or regional paycheck protection funds. Many online initiatives were driven by the theaters' marketing and communication teams. The internet has become the most obvious medium for many organizations to survive difficult economic times (Rae, 2020). It provides a source of income and permanent employment to employees of theater institutions, which might lead to prioritizing projects with funding, or overlooking the audience's needs. This could be observed in the low and decreasing number of views for many online performances offered by theaters across the world (Niedurny, 2020). Focus has now shifted to the central goal: "That the theater should exist in any form after all."[1]

The pandemic pushed creators operating in hybrid spaces to reconsider their approach to theater and implement new media language and tools. It will be interesting to observe the potential evolution of theatrical staging and fresh tactics for audience engagement which have emerged during this trying time.

REFERENCES

Auslander, P. (2006). The performativity of performance documentation. *PAJ: A Journal of Performance and Art*, *28*(3), 1–10. https://doi.org/10.1162/pajj.2006.28.3.1.

Bakhshi, H., & Throsby, D. (2013). Digital complements or substitutes? A quasi-field experiment from the Royal National Theatre. *Journal of Cultural Economics*, *38*(1), 1–8. https://doi.org/10.1007/s10824-013-9201-2.

Barriaud, N. (2002). *Postproduction: Culture as screenplay: How art reprograms the world*. Lukas & Sternberg.

Benjamin, W., & Underwood, J. A. (2008). *The work of art in the age of mechanical reproduction.* Penguin Books.

Berleant, A., & Kaprow, A. (1967). Assemblage, environments and happenings. *The Journal of Aesthetics and Art Criticism*, *26*(1), 136. https://doi.org/10.2307/429261.

Betzler, D., Loots, E., Prokůpek, M., Marques, L., & Grafenauer, P. (2020). COVID-19 and the arts and cultural sectors: Investigating countries' contextual factors and early policy measures. *International Journal of Cultural Policy*, 1–19. https://doi.org/10.1080/10286632.2020.1842383.

Bishop, C. (2004). Antagonism and relational aesthetics. *October*, *110*, 51–79. https://doi.org/10.1162/0162287042379810.

Brown, A. (2020). Life after covid: Who will survive? *ArtsProfessional*. https://www.artsprofessional.co.uk/magazine/article/life-after-covid-who-will-survive.

Brown, A., & Novak-Leonard, J. (2013, January 31). *Getting In on the Act: How Arts Groups are Creating Opportunities for Active Participation*. Arizona Commission on the Arts. https://azarts.gov/resources/getting-in-on-the-act-how-arts-groups-are-creating-opportunities-for-active-participation/.

Brown, L. (1997). Phonography. In D. Goldblatt & L. Brown (Eds.), *Aesthetics: A reader in philosophy of the arts*. essay, Prentice Hall.

Buchner, A., Fereniec-Błońska, K., Kalinowska, K., & Wierzbicka, M. (2021). *Obecność teatrów w przestrzeni online w trakcie pandemii*. Instytut Teatralny im. Zbigniewa Raszewskiego. https://issuu.com/instytut.teatralny/docs/obecno___teatr_w_w_przestrzeni_online_w_trakcie_pa.

CARES Act. (2020, June 3). *116th Congress (2019–2020): CARES Act*. Congress.gov. https://www.congress.gov/bill/116th-congress/senate-bill/3548.

Casetti, F. (2015). *The Lumière Galaxy: Seven key words for the cinema to come*. Columbia University Press.

Cerratto-Pargman, T., Rossitto, C., & Barkhuus, L. (2014). Understanding audience participation in an interactive theater performance. *Proceedings of the 8th Nordic Conference on Human-Computer Interaction: Fun, Fast, Foundational*. https://doi.org/10.1145/2639189.2641213.

Davies, S. M. (2010). The co-production of temporary museum exhibitions. *Museum Management and Curatorship*, *25*(3), 305–321. https://doi.org/10.1080/09647775.2010.498988.

DMED Media. (2020). The Walt Disney Company to fast-track premiere of the Tony Award®-and Pulitzer Prize-winning musical *Hamilton*. *Disney News*. https://dmedmedia.disney.com/news/hamilton-streaming-july-3.

Eco, U. (1986). *Semiotics and the philosophy of language*. Indiana University Press.

Govier, L. (2009). *Leaders in co-creation? Why and how museums could develop their co-creative practice with the public, building on ideas from the performing arts and other nonmuseum organisations*. University of Leicester. https://le.ac.uk/rcmg/research-archive/leaders-in-cocreation.

Greenblatt, S. (2012). *Shakespearean negotiations the circulation of social energy in Renaissance England*. Univ. of California Press.

Greenblatt, S. J. (1992). *Shakespearean negotiations*. Oxford University Press.

Grundström, H. (2018.). What digital revolution? Cinema-going as practice. *Participations. Journal of Audience and Reception Studies*, *15*(1), 5–22.

IDEA Consult. (2021). *Cultural and creative sectors in post-COVID-19 Europe*. Research for CULT Committee. https://www.europarl.europa.eu/RegData/etudes/STUD/2021/652242/IPOL_STU(2021)652242_EN.pdf.

Leadbeater, C. (2009). *The art of with.* Cornerhouse.

Leadbeater, C., & Powell, D. (2010). *We-think*. Profile.

Lim, S., Cha, S. Y., Park, C., Lee, I., & Kim, J. (2012). Getting closer and experiencing together: Antecedents and consequences of psychological distance in social media-enhanced real-time streaming video. *Computers in Human Behavior*, *28*(4), 1365–1378. https://doi.org/10.1016/j.chb.2012.02.022.

Loewenstern, M. (2020, October 15). How live theater is innovating its way through the pandemic. *Barrons*. https://www.barrons.com/articles/how-live-theater-is-innovating-its-way-through-the-pandemic-51602599501.

Macdonald, S. (2007). Interconnecting: Museum visiting and exhibition design. *CoDesign*, *3*(1), 149–162. https://doi.org/10.1080/15710880701311502.

Morawski, P. (2020). *Musimy zwolnić*. Dwutygodnik. https://www.dwutygodnik.com/artykul/8826-musimy-zwolnic.html.

Newell, J., Pilotta, J. J., & Thomas, J. C. (2008). Mass media displacement and saturation. *International Journal on Media Management*, *10*(4), 131–138. https://doi.org/10.1080/14241270802426600.

Niedurny, K. (2020). *Teatr w czasie epidemii: Między nadprodukcją, troską a wynagrodzeniem*. E-teatr.pl. https://e-teatr.pl/teatr-w-czasie-epidemii-miedzy-nadprodukcja-troska-a-wynagrodzeniem-a285009.

Ponte, B. (2020). *International arts management & COVID19 - The cultural ecosystem endangered*. www.artsmanagement.net. https://www.artsmanagement.net/Articles/International-Arts-Management-und-COVID19-The-cultural-ecosystem-endangered,4137.

Pszczołowski, T., & Kougan, E. (1959). *Na telewizyjnym ekranie*. Wydawnictwa Artystyczne i Filmowe.

Rae, P. (2021, June 21). How will the arts recover from COVID-19? *Pursuit.* https://pursuit.unimelb.edu.au/articles/how-will-the-arts-recover-from-covid-19.

Spolin, V. (2017). *Improvisation for the theater: A handbook of teaching and directing techniques*. Northwestern University Press.

Walmsley, B. (2013). Co-creating theatre: Authentic engagement or inter-legitimation? *Cultural Trends*, *22*(2), 108–118. https://doi.org/10.1080/09548963.2013.783176.

Walmsley, B. (2016). From arts marketing to audience enrichment: How digital engagement can deepen and democratize artistic exchange with audiences. *Poetics*, *58*, 66–78. https://doi.org/10.1016/j.poetic.2016.07.001.

Willis, S. (2009). *The BBC Shakespeare plays: Making the televised canon*. University of North Carolina Press.

Wiśniewski Snerg, A. (1987). Manifesto. My conception of decentrism. Retrieved February 22, 2021, from http://www.decentryzm.com/.

Zaporah, R. (1995). *Action theater: The improvisation of presence*. North Atlantic Books.

NOTES

1. The quote comes from the interview with an actress of National Old Theater in Cracow Ewa Kolasińska-Szremel, performed by Paulina Karcz for her master's thesis "At the interface between theater and the Internet. Blogs and chat as inspiration for scenic works."

Chapter Nine

Projecting Through the Mask

Theatre Techniques in the Hybrid Classroom

Alicia Corts

The 2020 global pandemic thrust many instructors into strange new classrooms with half of their students in the room and half on a teleconferencing platform such as Zoom. These hybrid classrooms felt odd and distanced to students and faculty alike. Face masks and social distancing became the norm for those in the classroom, while some of the class remained virtually present on a screen. The classroom shifted as instructors had to teach with a face mask present to stop the spread of the novel coronavirus. Professors could no longer perform many of the subtle, nonverbal cues that instructors previously relied on to communicate to a classroom, and students had to relearn how to read each classroom performance. The shift left many educators feeling frustrated without the tools to cope with the new constraints.

One kind of actor training specifically speaks to the problem of teaching with a face mask. Commedia dell'Arte, the Italian theatre form that began in the Renaissance, offers the acting challenge of portraying a character without the use of full facial expressions (Napier, 1986). The stock characters—such as Il Doctore, Pantalone, and Il Magnifico—use the mask as a part of the character rather than a hinderance. Laura Ewald, long before the pandemic, declared that teaching "can be enhanced using the same preparation, rehearsal, and audience analysis techniques utilized by [these] actors" (2005, p. 115). Commedia begins with the understanding that "all mankind wears or has worn a mask" (Callois, 1964, p. 106), then moves actors away from viewing the mask as a blockage to communication and towards seeing the mask as an extension of their character.

This chapter explores the origins and history of Commedia, looking specifically at how the RSVP (resources, score or arrangement of the resources, valueactions, and performance) method for performance and ENVoY (Educational Nonverbal Yardsticks) teaching techniques could be used in tandem to enhance the hybrid classroom experience for students and professors alike. Using specific examples from my own pandemic experiences as both a college professor as well as a professional development facilitator for fellow faculty, I will illustrate the efficacy of these theatrical techniques in the classroom. Rather than a moment of reflecting on what higher education lost in the transition to the new hybrid classroom, these techniques offer insight into how mask work can enhance teaching through the use of physicality. The pandemic represents a changing of resources, from in-person to virtual, and while we mourn the loss of the known, it is an opportunity for further pedagogical techniques that can serve instructors long after the mask is put away.

CENTERING COMMEDIA TRAINING IN HISTORY

Masks have been a part of many ancient theatrical artforms such as Indian Bhoana, Japanese Noh, and Greek and Roman theatre (Napier, 1986). In the context of the theatre, the mask becomes a sign of the character, a putting on of a different face. Indeed, actor training teaches us that "the mask is the reality" (Eldredge, 1996, p. 41), the center focus of our training and objective in performance. Commedia training often turns an actor's attention away from their facial expressions to a more physically demanding performance. In this way, the body becomes a communication vehicle, a tool the actor uses to tell a story to an audience. Commedia dell'Arte, the masked comedic form, grew from ancient Roman pantomime and comedy, reaching back to those ancient performances for "buffooneries" that audience regularly clamored for (Ducharte, 2012, p. 17).

Ancient pantomime was popular for many reasons, not the least of which was the simplicity with which it was represented (Hall, 2008). The pantomime was a dance form, highly physical, in which masks and movement worked together to present a simple comic scenario, often by a single dancer. There were no scripts or text to preserve. Each dancer/actor developed a set of evocative gestures designed to pull the audience in, emphasize important points of the story, and create a theatrical spectacle of movement. Movement replaced words in this performance; there were no words in a pantomime (Jory, 2008). To heighten the effect even further, the dancer would use different masks to indicate different characters, but all of the meaning was conveyed through the movement itself (Hall, 2008). The dancer made people understand the story with carefully coordinated, intricate movements. After the fall of Rome, these popular comedic techniques remained in the cultural consciousness until the beginning of the Renaissance, where they were revived as an improvised comic form with masks (Ducharte, 2012, pp. 18–19).

When Commedia revived the physicality of the ancient Roman pantomime, the gesture and the mask carried forward into improvised scenarios. A set of stock characters interacted with each other in increasingly comedic but simple stories, using movement and exaggerated masks to create a complete character (Vianello, 2018). Actors didn't rely solely on the mask or the movement, but rather, they carefully crafted a persona that merged movement and mask together to create a fully formed character (Ducharte, 2012). The mask covered the upper half of the face, blocking out the subtle movement of the eyes, nose, and forehead areas normally used for facial expression. Commedia actors blended the mask and the movement together to make up for this loss of facial expression. If a non-actor hears a person enter the room, for example, they might indicate the moment by a slight tilt of the head, moving their eyes toward the sound, and raising their eyebrows in surprise. For a Commedia actor, hearing a person enter the room might result in a full-body head turn, followed by hands thrown into the air in surprise. The motion, however, would begin with the mask, always allowing the absurdity of the mask to guide the actor in the movement. In this way, the actors guide the audience through the story, improvising their way through the scenario specifically marrying vocal work with nonverbal gestures and physicality to keep the audience's attention through the story, just as a professor guides students through specific content.

It is through these exaggerated moments that the stock characters of the Commedia draw laughter from an audience, but it is also to express specific, exaggerated emotions. Training for Commedia involves mask work, and actors learn to reflect on their own physicality to make their work clear and engaging for their audiences. The mask is immobile, and while that eliminates the ability for full facial expressions, the actor finds more freedom from the marriage of movement and mask (Mazzone-Clementi & Hill, 2003).

THE POSSIBILITY OF COMMEDIA'S POWER IN THE CLASSROOM

Putting Commedia into conversation with pedagogy challenges university professors to consider how they marry verbal and nonverbal performance. Clear research exists that indicates that instructors who use nonverbal techniques in the classroom are more effective (Baylor & Kim, 2009; Stamatis, 2011; Jordan, 2001; Melser, 2009). While the importance of nonverbal techniques existed prior to the start of the COVID-19 pandemic in 2020, the addition of masks in the classroom took away a major means of nonverbal communication: the lower half of the face. Just as the Commedia actor works with only half the face, instructors were now called upon to communicate the same amount of information without being able to use smiles, frowns, and the millions of other expressions they unconsciously rely upon to communicate.

Lawrence and Anna Halprin's RSVP method of devising a performance demonstrates how this loss can be turned into an opportunity. In the RSVP method, resources, score (the arrangement of resources), valueactions (the action the performer wants the audience to take based on the value they have established for the performance), and the actual performance itself work equally to create a performance (Halprin, 2014). A change in any of the four pillars necessitates a change in the others. If, for example, we were using an outdoor space for a show, we are assuming it will be clear and sunny. The resource is good weather. If it starts to rain, the resource has changed, which may necessitate altering how the resources are arranged by placing it indoors, a change in the score. If the valueaction was to want the audience to be amazed by good weather and spend more time outdoors, the performance troupe would have to reevaluate what action they want the audience to take based on the absence of the good weather resource. Perhaps the valueaction would change to a value of appreciating the protection of a building in inclement weather that would result in the audience cleaning up the space after the performance and caring for the space more mindfully. Those changes to the original performance are significant, and it could feel like a loss to the troupe who wanted to do a show celebrating good weather. The rain, however, is not a negative change. A resource shift in the RSVP method is neutral. It presents both challenges and opportunities. In this example, the resource shift led to a different performance, but one that still engaged the audience and offered a level of meaning and value.

For the hybrid professor, the RSVP method sheds some light on the stress of the shift from the traditional classroom. Several resources shifted: masked facial expressions, social distancing, and teaching to cameras as well as students in the room. The instructor was left with a choice about what to alter in response to those resource changes. These changes are not in themselves negative or positive; they are neutral shifts that changed the landscape for the performance and demanded necessary adjustments. In the case of the pandemic and teaching, the value of learning the material remains the highest priority, which means that the score (arrangement of resources) and the performance itself would have to change in order to maintain high valueaction for the students. The professor had to change the method and space of the performance when switching to hybrid. Commedia performers are used to resources changing throughout the performance process, since the entire performance is built extemporaneously from a loose scenario. Physicality is particularly emphasized in Commedia actor training as a major resource to help communicate the story clearly as the actors improvise. Instructors who utilize these training methods add more nonverbal resources to their repertoire for both masked and non-masked classrooms.

By starting with the physicality required of Commedia characters, instructors discover a movement style that fits with their own teaching persona. This mask work leads to an intersection with Michael Grinder's ENVoY nonverbal classroom management techniques, a theory that uses breathing, stance, and position within the room to signal to students how the lesson will progress. By using nonverbal gestures that are consistent and aligned with the performance goals of the instructor, students feel more at ease during each class session (Grinder, 2011). With the mask as a part of their persona, instructors in this current season of masked teaching will alleviate some of the stress on themselves and their students by finding ways of communicating nonverbally.

To start this process, professors must first shift their perspective and objectively examine their own practice. While the need for nonverbal communication in the classroom has always existed, the addition of the mask made one truth very plain: "Audiences form impressions of you before you say a word. Your total presentation consists of more than just content: It includes your voice and your body language" (Rafe, 1990, p. 24). We have always been teaching with our vocal work and nonverbal communication at the forefront, yet often without reflection about how those two components work in tandem. The medically important use of facial masks has emphasized how much these resources matter. When a professor thinks of the mask as a role, a performance that they must inhabit, the mask becomes a vital part of their persona as an instructor. Commedia demands acting the mask, the role itself (Rudlin, 1994). We must, therefore, begin by defining the character the mask represents. In Commedia, these roles are clearly outlined with each different maschera, or masked, role (Ducharte, 2012). Il Dottore, Pantalone, and Il Capitano, to name a few, can be clearly identified not only by their masks but by their voice and gestures. Il Capitano carries himself with military bearing, his chest puffed out, preening as a serial seducer would (Perlman, 2017). Il Dottore and Pantalone are both grumpy old men, a feature of the often-intergenerational conflict of Commedia, and posture themselves in such a way that they're both leering and hunched over (Jordan, 2017). These movements are exaggerated and comical, yet when combined with gestures and the mask, the performance presents itself as a complete character. That unified performance is what I'm suggesting with the integration of Commedia techniques: rather than having students see either a masked instructor in the classroom or on a screen, Commedia offers a way to create a persona—the hybrid professor—capable of performing both in front of a camera and in person. Many professors, especially those who have been teaching for years, have already committed to a teaching persona: the kindly curmudgeon, the absent-minded professor, or the encouraging coach (Davis, 2011). Commedia insists on taking a role and making them larger than life, mainly to make the communication of the role to the audience crystal clear regardless of the medium.

To make this leap, professors have to first consider what it is they want to accomplish in the hybrid classroom. I propose that a successful hybrid professor crafts a role with three main components: a community-builder, an expert in the content area, and a character who exists in both the virtual and the physical worlds. A safe, respectful classroom seems a reasonable goal, so we must begin by "seeing hybrid education, blended learning, e-learning, distance education—or any of the other myriad names applied to the combination of a student and technology—as opportunities to build community and care for one another" (Friend, 2021, p.xii). When thinking about this task from the perspective of RSVP devising, the resource of smiles and other kinds of mouth-based facial expression no longer exists. At the same time, kind or cheerful vocal intonation is similarly dampened as a resource since the mask muffles the voice to some extent. The hybrid instructor, however, has untapped resources that are rarely used: facial expression above the mask, head movement, and body movement. Rather than change the valueaction of a community-based, safe classroom, the resources have to shift to include these alternate methods of communication in the performance.

To perform as a content expert, the instructor again loses a resource when we transfer to the hybrid format. Rather than just being able to stand in behind the lectern, the instructor must now perform as someone who can efficiently and capably run a virtual classroom while simultaneously being present in a physical classroom with new restrictions, such as social distancing and the need to remain in one spot for video and audio purposes. The many technical difficulties that can arise in a virtual classroom can take away from the impression of competence. By creating a Commedia-like character for the classroom, the professor creates a persona who surprises with subtle shifts of voice and movement; these performances are designed to draw attention toward and away from situations onstage, a type of bait-and-switch that keeps the students engaged regardless of technology errors. Commedia techniques also carefully emphasize the important parts of the scenario through movement and vocal intonation (Foley, 2017). In other words, using Commedia techniques in the classroom can steer students' attention away from the technology mishaps and focus them instead on the competence and knowledge of the instructor.

While understanding Commedia techniques is the first step, instructors must also arrange the new resources in a way that speaks to students both in the physical classroom and online. Actors know that acting for the camera and acting for stage are two very different techniques. Film acting is often a much more subtle affair, though it often depends on the proximity of the camera as well as the objective of the scene. Stage acting requires an understanding of audience proximity. Here again, Commedia offers solutions to this issue. Commedia techniques remain the same for large, small, or filmed audiences. The gestures and vocal work for each character remains consistent between the media and communicate the same message. That consistency allows students to quickly grasp what the gesture means and keeps them in the flow of the lesson. For example, in Commedia, Il Doctore might gesture towards El Capitano when he wants to accuse him of a crime. The gesture shows the audience where to direct their attention. A masked instructor can work with the class to develop a gesture—perhaps a hand motion combined with body lean toward a particular student—to show where they want the attention of the class to go. This gesture then becomes the norm for the class, and it can be directed toward the camera or the in-person students equally. Because it uses the dramatic quality of Commedia, students are more likely to watch for and engage with the performance. Commedia audiences look for consistency in gestures to identify characters and important events (Callois, 1964), and students watch the hybrid professor for the gestures that lead them through the content.

While this theoretical discussion of how Commedia could work in the classroom may sound fantastical, current work in pedagogy and nonverbal techniques demonstrates that this concept is not new. Rather, bringing the nonverbal technique into a classroom has been a focus of study in education. Michael Grinder's (2011) ENVoY technique gives insight into how nonverbal work can be used within a lesson, and when put into conversation with Commedia, we can see how these educational notions are enhanced with the components of theatre.

ENGAGING STUDENTS WITH THE NONVERBAL GESTURES

Long before the pandemic, instructors were already using the idea of using vocal cues and movement to enhance their teaching. ENVoY, a classroom practice used across the United States, is one practical method of adding gesture into the classroom. Through several decades of research in high school classrooms, the use of nonverbal techniques shows a more than 57% increase in student engagement and an additional hour and a half of instruction time, and an 84% decrease in student suspensions (Grinder, 2020). All of this work, however, was done ahead of the pandemic, when facial expressions were automatically assumed to be a part of the performance. When combined with

Commedia techniques, ENVoY nonverbal pedagogy adds a level of consistency and purpose to the hybrid professor's performance.

One of the areas that nonverbal techniques helps with is the flow of the classroom experience, an essential part of student learning. Technology disrupted how instructors managed their classrooms when classrooms went online. Most professors have established comfortable patterns of teaching in their classroom, a collection of activities and content that guide students' attention through the topic. For experienced master teachers, most attribute their ability to engage students to excellent lecture abilities and/or deep content knowledge. What we know about flow theory, however, is that students require a narrow field of stimulus that guides them into a sense of deep focus and engagement. Mihaly Csikszentmihalyi, the originator of flow theory, describes flow as the careful consideration of how to move students from inertia to considered action (Whalen, 1999). When a student faces an obstacle, they may move into a state of inertia rather than pushing forward (Csikszentmihalyi, 1997). For example, if a virtual student in the hybrid classroom doesn't think the professor recognizes that they are present, they may find it difficult to overcome inertia and interact in the chat window or unmute their microphone to interact in the class. Professors who consider flow in the planning of their lesson take all potential obstacles into account in order to make learning more accessible for their students. The hybrid professor can use nonverbal gestures and body motion to quickly communicate with a wealth of emotion, and those nonverbal signals are the key not only to a seamless experience but student success as well (Babad, 2009).

In ENVoY, there are seven "gems" or techniques that are intended to guide the students into a seamless experience (Grinder, 1990). These performance-based techniques narrow the field of stimuli so that students are more likely to engage with the material effortlessly (Grinder, 2011). The first of these gems, Freeze Body, is a technique that easily comes into conversation with acting techniques. In this practice, an instructor stills their body, points the toes forward, and rests their weight evenly on both feet while maintaining a steady and even breath (Grinder, 2011). Actors, similarly, are taught to find a neutral state where their breath and body are ready for the next action (Eldredge & Huston, 2005). By stilling the body and breath, the actor/teacher takes away some visual and auditory stimuli that can take the student out of the flow of the lesson. Another of ENVoY's seven gems, Above Pause Whisper, similarly limits stimuli by using vocal volume and stillness:

> You want the volume of your voice to be slightly above the class' collective volume. Whatever your style is, once you have their attention, pause; then drop your voice to a whisper. The above process produces or increases an atmosphere that is quiet, receptive, and productive. (Grinder, 2011, p. 19)

The key to the above quote is that the performance results in student reception, which, in turn, results in better productivity. Instructors have to train themselves to reduce the stimuli in their own teaching so that they control when and how auditory and visual stimuli are directed toward the student.

Commedia and theatre in general similarly narrow the field of stimuli, and actors are trained to understand when to use their voice and body to direct the audience into the story and away from distracting factors. Mask training in Commedia is designed to help actors understand how they personally control each movement and sound, which is where actor training and pedagogical development differ (Eldredge, 1996, p. 50). The mask is there to help the actor control the character; the actor uses the mask to regulate the rhythm, tempo, and intonation of the character in order to bring the character to life and direct the audience's eye (National Theatre, 2011). Rather than suggesting a single technique that applies to every instructor, Commedia training asks the actor to find how the mask illuminates them as a performer. As an instructor begins to create a masked persona that works toward both camera and in-person students as a "hybrid professor," the results are dependent on what feels comfortable in their own skin. For some professors, that might mean sweeping arm gesture to indicate a shift in topic, followed by stillness. Whatever choice the professor makes, they must use those nonverbal techniques consistently for the performance to affect the class: as Michael Grinder emphasizes repeatedly, "When a teacher consistently uses certain nonverbals with a concept or idea, then the nonverbals and the concept are associated" (Grinder, 1991, p. 160). Students learn to follow the gestures of a performance because the expectations for their own performance—attention, engagement, and focus—are connected to the hybrid professor's performance through the classroom flow generated from the consistent nonverbal gestures.

Nonverbal communication shortens the time it takes for students to move into a task. When there is consistency in voice, body, and instruction, the students enter an "anticipatory state," a point where they know what will come next and how they are expected to interact with that next step (Grinder, 1991, p. 160). In my hybrid classroom, I have used this particular technique when it comes time to open up the room for questions. I take a step back from the microphone, make a sweeping, open gesture with my arms, then say in an upbeat voice, "It's time for you to weigh in with questions and thoughts." When I make that motion, I can see students in the physical space as well as on Zoom adjust their positions in anticipation of talking and being a part of the conversation. This set of nonverbal gestures anchors the students in classroom processes, eliminates obstacles, and guide the students into a positive classroom flow (Grinder, 1991).

Hybrid professors can use a mixture of the pedagogical techniques we know and use in concert with a Commedia persona created specifically for the hybrid professor that fits the individual instructor. By working through the exercises of a Commedia performer as well as investigating nonverbal pedagogy, the hybrid professor can create a dynamic flow in the classroom that focuses the student on the learning rather than the stimuli from the technology. The journey to incorporate these tools begins with mask exercises that encourage the hybrid professor to consider their persona in the classroom.

REFLECTING ON THE MASKED PERFORMANCE

Jaques Copeau taught his students that the mask does less to conceal the wearer than it does to reveal the wearer (Eldredge, 1996, p. 17). The primary thought for actors at the beginning stages of mask work is to focus too much on what the mask conceals, performing physically to over-or undercompensate for what is lost after the mask appears. Professors, similarly, may find that trying these techniques results in over-performing or not quite reaching what they want to accomplish. The key to any training is reflecting on what specifically works for each person's individual performance. Actor training takes time and discipline, which, if we follow what Michael Grinder suggests about discipline in the classroom, is a parallel course in the nonverbal classroom. As the hybrid instructor disciplines themselves in the pursuit of a persona augmented with gestures and vocal intonation, each person finds the more expressive physical technique easier.

The first step for the hybrid professor is to use the mask not for the medical reasons surrounding the pandemic but as an exercise in thinking about performance. One acting exercise for masked actors involves using a mirror to simply observe their own movements (Eldredge, 1996, pp. 132–133). In this exercise, the actor looks at the mask itself before putting it on and observing themselves in a mirror. When we were thrust into the global pandemic, the mask became a necessity without the time or space to consider how it might be used to enhance a performance. The hybrid professor needs to take a step away from the required nature of the mask to consider how other people view them in the mask. How does a slight head tilt say something different than nodding your head? How can combining hand and arm movements with head movements indicate acceptance, interest, curiosity, or a desire for more information? Does the professor's vocal tone match what the face and the mask are saying? The hybrid professor has to not only consider these questions, but they must also come up with the questions that are important for their own performance. Each individual professor has something that they miss about their style of teaching that was lost with the movement to a masked classroom. Remembering the RSVP process, nonverbal gestures that are practiced as a discipline can be the added new resource to maintain the style and efficacy of pre-pandemic teaching.

Nonverbal gestures in both Commedia and the ENVoY classroom work in tandem with vocal work, specifically marrying the two in patterns that students recognize. Commedia artists such as Jacques Lecoq, Dario Fo, and Giorgio Stehler focused on vocal intonation, small movements of the head and neck, and speech rhythms to give actors more freedom in how they express themselves (Rudlin, 1994, p. 192). The mirror exercise is one way to practice changing vocal pace and tone in a way that matches the nonverbal aspect of the performance. In the fall of 2020 and spring of 2021, I conducted faculty trainings in these techniques at Saint Leo University with a group of 37 professors from the Colleges of Business and Arts and Sciences. Several professors noted that what they thought they sounded and looked like didn't match what was happening in the mirror. Many commented that the feedback from the mirror exercise gave them the ability to play with their voice and body in a way that they had never given themselves permission to do prior to the pandemic. The first step in Commedia training is exactly that kind of work: giving yourself permission to play with the mask.

Just as the voice and body work together in Commedia to portray a character, vocal work in an ENVoY classroom establishes the pace for the lesson while the nonverbal movement keeps the class active, engaged, and focused (Grinder, 1991, p. 201). In the hybrid classroom, one of the benefits to combining the nonverbal and verbal is that once a professor has given themselves permission to playfully perform, they are better able to improvise when something goes wrong with technology. After rehearsing nonverbal techniques through the mirror exercise, the hybrid professor is aware of what can be substituted for vocal communication when the technology goes awry, keeping students engaged and in the flow of the lesson. One professor used a typing motion to indicate when a student's microphone wasn't working and needed to use the chat function in the virtual space, and eventually, the students used the same motion to indicate when the professor's microphone wasn't working. When there's a spirit of play in the room, students will begin to use nonverbal communication as well.

Another important benefit to the mirror exercise is the ability to test, strengthen, and rehearse a teaching persona. One professor commented after his first attempt at the mirror exercise that he had no idea that his eyebrows and vocal tone combined to make him seem more curmudgeonly than he intended. He had been known for his broad smile prior to the pandemic, so the issue hadn't been an issue for him before. He noted that his student evaluations for the fall semester prior to the training had been far less enthusiastic about his teaching style than they normally were, and he openly wondered if his unintentional performance as, in his words, a "crotchety old guy" were the cause of the dip in reviews. The mirror exercise asks the masked actor to objectively consider what they experience both as a spectator and a performer simultaneously, reflect on that experience, then play with their voice and body to attempt another outcome.

Just as the RSVP method of devised performance is agile and responsive, professors who use the mirror exercise are adding new physical tools that lead to an iterative, reflective loop that leads to a better awareness of their own teaching persona. These disciplined exercises not only strengthen the hybrid professor's performance, but they also work to help them realize a performance that feels like a second skin: a natural, easy, and repeatable one. When a professor returns to the mirror exercise regularly, it becomes a way of reflecting not just on a specific classroom experience but how to improve future interactions with students.

After many sessions of rehearsal, the hybrid professor will find themselves comfortable in the persona that they have created. Actors who have worked with masks report that working with a mask leads them to use their other capabilities, such as voice and movement, in new ways. Peter Brook, a director famous for his masked productions, speaks of this transformation actors go through in this work: "The great magic of the mask, which every actor receives from it, is that he can't tell what it looks like on him; he can't tell what impression he is making—and yet he knows" (Brook, 1981, p. 4). This quote should strengthen the heart of the hybrid professor. When you commit to the process of rehearsing with the mask and finding nonverbal ways of communicating, the work will eventually pay off in unconscious, spontaneous ability to use the tools of masked acting in the classroom to communicate with students.

AFTER THE PANDEMIC

With the approval of multiple vaccines around the world, there is hope that our time with the COVID-19 pandemic is coming to an end. We may be past the medical crisis that forced our classrooms into the hybrid mode, but as classroom resources return to what they were in the pre-pandemic era, we should consider what we want to keep from our time in the pandemic, hybrid classroom.

Eventually, the masks will disappear, and as they do, there will be a temptation to return to a reliance on facial expressions rather than nonverbal technique. The shift in resources, however, is an opportunity for us as higher education pedagogues to refine our practice. The flow of a lesson is enhanced when the students know what to expect and are guided in those expectations through clear communication, both verbal and nonverbal. Specific body movements, which professors can learn with basic Commedia training, allows for easy gestures that keep each lesson flowing. It takes practice and discipline to attain the skills, but when they are consistently used in each lesson, the practice becomes not only a stopgap measure during a pandemic but a mastered tool that can be used far into the future.

REFERENCES

Babad, E. (2009). Teaching and nonverbal behavior in the classroom. In H. Fives and M. G. Gill (Eds.), *International handbook of research on teachers and teaching* (pp. 817–827). Springer.

Baylor, A. L., & Kim, S. (2009). Designing nonverbal communication for pedagogical agents: When less is more. *Computers in Human Behavior*, *25*(2), 450–457.

Brook, P. (1981). Lie and glorious adjective. *Parabola* *6*(3), 1–17.

Caillois, R. (1964). *The mask of Medusa*. C.N. Potter.

Csikszentmihalyi, M. (1997). Flow and education. *NAMTA Journal*, *22*(2), 2–35.

Davis, J. S. (2011). Five secondary teachers: Creating and presenting a teaching persona. *Current Issues in Education*, *14*(1), 1–26.

Ducharte, P. L. (2012). *The Italian Comedy*. Dover.

Eldredge, S. A. (1996). *Mask Improvisation for Actor and Performance*. Northwestern University Press.

Eldredge, S. A. and Huston, H. W. (2005). Actor training in the neutral mask. In P. Zarrilli (Ed.), *Acting (re)considered: A theoretical and practical guide* (140–147). Routledge.

Ewald, L. A. (2005). Commedia dell'Arte academica. *College Teaching* *53*(3), 115–119.

Foley, B. (2017). Principles of comedy for Commedia dell'Arte. In J. Chaffee and O. Crick (Eds.), *The Routledge companion to Commedia dell'Arte* (177–184). Routledge.

Friend, C. (2021). Introduction to hybrid pedagogy: People, pedagogy, politics. In C. Friend (Ed.), *Hybrid teaching: Pedagogy, people, politics* (x-xvii). Hybrid Pedagogy Inc.

Grinder, M. (2020, June 16). *ENVoY nonverbal communication: Classroom management for educators*. Michael Grinder & Associates. https://michaelgrinder.com/envoy/.

Grinder, M. (2011). *ENVoY: A personal guide to classroom management*. Michael Grinder & Associates.

Grinder, M. (1991). *Righting the educational conveyor belt*. Metamorphous Press.

Hall, E. (2008). Introduction: Pantomime, a lost chord of ancient culture. In E. Hall and R. Wyles (Eds.), *New directions in ancient pantomime* (1–42). London: Oxford University Press.

Jordan, P. (2017). Pantalone and IL Dottore: The old men of Commedia. In J. Chaffee and O. Crick (Eds.), *The Routledge Companion to Commedia dell'Arte* (62–69). Routledge.

Jordon, S. (2001). Embodied pedagogy: The body and teaching theology. *Teaching Theology & Religion*, *4*(2), 98–101.

Jory, J. (2008). The pantomime dancer and his libretto. In E. Hall and R. Wyles (Eds.), *New directions in ancient pantomime* (157–168). Oxford University Press.

Mazzone-Clementi, C. and Hill, J. (2017). Commedia and the actor. In J. Schechter (Ed.), *Popular theatre sourcebook* (83–90). Routledge.

Melser, D. (2009). Verbal communication: From pedagogy to make-believe. *Language Sciences*, *31*(5), 555–571.

National Theatre [ntdiscovertheatre]. (2011, October 6). *Commedia dell'Arte: Character Shape* [Video]. YouTube. https://www.youtube.com/watch?v=JJEwuurzDe4.

Perlman, M. (2017). Reading and interpreting the Capitano's multiple mask shapes. In J. Chaffee and O. Crick (Eds.), *The Routledge companion to Commedia dell'Arte* (82–90). Routledge.

Rafe, S. C. (1990). *How to think on your feet*. Harper Collins.

Rudlin, J. (1994). *Commedia dell'Arte*. Routledge.

Stamatis, P. J. (2011). Nonverbal communication in classroom interactions: A pedagogical perspective of touch. *Education and Psychology* *9*(3), 1429–1442.

Vianello, D. (2018). Introduction: Commedia dell'Arte: History, myth, reception. In C. B. Balme, P. Vescovo, and D. Vianello (Eds.), *Commedia dell'Arte in context* (i-xxi). Cambridge University Press.

Whalen, S. P. (1999). Finding flow at school and at home: A conversation with Mihaly Csikszentmihalyi. *Journal of Secondary Gifted Education*, *10*(4), 161–165.

Chapter Ten

Cultivating Student Creativity during the Pandemic

Short-Term Remedy with Long-Term Value

Heather J. Hether

The COVID-19 pandemic, along with other pressing social issues, challenged students' mental health and their ability to pursue higher education. Consequently, administrators and faculty applied multiple strategies to support students, including bolstering mental health services and providing additional accommodations for coursework (Johnson et al., 2020; Turk et al., 2020). Alongside these critical strategies, creative activities offered another avenue by which students could reduce stress, manage negative emotions, and connect with others (Jensen & Bonde, 2018; Stuckey & Nobel, 2010; Tan et al., 2019). This chapter presents an analysis of such an opportunity with a case study examining a new undergraduate course on creativity offered during the pandemic. Informed by creativity scholarship, the course curriculum was designed to support students' critical and creative thinking skills and provide opportunities for them to cultivate their creativity. However, as the analysis illustrates, the course supported more than the achievement of course learning outcomes: it also helped students cope during the pandemic.

DEFINING CREATIVITY

Researchers agree that creativity consists of two essential elements: 1) novelty or originality and 2) value or task-appropriateness (Kaufman &

Sternberg, 2007; Runco & Jaeger, 2012; Sawyer, 2012). Together, these two elements suggest, "creativity does not [just] happen inside people's heads, but in the interaction between a person's thoughts and a sociocultural context" (Csikszentmihalyi, 2013, p. 23). More specifically, Csikszentmihalyi (2013) describes a systems model of creativity consisting of three main elements: 1) the domain (an area of expertise), 2) the field (the individual gatekeepers to the domain), and 3) the individual person (who devises a novel contribution to the domain that is approved by the field). The author suggests that creativity is exhibited when an individual changes a domain with the consent of its gatekeepers. Thus, creativity is more than a personal ability it also includes a social dimension.

While this systems model of creativity has garnered support from researchers, there is no agreement on how best to study creativity. Instead, researchers have approached the topic from a myriad of perspectives. More than a half century ago, Rhodes (1961) summarized the different approaches to creativity research with a Four P framework that remains relevant today. Rhodes suggested that creativity has been studied from four different perspectives, each with a different focus, including the: 1) person, 2) process, 3) product, and 4) press. Research on the person addresses aspects of the individual that may be associated with creativity including personality, intelligence, temperament, traits, attitudes, and values. Research on the process examines how motivation, perception, learning, thinking, and communication are associated with creativity. This approach focuses on the cognitive processes and stages of creativity. Research on products examines the artifacts, or tangible outcomes, of creative thought. Lastly, press refers to the environmental and contextual pressures and influences on creativity.

In addition to the Four P framework that identifies areas of creativity research, another well-known typology segments creativity into different levels based on its outputs. This was initially a dichotomous distinction of Big-C and little-c, which was subsequently expanded with the additions of pro-c and mini-c creativity. Big-C creativity refers to the legacy of a significant creative figure who has left an imprint on society (Kaufman & Glaveanu, 2019). Whereas, little-c creativity refers to a lived creativity that is reflected in everyday activities, such as cooking a nice meal, creatively decorating the home, and working in the garden. The addition of pro-c refers to creativity that is practiced in a professional context by the professional or expert. Lastly, mini-c creativity refers to "the novel and personally meaningful interpretation of experiences, actions, and events" (Beghetto & Kaufman, 2014, p. 73). This kind of creativity is related to intrapersonal judgement and interpretation. It is reflected when individuals reorganize existing knowledge to accommodate new information, similar to learning but not synonymous with it. Mini-c creativity is the beginning of the creative process that can lead to little-c creativity and, over time and with practice, it can develop into higher levels (Beghetto & Kaufman, 2007; Beghetto & Kaufman, 2014).

While creativity is valuable for the tangible outcomes it produces, such as beautiful artwork and technological innovation, its impacts are bigger than its products. Instead, creativity is so important because it provides "a central source of meaning in our lives" (Csikszentmihalyi, 2013, p. 1). Moreover, engaging in creative activities is associated with a range of positive effects that include physical, emotional, social, and intellectual benefits.

THE BENEFITS OF CREATIVITY

Throughout history and across different cultures, people have engaged in the arts to promote the healing process. This includes the use of pictures, stories, dances, and chants as healing rituals (Stuckey & Nobel, 2010). More recently, creative arts therapies have been studied for their positive effects for patients coping with a range of illnesses (Jensen & Bonde, 2018). Thus, in both clinical and non-clinical contexts, there is a growing body of evidence identifying the positive influence of creativity on a variety of outcomes.

Increasingly, public health agencies and other researchers are exploring how the arts are associated with public health. Recently, the World Health Organization (WHO) conducted a scoping review in which they concluded that arts engagement is positively associated with both physical and mental health (Fancourt & Finn, 2020). The impact of the arts on mental health is particularly relevant for higher education because students face a range of stressors that were exacerbated during the COVID-19 pandemic (Turk et al., 2020). Fortunately, research indicates that creativity—whether it be the consumption or creation of art or creative products—can support psychological functioning, which further underscores its value in higher education.

Researchers have found the arts and creativity promote health and well-being (Burt & Atkinson, 2012; Jensen & Bonde, 2018; Tamannaeifar & Motaghedifard, 2014; Tymoszyj et al., 2021). More specifically, studies have shown that being creative predicts happiness and positive affect (Conner et al., 2018; Stuckey & Nobel, 2010; Tan et al., 2019). However, the reverse is also true: positive affect predicts creativity (Amabile et al., 2005). Thus, scholars have suggested a reciprocal relationship between creativity and positive affect that may result in "an upward spiral for well-being and creativity" (Conner et al., 2018, p. 186). Positive affect predicts creative activity and creative activity then predicts more positive affect, and so on.

Creativity has also been associated with a range of other psychological benefits, including resilience and an ability to cope. Researchers have suggested that some of the characteristics inherent in creativity are also important for resilience (Metzl & Morrell, 2008). A tolerance for ambiguity, an aptitude for divergent thinking, and problem-solving capacities are often associated with creativity and these qualities may cultivate resilience too (Metzl, 2009; Metzl & Morrell, 2008; Parr et al., 1998). Additional psychological characteristics of creativity include openness, autonomy, and flexibility—all characteristics that are favorable to mental health (Cropley, 1990). Thus, supporting students' creativity is likely to support their mental health, too.

In addition to the psychological benefits, arts and creative activities also support new social relationships and individuals' sense of being part of a community (Jensen & Bonde, 2018). People can enjoy creative activities together, which can provide support and encouragement to participants (Burt & Atkinson, 2012). Pachucki et al. (2010) also found that students identified social interactions as a primary context for creativity. Through humor, self-expression, relationship negotiation, and interpersonal communication students found they could be creative through their peer interactions.

Beyond the health-related benefits of creativity, creative thinking also supports higher levels of learning and is valuable for students' future careers. Higher levels of learning require cognitive skills that depend on many of the same aptitudes that facilitate creativity, such as openness and curiosity (Lin, 2011; Livingston, 2010; Sawyer, 2015). Moreover, in the updated Bloom's (1956) taxonomy of learning objectives, "creating" is identified as the most complex level of cognitive activity (Anderson, et al., 2001 as cited in Wilson, 2016). In addition, a growing chorus of voices has argued that creativity is important for students' future professional success. Experts assert that creative professionals are needed to make productive contributions and solve thorny, social problems; thus, cultivating students' creativity has important implications for a variety of outcomes (Livingston, 2010; Wagner, 2012; Sawyer, 2015, 2019).

Overwhelmingly, the evidence suggests that engaging in creative activities can facilitate positive effects for students across a range of variables. Some of these positive effects may be associated with flow states that individuals may experience during creative activities. Flow states are optimal experiences that individuals pursue for their enjoyment (Beard, 2015; Nakamura & Csikszentmihalyi, 2009). Csikszentmihalyi (2013) describes a flow experience as an "effortless, yet highly focused state of consciousness" (p. 110). Flow states are also associated with outcomes that are important to educators, such as concentration, engagement, and learning (Beard, 2015; Csikszentmihalyi, 2013; Guo & Ro, 2008). Not surprisingly, educators are encouraged increasingly to integrate more creativity into their classrooms (Livingston, 2010; Sawyer, 2015, 2019; Wagner, 2012).

CREATIVITY IN THE CLASSROOM

Encouraging student creativity reflects the perspective that students can learn to be creative. McWilliam (2009) suggests that creativity has become unhinged from "artiness, individual genius and idiosyncrasy, rendering it . . . observable and learnable" (p. 282). In fact, research going back to the 1950s has examined how creativity can be taught, as opposed to viewing it as a trait restricted to the sole purview of the gifted and talented (Sawyer, 2012). Since then, two primary approaches to creativity training have developed.

The two approaches to creativity training differentiate between a general versus a domain specific focus (Sawyer, 2015). General creativity training programs focus on teaching participants general skills to facilitate creative thinking. Many programs, for example, focus on teaching participants strategies to facilitate divergent thinking. Divergent thinking refers to generating original ideas around a particular issue or problem and it has been recognized as an "essential constituent of creativity" (Weiss et al., 2020, p. 292). Moreover, divergent thinking tests are often used to measure creativity or creative potential (Runco, 2008).

In addition to divergent thinking, creativity training often teaches a staged approach to creative thinking. In this approach, participants learn how to move through the various stages of cognitive activity to help them think more creatively. Often these programs involve stages of problem identification, knowledge gathering, and divergent and convergent thinking (Sawyer, 2012). One of the most well established programs is the creative problem solving (CPS) model. This approach includes three main components, broken down into six steps. These components broadly focus on understanding the challenge (problem identification), generating ideas (divergent thinking), and preparing for action (convergent thinking). The core of this system is a balance between generating ideas (divergent thinking) and focusing ideas (convergent thinking) (Treffinger, Isaksen, & Stead-Dorval, 2006).

While general creativity training programs can be effective at boosting creativity, research suggests that creativity training specific to a particular context or domain is more effective (Sawyer, 2015). Domain-specific creativity education is likely more effective because creativity requires novelty of thought that advances the domain into new, innovative areas. To do so requires a deep understanding of the domain (Csikszentmihalyi, 2013). Thus, while the principles and practices from general creativity training programs are effective, they may be most valuable when applied within a specific content area (Sawyer, 2015).

In further considering the role of education in developing creativity, Lin (2011) offers a tripartite model of creative pedagogy that illustrates how creativity can be applied in the classroom. While Lin frames her discussion within the K-12 context, her model is also valuable in higher education. Lin suggests that students' creativity can be facilitated through three interrelated elements: 1) creative teaching, 2) creative learning, and 3) teaching for creativity. Creative teaching highlights instructor strategies and practices. This element of the model focuses on what instructors can do to teach the material creatively to their students; it focuses on the instructor's approach to teaching. Creative learning focuses on the learner's role and their agency in the learning process. This element of the model focuses on what learners can do to support their learning in creative ways, such as through questioning, exploring, collaborating, experimenting, etc. Lastly, teaching for creativity is the reciprocal of creative teaching. This element reflects learning outcomes; it focuses on the creative abilities that instructors strive to cultivate within their students, such as imaginative thinking and innovative approaches to problem solving.

A critical aspect of Lin's (2011) model is that it is not a linear model. Instead, "the three elements of creative pedagogy interplay and contribute to each other, forming a dialogic and improvisational process" (p. 153). Informed by Sawyer's argument that the most effective teaching is improvisational and emergent, this model reflects the dynamism of creative pedagogy (Sawyer, 2015; 2019). In the creative classroom, the three elements of this model are in constant interaction with each other. Thus, Lin (2011) urges educators to adopt a more holistic perspective of creative pedagogy that recognizes the constant interplay of these three elements.

THE CREATIVE LIFE

Creative Pedagogy

The Creative Life is a first-year seminar that was offered for the first time during the pandemic. First-year seminars are small enrollment, general education courses intended especially for new students, but open to all. They are designed to support conversation and community while students explore subjects of interest. This course was planned initially for the classroom but when the pandemic reached the United States, it was shifted to remote/online delivery.

The course learning outcomes are oriented around two key instructional goals: 1) introduce students to the dominant themes and ideas within seminal creativity scholarship and 2) encourage the development of students' creativity and creative thinking. Instructional goals and related learning outcomes are supported by short, weekly assignments and two longer assignments. Every week, students do readings, participate in discussion, complete creativity challenges, and write a blog post. The two longer assignments include: 1) a biography of a creative legend (i.e., Big-C creativity), presented in an infographic /visual format, and 2) a creative project proposal (i.e., "aspirational" pro-c creativity).

The course design encourages students to reflect upon their creativity by engaging with some of the major ideas within creativity scholarship. Rather than working through a thick, academic text, the primary reading for the course is a book written by an academic and a practitioner for a general audience (Kaufman & Gregoire, 2015). This book is accessible for new college students and it reflects both the theory and practice of creativity. Students are also assigned videos to watch. These videos examine creativity either through profiling accomplished creators (e.g., Twyla Tharp, Elizabeth Gilbert, Pixar founders) or elaborating on another topic from the course (e.g., flow theory, cultural perspectives of creativity, idea generation).

The readings and videos introduce students to key ideas from the creativity research in an accessible way and students develop their fluency with these ideas and perspectives through class discussion. During the pandemic, discussion took place primarily asynchronously through an online discussion board on the course learning management system (LMS). Individual students lead the discussion every week by posting their reflections on the material along with discussion questions. The discussions provide a forum for students to learn creatively through dialogic communication, questioning, and exploring. While not unique to creative pedagogy per se, this course structure creates opportunities for students to cultivate new insights (e.g., mini-c creativity) about creativity scholarship and their creative interests.

In addition to the weekly reading and discussion, another ongoing course assignment consists of creativity challenges. Every week, students are assigned novel creativity challenges that are informed and inspired by various contemporary sources (e.g., Bell, 2019; Cameron, 1992; Kaufman & Gregoire, 2015). The challenges reflect activities of renowned creative practitioners and include practices like daily journaling, daily walking, daily meditation as well as more explicit imaginative and creative exercises that facilitate divergent and convergent thinking. After completing the weekly challenge, students reflect on their experiences in their blogs that they share with the class. These challenges reflect all three elements of Lin's (2011) creative pedagogy. The instructor must think creatively in terms of identifying a novel challenge that will stimulate students, connect with that week's topics, and support course learning outcomes (creative teaching) and students are challenged with doing something novel and reflecting on it and its impact on them (creative learning). Moreover, many of the challenges also include opportunities for students to be creative (e.g., teaching for creativity) either through divergent thinking challenges (e.g., describe 100 uses for object X) or artistic activities (e.g., cook a new meal or draw a cartoon). The challenges are often little-c creativity exercises that are intended to facilitate mini-c creativity through blog reflections and online discussion.

While teaching for creativity (Lin, 2011) is supported through the creative challenges, it is most explicitly supported in the longer assignments, particularly the infographic biography. In this assignment, students identify someone who has led an exemplary creative life. They conduct research on this person and then share their findings in a visual presentation (i.e., infographic) to the class. Students are encouraged to identify a Big-C legend or an accomplished, pro-c figure who has made a significant impact on their field. Prior to conducting their research, all students share their selected figure with the instructor to ensure there are no duplicate figures among students. Students then apply the Four P framework of creativity (Rhodes, 1961) to learn more about the background, habits, personality, cultural context, and art of productive, creative people. The assignment supports course learning outcomes on multiple levels. First, students develop their critical and creative thinking skills through research, analysis, and synthesis of their findings. In addition, they develop their applied skills by creatively communicating their research to the class. Moreover, by sharing their work students are encouraged to look for commonalities across the biographies—a practice that further develops their understanding of creativity, creative expression, and creative leaders.

For the final project, students create a proposal that identifies an aspirational, yet achievable, creative project and formulates their plans for realizing it. The overall structure and purpose of the plan reflects the three major aspects of the creative problem solving (CPS) framework including understanding the challenge, generating ideas (divergent thinking), and preparing for action (convergent thinking) (Treffinger et al., 2006). Students are asked to think deeply about what they want to accomplish and how they can do so.

Alongside the CPS framework, students apply the Four P model of creativity (Rhodes, 1961) when describing their project and the skills needed to complete it. In their analysis, students provide a description of the context, or field, to which their project would contribute (i.e., "press"). This requires background research on the domain of interest—whether it be food photography, cookbooks, or small art galleries. Through their research, students identify and consider potential barriers to their success. They also describe the work of two to three inspirational Creatives working in the relevant context. Students analyze the characteristics and behaviors of these leaders and, thus, identify the skills and aptitudes that support success in this field (i.e., the person). Students describe the product they want to create and, in doing so, they describe how their work will reflect the two key dimensions of creativity: novelty/originality and task appropriateness (Kaufman & Sternberg, 2007; Runco & Jaeger, 2012; Sawyer, 2012). The last major section of their paper outlines the key milestones students envision for completing the work (i.e., the process). The proposed timeline for their project has a finish date within one to five years. Students submit their proposals to the instructor and share them with the class in visual presentations so that students may learn from each other.

ANALYSIS

The Creative Life seminar was offered twice during the pandemic, with enrollment less than 10 each time.[1] Across both classes, students represented a range of academic majors, class standing, and creative interests. Students' interests included fine arts, commercial arts, culinary arts, cinema, writing, fashion, music, and more. Throughout the course, the ongoing assignments supported students' achievement of course learning outcomes and ensured their learning was observable.

All of the assignments encouraged students' creative and critical thinking; in addition, many of the assignments also encouraged students' creative expression. For example, students were encouraged to cultivate their creativity through both the weekly challenges and the longer assignments. The creative challenges often included prompts to engage in explicit creative activities, such as drawing or cooking a new meal. Typically, students' creative output was not shared from these challenges, but they discussed their experiences with the activity on their blogs. The longer-form assignments, however, provided students with opportunities to engage in creative expression through the visual presentations they shared with the class. In the infographic assignment, students found creative ways to visually connect their infographic to their subject, such as using the color palette or visual style that was similar to their selected artist. Students enjoyed the opportunity to present their work creatively. In fact, one student suggested he had entered a flow state when designing the infographic. He explained in class that he had enjoyed the process so much that he had probably spent too much time on his infographic, relative to the overall contribution of the assignment toward his final grade.

In the creative project proposal students identified their creative interests and developed a plan to produce something tangible in this domain. These proposals reflected a range of interests including photography, graphic novels, short stories, artistic shows, new business ventures, and even a cookbook. In this proposal, students applied some of the key ideas from creativity scholarship while describing their vision for their own contribution to a particular domain.

Overall, student work reflected a high level of achievement of course learning outcomes. Students engaged thoughtfully with the scholarship and with their own creativity throughout the term. In addition, there was evidence that the course supported students in ways that went beyond learning outcomes. The course also seemed to provide students with a sense of connection and community that was lacking during the pandemic. This was most apparent in both the online discussions and the anonymous course evaluations.

Students were primarily responsible for initiating and moderating the online discussion of the weekly readings and videos. In this context, students asked thoughtful questions related to the course material, such as questions about flow theory, culture and creativity, characteristics of creative people, and creativity across the lifespan. However, alongside these scholarly questions, students also posed personal discussion questions that required some vulnerability from their peers. For example, students asked about their classmates' emotional lives, "When was the last time you felt happy about something?," their memories, "Can you recall a specific time where a song [brought] you back to a time period in your life?," and managing their emotions, "If you don't meditate, what do you do to calm yourself?"[2] Students responded to these questions in ways that were personally revealing, such as reflecting on their current emotional state or sharing that that they cannot listen to a particular song because it is associated with bad memories.

In one of these discussions, a student asked whether their peers used creative work as a "refuge from" or as "a way to process the struggle" of the pandemic. There was a range of responses, with several students indicating that creative work provided them with an escape from the pandemic for a little while, ". . . it makes your mind and stress of what you are thinking and feeling go away for awhile" wrote one student. Other students suggested that creative work was a way to both process the pandemic and seek refuge from it. For example, another student wrote, "I definitely think that this class has been both a refuge and a way to process the pandemic. Creativity has been an amazing way to escape the world that we live in, whether it be through the exercises for this class or a creative project that I'm working on . . . " Thus, most students found there were benefits to creative work particularly during the pandemic. Students appreciated the distraction the work offered from real-life events, the opportunities it provided to enter flow states and be wholly "in the moment," and the inspiration it provided them during a difficult time.

The logistics of creative work—the fact that it can be done at home, in isolation—were also helpful with stay-at-home orders in effect. However, a few students suggested more nuanced impacts of creative work. For example, one student indicated they could see the benefits of creative work in general during stressful times, but they also found getting to the store to get creative supplies was difficult, resulting in them being less creative during the pandemic. However, this student concluded that, "Overall . . . creativity helps people get through hard times." In addition, another student suggested that assigned creative work could "be detrimental to my mental health during tough times" because it adds to their existing workload. This student's response indicated they were not necessarily referring to this particular course; nonetheless, their comments suggest there may be differential impacts of creative work that is assigned versus creative projects that students pursue on their own.

While few students (n = 5) completed the anonymous course evaluations across both terms, many of those students that did reflected on the importance of creativity during the pandemic. Interestingly, one student commented on the value of having a creative community, "The seminar . . . provided a great creative community that I'd been missing. This was pretty much exactly what I needed in a pandemic." While another student noted, "This course was valuable especially in the time of the COVID-19 pandemic because it allowed me to have an outlet for my creativity, and to learn more about creativity overall."

The course evaluations also reflect students' critical thinking related to the scholarship introduced in the course. For example, one student wrote that they learned, " . . . creativity needs to be nurtured. Dedication is just as important as raw talent." Another student also reflected on the theme of raw talent versus environmental influence, by writing, "I learned . . . how being creative is not only based on our capabilities but also the environment." Another student seemed to summarize these perspectives by saying, "Creativity is a spectrum and cannot be thought of in one basic way." These comments reflect research that suggests creativity can be cultivated and, thus, is important to include in higher education curricula (Sawyer, 2015).

DISCUSSION

A large body of scholarship explores creativity from a range of perspectives, such as those reflected in the Four P (Rhodes, 1961) and 4-C models (e.g., Kaufman & Glaveanu, 2019), as well as the systems model proposed by Csikszentmihalyi (2013). While scholars have explored the scope and processes of creativity as reflected in these models, researchers have also identified a myriad of benefits associated with creativity, including physical health, social connection, resilience, and problem-solving skills (e.g., Fancourt & Finn, 2020; Jensen & Bonde, 2018; Metzl, 2009; Metzl & Morrell, 2008; Parr et al., 1998; Stuckey & Nobel, 2010). Moreover, educators have been encouraged to integrate more opportunities for student creativity into the curriculum because it facilitates learning at the highest levels and it embodies skills that are increasingly in demand in the professional context (Anderson et al., 2001 as cited in Wilson, 2016; Wagner, 2012).

The Creative Life is a first–year seminar informed by creativity scholarship whose instructional goals support students' critical and creative thinking, and creative expression. Through course assignments, students reflect on and apply some of the major ideas from creativity scholarship to their work. They also learn more about the contributions, habits, and skills of accomplished creative figures while exploring their own creative interests.

While evidence indicates student achievement of course learning outcomes, comments from students suggested the course might have facilitated something more than learning: it also offered a sense of community and connection that some students missed during the pandemic. In addition, the opportunities for creative expression provided by the course facilitated flow states and provided a welcome distraction from the stress caused by the pandemic. Thus, the course may have benefitted students' emotional health in unanticipated ways.

While the pandemic highlights how such a learning community can benefit students' mental health by fulfilling unmet social and emotional needs, it is worthwhile to remember that students face ongoing stressors even without a pandemic. Therefore, providing space within our course curricula that encourages creativity, connection, and community has the potential to provide benefits to students even in more routine social conditions. However, it is also important to recognize that instructors can provide these opportunities but students must embrace them to realize their full potential. As one student suggested, opportunities for creativity that are extrinsically motivated may inadvertently also cause stress as they may add to students' existing workload. Nonetheless, the consensus of students during this course was that engaging in creative expression is beneficial to students' mental health during difficult times.

IMPLICATIONS AND FUTURE DIRECTIONS

Moving forward, this course will shift to a face-to-face context and the stressors of the pandemic will fade. Both of these changes will influence how students engage with the course material and each other. In anticipation of these changes, the instructor will reevaluate how the course can continue to facilitate thoughtful reflection and authentic engagement, outside of a global health crisis.

One central aspect of the course is discussion. While seminar-style classes typically have face-to-face discussion as a central pedagogical element, this recent course experience suggests that maintaining an online space for conversation is also important. This provides opportunities to nurture connectivity and authentic exchange in an environment where students may feel more comfortable. Thus, the instructor will likely maintain online discussion forums to supplement the face-to-face (F2F) conversation. This could be a pre-cursor to the F2F conversation or separate threads altogether, but the main goal will be to create online spaces for engagement where students may feel more comfortable to reflect and connect (e.g., Hamann et al., 2012; Poole, 2000).

Consequently, classroom time that may have been allocated toward F2F discussion can be repurposed for the class to engage in creative activities together. This can support students' creative development and provide opportunities for them to enter flow states (Csikszentmihalyi, 2013). Moreover, these experiences can facilitate authentic conversations that support student learning, as well as their sense of community and connection.

Additional refinements to the course may include changes to the reading and the scope of assignments. The current reading is accessible and reflects both an academic and practitioner perspective. However, the text predominantly reflects an individualist approach to creativity (e.g., traits, characteristics, habits), leaving a large area of scholarship excluded from the course readings. Rather than relying on one text, a selection of readings from both academic and general sources may support a broader introduction to creativity scholarship. Similarly, the assignments may be further refined to align more closely with the readings and course learning outcomes.

CONCLUSION

This case study describes the unanticipated benefits that a course on creativity offered students during the pandemic. While the course effectively supported learning outcomes, it also provided students with authentic social connections and a peer community that may have been lacking during the pandemic. Moreover, engaging in creative activities provided students with opportunities to enter flow states, which took their minds off stressful, global events. Thus, this course was valuable to students, not only as a learning experience but also as a coping mechanism during a difficult time.

REFERENCES

Amabile, T. M., Barsade, S. G., Mueller, J. S., & Staw, B. M. (2005). Affect and creativity at work. *Administrative Science Quarterly, 50*(3), 367–403. https://doi.org/10.2189/asqu.2005.50.3.367.

Anderson, L. W., Krathwohl, D. R., & and Bloom, B. S. (2001). *A taxonomy for learning, teaching, and assessing: A revision of Bloom's Taxonomy of Educational Objectives*. Longman.

Beard, K. S. (2015). Theoretically speaking: An interview with Mihaly Csikszentmihalyi on flow theory development and its usefulness in addressing contemporary challenges in education. *Educational Psychology Review, 27*(2), 353–364. https://doi.org/10.1007/s10648-014-9291-1.

Beghetto, R. A., & Kaufman, J. C. (2007). Toward a broader conception of creativity: A case for "mini-c" creativity. Psychology of Aesthetics, Creativity, and the Arts, 1(2), 73–79. https://doi.org/10.1037/1931-3896.1.2.73.

Beghetto, R. A., & Kaufman, J. S. (2014). Classroom contexts for creativity. *High Ability Studies, 25*(1), 53–69. https://doi.org/10.1080/13598139.2014.905247.

Bell, E. (2019). *The 30-Day Creativity Challenge.* The Song Foundry.

Bloom, B. S. (1956). Taxonomy of educational objectives. Vol. 1: Cognitive domain. *McKay*, *20*(24), 1.

Burt, E. L., & Atkinson, J. (2012). The relationship between quilting and wellbeing. *Journal of Public Health, 34*(1), 54–59. https://doi.org/10.1093/pubmed/fdr041.

Cameron, J. (1992). *The artist's way: A spiritual path to higher creativity*. Penguin Putnam.

Christensen, T. (2015). *The creativity challenge.* Adams Media.

Conner, T. S., DeYoung, C. G., and Silvia, P. J. (2018). Everyday creative activity as a path to flourishing. *The Journal of Positive Psychology, 13*(2), 181–189. https://doi.org/10.1080/17439760.2016.1257049.

Cropley, A. J. (1990). Creativity and mental health in everyday life. *Creativity Research Journal, 3*(3), 167–178. https://doi.org/10.1080/10400419009534351.

Csikszentmihalyi, M. (2013). *Creativity*. Harper Perennial Modern Classics.

Fancourt, D., & Finn, S. (2020). *What is the evidence on the role of the arts in improving health and well-being? A scoping review.* World Health Organization (WHO). https://www.euro.who.int/en/publications/abstracts/what-is-the-evidence-on-the-role-of-the-arts-in-improving-health-and-well-being-a-scoping-review-2019.

Guo, Y. M., & Ro, Y. K. (2008). Capturing flow in the business classroom. *Decision Sciences Journal of Innovative Education, 6*(2), 437–462. https://doi.org/10.1111/j.1540-4609.2008.00185.x.

Hamann, K., Pollock, P. H., & Wilson, B. M. (2012). Assessing student perceptions of the benefits of discussions in small-group, large-class, and online learning contexts. *College Teaching*, *60*(2), 65–75. https://doi.org/10.1080/87567555.2011.633407.

Jensen, A., & Bonde, L. (2018). The use of arts interventions for mental health and wellbeing in health settings. *Perspectives in Public Health*, *138*(4), 209–214. https://doi.org/10.1177/1757913918772602.

Johnson, N., Veletsianos, G., & Seaman, J. (2020). U.S. faculty and administrators' experiences and approaches in the early weeks of the COVID-19 pandemic. *Online Learning, 24*(2), 6–21. https://doi.org/10.24059/olj.v24i2.2285.

Kaufman, J. C., & Sternberg, R. J. (2007). Creativity. *Change: The Magazine of Higher Learning 39*(4), 55–60.: https://doi.org/10.3200/CHNG.39.4.55-C4.

Kaufman, J. C., & Glaveanu, V. P. (2019). A review of creativity theories. In J. C. Kaufman & R. J. Sternberg (Eds.), *The Cambridge handbook of creativity,* (pp. 27–43). Cambridge University Press.

Kaufman, S. B., & Gregoire, C. (2015). *Wired to create: Unraveling the mysteries of the Creative mind.* TarcherPerigee.

Lin, Y. (2011) Fostering creativity through education—A conceptual framework of creative pedagogy. *Creative Education, 2*, 149–155. https://doi: 10.4236/ce.2011.23021.

Livingston, L. (2010). Teaching creativity in higher education. *Arts Education Policy Review, 111*(2), 59–62. https://doi.org/10.1080/10632910903455884.

McWilliam, E. (2009). Teaching for creativity: From sage to guide to meddler. *Asia Pacific Journal of Education, 29*(3), 281–293. https://doi.org/10.1080/02188790903092787.

Metzl, E. S. (2009). The role of creative thinking in resilience after hurricane Katrina. Psychology of Aesthetics, Creativity, and the Arts, 3(2), 112–123. https://doi.org/10.1037/a0013479.

Metzl, E. S., & Morrell, M. A. (2008). The role of creativity in models of resilience: Theoretical exploration and practical applications. *Journal of Creativity in Mental Health, 3*(3), 303–318. https://doi.org/10.1080/15401380802385228.

Nakamura, J., & Csikszentmihalyi, M. (2009). Flow theory and research. In S.J. Lopez & C.R. Snyder (Eds.), *Handbook of positive psychology* (2nd ed., pp. 195–206).

Pachucki, M. A., Lena, J. C., & Tepper, S. J. (2010). Creativity narratives among college students: Sociability and everyday creativity. *The Sociological Quarterly, 51*(1), 122–149.

Parr, G. D., Montgomery, M., & DeBell, C. (1998). Flow theory as a model for enhancing student resilience. *Professional School Counseling, 1*(5), 26–31.

Poole, D. M. (2000). Student participation in a discussion-oriented online course: A case study. *Journal of Research on Computing in Education, 33*(2), 162–177. https://doi.org/10.1080/08886504.2000.10782307.

Rhodes, M. (1961). An analysis of creativity. *The Phi Delta Kappan, 42*(7), 305–310.

Runco, Mark A. (2008). Commentary: Divergent thinking is not synonymous with creativity. *Psychology of Aesthetics*, Creativity, and the Arts, 2(2), 93–96. https://doi.org/10.1037/1931-3896.2.2.93.

Runco, M. A., & Jaeger, G. J. (2012). The standard definition of creativity. *Creativity Research Journal, 24*(1), 2–96.

Sawyer, K. (2012). *Explaining creativity: The science of human innovation.* Oxford University Press.

Sawyer, K. (2015). A call to action: The challenges of creative teaching and learning. *Teachers College Record, 117*(10), 1–34.

Sawyer, K. (2019). *The creative classroom: Innovative teaching for 21st-century learners.* Teachers College Press.

Stuckey, H. L., & Nobel, J. (2010). The connection between art, healing, and public health: A review of current literature. *American Journal of Public Health, 100*(2), 254–263.

Tamannaeifar, M. R., & Motaghedifard, M. (2014). Subjective well-being and its sub-scales among students: The study of role of creativity and self-efficacy. *Thinking Skills and Creativity, 12*, 37–42. https://doi.org/10.1016/j.tsc.2013.12.003.

Tan, C. S., Tan, S. A., Hashim, I. H. M., Lee, M. N., Ong, A. W., & Yaacob, S. N. B (2019). Problem-solving ability and stress mediate the relationship between creativity and happiness. *Creativity Research Journal, 31*(1), 15–25.

Treffinger, D. J., Isaksen, S. J., and Stead-Dorval, B. K. (2006). *Creative problem solving: An introduction*. Prufrock Press.

Turk, J. M., Soler, M.C., Chessman, H. M., & de Jesus Gonzalez, A. (2020). *College and university presidents respond to COVID-19: 2020 fall term survey, part II.* American Council on Education. https://www.acenet.edu/Research-Insights/Pages/Senior-Leaders/College-and-University-Presidents-Respond-to-COVID19–2020-Fall-Term-Part-Two.aspx.

Tymoszuk, U., Spiro, N., Perkins, R., Mason-Bertrand, A., Gee, K., & Williamon, A. (2021) Arts engagement trends in the United Kingdom and their mental and social wellbeing implications: Hearts survey. *PloS One, 16*(3)3, Article e0246078. https://journals.plos.org/plosone/article?id=10.1371/journal.pone.0246078.

Wagner, T. (2012). *Creating innovators: The making of young people who will change the world*. Simon and Schuster.

Weiss, S., Steger, D., Kaur, Y., Hildebrandt, A., Schroeders, U., Wilhelm, O., & Kandler, C. (2020). On the trail of creativity: Dimensionality of divergent thinking and its relation with cognitive abilities, personality, and insight. *European Journal of Personality, 35*(3), 291–314. https://doi.org/10.1002/per.2288.

Wilson, L. O. (2016). *Anderson and Krathwohl–Bloom's Taxonomy revised: Understanding the New Version of Bloom's Taxonomy*, Last modified 2016, http://www0.sun.ac.za/ctlresources/wp-content/uploads/2018/11/Anderson-andKrathwohl.-2001.-Extract-from-A-taxonomy-for-learning-teaching-and-assessing-arevised-Blooms-Taxonomy.pdf.

NOTES

1. IRB review was not required. IRB ID: 1785010–1
2. Student quotes are included anonymously with student permission.

Chapter Eleven

Creativity and Consolation in *The Golden Girls*

How Revisiting an Old Show Was a Balm for the New Hard Times

Lauren Kelly and Sarah Royal

Picture it: Brooklyn, March 2020.

A coronavirus pandemic creeps across oceans and reaches New York City. Businesses shutter. Toilet paper is nowhere to be found. Hospitals are overrun. The situation is extremely bleak and unprecedented for nearly everyone worldwide. Two young women decide that the way to both cope with living in a time of chaotic uncertainty and alleviate their stress is to delve into what they know best. They turn to a longstanding comforting presence in their lives: Dorothy Zbornak, Blanche Devereaux, Rose Nylund, and Sophia Petrillo: *The Golden Girls.*

Nearly 40 years after its premiere on NBC, *The Golden Girls* maintains a cultural relevance rarely enjoyed by network sitcoms, and especially impressive for a show with four female leads over the age of 50. Intrepid actresses Betty White, Bea Arthur, Rue McClanahan, and Estelle Getty brought depth and determination to these four characters back in the '80s to prove that anyone can start over, even when life brings along major upheaval—and it has resonated ever since. Turn on Hulu, the Hallmark Channel, or TV Land and one can binge-watch all seven seasons, which originally ran from 1985–1992. Click on Instagram and one will unearth a batch of late millennials and Gen-Zers who run fan accounts dedicated to this show that went off the air before they were born. Hop over to Etsy and one can find anything from cross stitch patterns featuring Rose's St. Olaf quotes, to Shady Pines retirement home keychains, to lingerie emblazoned with "Dorothy in the streets, Blanche in the sheets." In short, it is everywhere. And for us, two thirty-somethings, it has been everywhere our entire lives. There is no episode we have not seen, no line we cannot recall off the top of our heads, no joke we do not anticipate—much to the chagrin of anyone watching along with us.

Despite admonishments to stop trying to be productive circulating in the *New York Times* (Lorenz, 2020) and other places, we started discussing ways to explore and augment this new hobby of digesting an old show. As Sörqvist and Marsh (2015) found, concentration is a shield against distraction and in our case, it served as an incredible tool to counteract the effects of the daily COVID-19 death statistics, or yet another report of an extrajudicial shooting of an unarmed Black person, or whatever fresh horrors presented themselves on the newsfeed. It is natural to lean on a creative project as a means to process, or pay little attention to, exigent traumas. It is why art therapy has proven to be so successful (Leckey, 2011). Thus, we adopted a maxim: When the world takes something away from you, put something back in and create.

Through the established notions of volitional reconsumption, experience-taking, and parasocial interactions, we will explain how revisiting a 1980s network sitcom can produce grounding comfort in difficult times, spark creativity through the development of a scholarly podcast, and how relating to these particular characters impacts real-life intrapersonal and interpersonal growth for ourselves and so many viewers. Simultaneously, we imagine how *The Golden Girls* themselves might have coped with the lamentable events of 2020 in the form of interspersed bits of dialogue prior to each section of this essay. If we can fully attest to one thing, it is that there is nothing better to break up hefty spurts of serious thought than a punchy bit of *The Golden Girls* dialogue.

ROSE: NOW THAT WE HAVE TO STAY HOME ALL THE TIME, I THINK I NEED A NEW HOBBY.

SOPHIA: YOU HAVE A FACE FOR RADIO.

BLANCHE: YOU KNOW WHAT, ROSE, THAT'S NOT A BAD IDEA. WHY NOT START A PODCAST? THERE'S AN AUDIENCE OUT THERE FOR ANYTHING THESE DAYS.

DOROTHY: RIGHT, BLANCHE. I'M SURE A PODCAST ABOUT THE COLORFUL PEOPLE OF ST. OLAF AND THEIR FARM ANIMAL COMPANIONS WILL TOP THE ITUNES CHARTS.[1]

Sitting on our couches back in March 2020, we were already delving into our comfort reruns of *The Golden Girls* and delighting in Sophia's snarky one-liners, Dorothy's morose staring, Blanche's vibrant zeal and salaciousness, and Rose's at-times admirable quality of thinking the world is a wonderful place. Naturally, we found ourselves incessantly texting each other funny lines out of context, and chatting about various scenarios that hit a little differently as we were watching this time around. It eventually occurred to us: Why not, in this age of digital documentation, record ourselves discussing the show and share it with the world in the process? Like experimenting with sourdough starters, it was not a unique idea to record ourselves in conversation during this troubling moment in time. According to data aggregated by Listen Notes (2020), more new podcasts launched in the first half of 2020 than all of 2019, as podcasting offers that beautiful intersection of creative project, personal connection, and wholly virtual setup.

Our nostalgic passion for this antiquated TV show laid a foundation, and all we had to do was build the new atop. In order to create something unique and worth consuming, we found the need to differentiate our project from all of the other excellent *Golden Girls*-focused podcasts already in existence, and decided to approach the show from an academic angle. As Joanne Morreale (2003) explains in her introduction to the collection *Critiquing the Sitcom: A Reader,* "television, like all forms of social discourse, helps to shape not only beliefs, values, and attitudes, but also subjectivities, people's sense of themselves and their place in the world" (p. xi). Our conversations still involved reciting the one-liners in a way that pales in comparison to the legendary actresses, but began to delve more deeply into themes such as feminist representation on television, sexuality, and aging, adhering to—and flouting—female archetypes, and what it means to be an old woman in America (Macey, 2012). As our plan for research evolved from simply taking notes on episodes to immersing ourselves in scholarly analysis of *The Golden Girls*, the fully-formed idea for *Enough Wicker: Intellectualizing the Golden Girls* came to be.

As we went about this background research, we were struck by the quantity of scholarship that referred to this singular sitcom from the 1980s. Today, JSTOR lists 545 references of *The Golden Girls,* many of which we have used (and will use here) as citations. Additionally, we found that many scholars of media such as Deborah A. Macey, an editor of this book, had written dissertations about the show and its impact on television, pop culture, and women in media. We decided that beyond reading these works and providing our own commentary and analysis on each episode, it could be interesting to have the authors on as guests, and we were delighted to find that many of them (including Macey, thankfully) were excited by the opportunity to discuss the show with fellow students and super fans. These conversations with scholars who had spent years researching the show challenged us to elevate our own critiques and observations, which ranged from drawing parallels and distinctions between *The Golden Girls* and *Living Single* (Macey, 2012), to reading Rose Nylund's faith in America as endemic to a Midwestern member of the Greatest Generation (Browne, 2020), to imagining how the Girls would handle the tumultuous circumstances that began in 2020—the last a playful speculatory exercise that emerged again and again with our podcast guests.

This method of intellectualizing *The Golden Girls* allowed us to merge repeated comfort viewing with a new academic pursuit that had the added benefit of self-reflection. The concept of volitional reconsumption illuminated by Cristel Antonia Russell and Sidney J. Levy (2012) quite literally refers to reconsuming the exact same piece of media, over and over again. When one engages in volitional reconsumption, as we were doing, it is immensely soothing; there is no anticipation or deduction necessary, but the jokes remain funny and the plots are still entertaining. But as Andrew Goodwin and Garry Whannel (2016) explain in *Understanding Television*, sitcoms, or at least the good ones, one cannot enjoy mere escapism without being affected by the content. It is precisely the nature of the soothing jokes and flowing plots that act as a comforting lure to immerse viewers into the show's environment—at which point a show is able to imprint its dialogue, point of view, philosophy, and unique content into hearts and minds.

Additionally, consuming the same show over and over helps mark the passage of time in our own lives. Russell & Levy (2012) elaborate:

> The dynamics in time and focus fueled by the reconsumed object allow emotional efficiency, as consumers optimize the search for and attainment of the emotional outcomes sought in volitional reconsumption, and facilitate existential understanding, as the linkages across past, present, and future experiences enable an active synthesis of time and promote self-reflexivity. (p. 341)

This idea of "emotional efficiency" served as a eureka moment for us, the linkage between our analogous individual relationships with the show, and eventually the public-facing podcast. What we related to as teenagers when we watched the show during high school is different from what we relate to now with the compounded life experiences as 30-somethings (and assuredly will be different as 60-somethings), even as we consume the exact same sitcom. Understanding the evolution of our perception of this singular TV show enabled us to use it as an anchor point to zoom out and ponder the entirety of our own personal growth.

BLANCHE: DOROTHY, WE NEED TO ENABLE PARENTAL CONTROLS ON THE TV.

DOROTHY: WHY? IS MA RENTING DIRTY MOVIES AGAIN?

BLANCHE: I WISH. ROSE INSISTS ON WATCHING THE SAME 3 EPISODES OF *LITTLE HOUSE ON THE PRAIRIE* EVERY WEEK. SHE SAYS IT'S COMFORTING. WHAT'S COMFORTING? THEY LIVE ON A FARM WITH NO ELECTRICITY, NO RESTAURANTS, AND NO ELIGIBLE MEN IN A 50-MILE RADIUS.

We were far from alone in our pursuit of comfort viewing and "emotional efficiency" of this particular show. In April 2020 alone, Hulu viewers watched nearly 11 million hours of *The Golden Girls* (Koblin, 2020). With nearly limitless streaming options, it is natural to wonder why this show, with its dated references to box-office flop *Ishtar* and iconic '70s homophobe Anita Bryant, resonates so deeply with newer and younger audiences. First, as we have alluded to, it is still an incredibly funny and well-crafted sitcom. Secondly, and more interestingly, it appears that *The Golden Girls,* specifically, encourages community, and what is the foundation of community, if not comfort? The initial vision was that the *Enough Wicker* podcast would end up satisfying approximately less than 10 individuals, perhaps a handful of die-hard nerdy fans who wanted to move past the run-of-the-mill 'Which Golden Girl Are You?' *Buzzfeed*-style internet quizzes in the cultivation of their fandom, but we have discovered hundreds—hopefully by the time you are reading this, thousands—of enthusiastic listeners.

As they have since the earliest days of the internet, people continue to flock to online fan groups to swap favorite episodes or dissect scenes with friends they have never met, and in most cases never will. *Enough Wicker*'s own social media accounts engage every day with followers from all over the world who exchange personal interpretations of life advice, extrapolate modern political guidance, and consistently unearth new readings or angles from episodes, characters, and individual lines of dialogue. As Wendy Burns-Ardolino (2013) finds, fans are not passive, but rather "engage in the development of resistant, oppositional and negotiated readings and the construction of an online fan imaginary that has the capacity to empower members of the fandom and to support re-visioning of historical and contemporary female foursome shows" (p. 180). Jared Clayton Brown (2013) draws a comparison between fans of the show and sports fans, describing the "feeling of a sense of identity and an ability to feel the positive emotions found in fan experiences" (p. 6). This theory is grounded in interaction ritual theory, where positive emotion is socially emergent (Brown, 2013). In other words, the show only gets better when you share it with friends—which brings us right back to the origin of the podcast. Even our original community, population: 2, shaped the way we each viewed the show for the better.

The plot of *The Golden Girls* is, at its core, about forging community. Three widows and a divorcée find themselves thrust into the latter years of life, wondering what to do next to both financially and emotionally survive. They join together as strangers and roommates and end up discovering a sisterhood and chosen family that rivals any prior relationships or kinships they'd each had previously in life. When the show shines a spotlight on building community for marginalized people—such as women of a certain age who are not defined by their relationships to men—it shines a spotlight, however purposefully or inadvertently, for all marginalized people, invites alternative readings, and allows viewers to decide for themselves how they can live their fullest and best life as whole people. Understood this way, it is little wonder that *The Golden Girls* has fans from a wide variety of communities, such as Facebook groups, Instagram parody accounts, or pontificating Twitter users. The reconsumption of the show not only expands fans' understanding of themselves, but necessarily broadens fans' readings of, and deepens fans' insight into, the object of reconsumption—the show itself. What may help to understand fans' desire to build relationships with each other is to understand the relationships we have with the characters themselves. These characters are, in effect, role models, presenting the same admirable qualities of real-life mentors. We constantly find ourselves citing the most admirable traits about each of these women: Dorothy's steadfast commitment to fairness, feminism, and intelligence; Rose's inherent belief that goodness and kindness matter most in the world; Blanche's conviction, confidence, and ability to remain self-aware even through trying times; and Sophia's refusal to be boxed into simply being "an old person" and her commitment to adapt whenever circumstances call for it.

There is a body of evidence to suggest that the relationships we create with fictional characters can, and often do, fulfill us in the same way as those we create with real people. The term "parasocial interaction" was coined in 1956 by social scientists Donald Horton and R. Richard Wohl to describe the one-sided imagined interactions between real people and media characters. These relationships have been shown to help shepherd people through traumatic situations, as well as to satiate the need for connection in situations where real-life socialization is not possible (Derrick, Gabriel & Tippin, 2008). Considering this, it is no wonder that the desperation for connection created by lockdowns and a daily barrage of bad news motivated so many of us to lean into our existing parasocial relationships with Dorothy, Blanche, Rose, and Sophia.

In addition to simply making us feel better, parasocial interactions often turn people into better versions of themselves, echoing the hoped-for effects of real-life relationships. A moral compass has many architects, and if interaction can be imagined, reasonably so can influence. Identification refers to viewers perceiving a story from the perspective of a character while taking that character's beliefs, values, and goals into account (Cohen, 2006). It is why—even after watching the finale of *The Golden Girls* more times than we can count—it still makes us tear up when Dorothy utters the line she "couldn't have asked for a better surprise" than such a fierce friendship at this point in her life (S07E23; Hurwitz et al., 1992). It is not just that we are sad our favorite show is over, it is that we can feel the conflicting wave of emotion of leaving a home you built with one family to build another. This ability to put ourselves in another's shoes—even those of a fictional character—makes everyday empathy more accessible, and it is difficult to remember a time when empathy was more necessary than 2020.

> DOROTHY: MA, YOU ARE 85 YEARS OLD, YOU ARE NOT GETTING A JOB AS AN INSTACART SHOPPER.
>
> SOPHIA: IT'S PRACTICALLY FREE MONEY, DOROTHY! I ALREADY LIVE WITH THE RISK OF IMMINENT DEATH.

Living these experiences oneself is different than empathizing with a fictional character who is living them, but that does not discount the fact that identifying with and forming an attachment to a character can alter behavior and viewpoints. A 2012 study at Ohio State University found that subjects who read a fictional story could actually feel the emotions, beliefs, and thoughts of the character in the story, a phenomenon known as experience taking (Kaufman & Libby, 2012). Perhaps obviously, the study found participants had the easiest time identifying with characters that reminded them of themselves. By that logic, only older, white, straight women should have been able to identify with *The Golden Girls*. However, another finding of the study was that when the white, straight participants found out a character was gay or Black later in the story rather than at the beginning, they had higher levels of experience-taking, lower levels of stereotype application, and more favorable attitudes toward the group to which that character belonged—suggesting that if you can make audiences like a character first, and then reveal that they are in some way different than expected, audiences will stick by that character (Kaufman & Libby, 2012).

This empathy technique partly explains why *The Golden Girls* was so successful in eliminating stereotypes about older women, why the show was able to insert incredibly progressive storylines into the show without being dismissed as "preachy," and how the show maintained favorable ratings throughout its seven-season run. The show made a point of getting viewers invested in common ground, such as chosen family or a sarcastic sense of humor, before running the risk of alienating them with a homosexual character, a teen pregnancy storyline, or a joke knocking George H. W. Bush. Further, the storied combination of four star performers, clever writing, and older women characters, a demographic often portrayed as completely harmless, helped relax a perhaps more conservative viewer's guard, and encouraged them to consider a potential progressive point being made. This is especially impressive when we consider the constraints of network standards; *The Golden Girls* could not be as subversive as HBO's *Sex and the City*, for example, but it was essentially tasked with conveying the same message and by all accounts, did so successfully (Macey, 2012).

Consider how the show famously addressed the HIV/AIDS crisis. Despite thousands of people dying from what was then a mysterious illness, President Reagan's administration did not publicly acknowledge AIDS until 1985 (Bennington-Castro, 2020). Perhaps equally as disturbingly, there are recorded incidents of Reagan's press secretary, Larry Speakes, joking about the epidemic (Lopez, 2016). It is against this backdrop, albeit slightly removed from the panic of HIV/AIDS, that an episode of *The Golden Girls* called "72 Hours" (S05E19) aired in 1992. In it, the most naive and innocent of the characters, Rose Nylund, finds out she may have been exposed to HIV through a blood transfusion (Gamble & Vaczy, 1990). The decision to have Rose deal with the scare, rather than much more sexually active Blanche, is purposeful. Rose even says "this isn't supposed to happen to people like me," implying that this is supposed to happen to some people, just not her (Gamble and Vaczy, 1992). In her book, *The Golden Girls: TV Milestone Series*, Kate Browne (2020) highlights that episode's heated exchange between Rose and Blanche, wherein Blanche says "AIDS is not a bad person's disease," as a direct challenge to the at-the-time pervasively held belief that AIDS was a punishment for gay men and anyone who contracted the illness had done something bad (pp. 62–63). According to Nielsen ratings, "72 Hours" had an audience of 31.3 million American households. While there is no way to measure the number of conversations started, it seems reasonable to assume it had an impact on at least a few hearts and minds.

Bringing this subtle primetime proselytizing back to 2020: It wasn't like we found ourselves marching at Black Lives Matter protests solely because we think that's what Dorothy Zbornak would have done. We inherently knew from our own personalities and sense of right and wrong that we chose to take that action to stand up against police brutality and white supremacy. But it is difficult to parse the parts of us not directly affected by this television show, given our reconsumption habits. *The Golden Girls* is so entrenched in and entangled with our personal development that it is fair to say that this show both provided us a guide to right and wrong as girls, and continues to reflect the values we hold as women.

BLANCHE: DOROTHY, I WANT TO THANK YOU FOR EDUCATING ME. WHY, I WAS SO MOVED BY THAT ARTICLE ON BLACK EXCELLENCE, I DECIDED TO HANG A REPLICA OF BARACK OBAMA'S PRESIDENTIAL PORTRAIT IN MY BEDROOM.

DOROTHY: BLANCHE, BARACK OBAMA WAS NOT SHIRTLESS ON A BEACH IN HIS PRESIDENTIAL PORTRAIT.

Just prior to the 2020 presidential election, renowned *Golden Girls* scholar Jim Colucci penned an opinion piece for CNN titled "How 'The Golden Girls' Would Handle Donald Trump." In it, he laid out a solid argument for how *The Golden Girls* embodies love, and how Trump—a large part of why 2020 ended up being so tumultuous—embodies fear (Colucci, 2020). In short, *The Golden Girls* confronted their own prejudices, supported queer people, stood up for women, gave to the homeless, advocated for care for the elderly, questioned unfair immigration policies, rejected anti-semitism, respected all Americans, learned from people who were different than them, and changed their minds when presented with the truth. And yes, Dorothy even compliments producer Merv Griffin back in Season 7's Questions & Answers (S7E17) episode by telling him that he's the "anti-Trump" (Seigel & Perzigian, 1992).

Beyond simply taking swipes at individual political and pop-cultural figures, *The Golden Girls* continuously illustrated a concept that the two of us (and many other Americans) have always held true, which is that politics are morals. The aforementioned "72 Hours" is cited frequently as a significant moral moment in the series, but the truth is there are these a-ha moments surrounding political discourse and collective social responsibility all throughout the series, which are almost never called out as "very special episodes." The choice to show, rather than tell, makes the points that much more effective. For example, an episode called "Sophia's Choice" (S04E22) centers on a friend of Sophia named Lilian and her stay at an ill-equipped and underfunded nursing home, which is the only place she can afford to live. In a particularly powerful scene, Dorothy and Sophia meet with the well-intentioned yet bumbling manager of the facility, who fully acknowledges that a lack of federal funding has led to sub-par care for his residents (Gamble & Vaczy, 1989). This episode, while completely fictional, represented a very real situation for millions of Americans at the time, especially as the Reagan administration endorsed repealing standards such as the requirement that nursing homes must not employ people with communicable diseases in favor of slashing budgets (Pear, 1981). One is able to draw a line directly from this Reagan administration policy to the disproportionate disastrous effects of COVID-19 on nursing homes in 2020, with a study in the *New England Journal of Medicine* stating that the "tragedy unfolding in nursing homes is the result of decades of neglect of long-term care policy" (Werner, Hoffman & Coe, 2020).

While distinct from the tumultuous times of the 1980s, the tumultuous times of 2020 forced us to confront our thoughts and feelings about impending fascism, immigration concerns, economic inequality, systemic racism, coping mechanisms, socialization, public health, and collective responsibility. Part of that confrontation included turning over these deeply relatable and, in some ways, newly applicable storylines from *The Golden Girls* in our minds. We recognized that Rose has her volunteering, Sophia has her cooking, Dorothy has her reading, and Blanche has her flirting as activities that serve as comfort mechanisms and easy ways to experience pleasure during difficult times. We recalled moments when the girls gave up their own pleasure in service to the greater good of their community, such as when the notoriously selfish Blanche reallocates money she planned to spend on plastic surgery to help pay for better care for Lilian in the oh-so-sitcom-y conclusion of Sophia's Choice (S04E22) (Gamble & Vaczy, 1989). We reflected on the immense pride that Sophia, an immigrant, has in America and its proclaimed freedoms for all, which in turn reignited the passion in us to fight to make good on that promise. As Rose naively says to Dorothy's communist cousin-in-law in defense of the U.S., "Well, sure there are inequities, but at least we treat everybody the same" (Cherry & Wooten, 1990).

The Golden Girls is a progressive show, but it is imperfect. Like many progressive movements in the U.S., intentions are almost always noble but do occasionally miss the mark. It bears repeating that to love something does not mean a refusal to find fault. Criticism, after all, is part of viewing a show critically. Finding reflections of ourselves in, and maintaining a fascination with, our favorite television show doesn't mean we find either the show or ourselves beyond reproach. In fact, that's another matter of contention we processed in 2020, with regard to our own whiteness and the privilege it has afforded us. Flaws in the show include the fact that *The Golden Girls* doesn't feature many Black characters at all, despite being 20 percent of the population of Miami at the time (Metropolitan Center at Florida International University, 2007), and often resorts to stereotyping—or inviting a racist comment—when depicting a character who happens to be Asian or Latino. Despite defending against abusive relationships through one storyline, fat-phobic and demeaning comments abound throughout several others, and sometimes even in the same episode. And as scholar Steven Thrasher (2020) pointed out, there is an incredibly pointed "joke" in the series about Stan drugging Dorothy, and raping her while she was unconscious. Even its representation of queerness, while generally celebrated, is relatively one-dimensional, mostly featuring white, cis-gender people who happen to be gay and in monogamous relationships. We were lucky enough to speak with scholar Elliot H. Powell, whose paper elaborated on this last point. Citing Gayle Rubin's famous 1984 essay *Thinking Sex*, Powell (2018) points out that being monogamous is used multiple times as a key pillar in the show's argument for gay acceptance, which—while likely unintentional—implies that there is a right way, and thus a wrong way, to be queer.

For the progressive blind spots in this show, we take care to process our own feelings about them, call them out, and point out why they are wrong—all publicly on the podcast. As processing the presidency of Donald Trump has taught perhaps a larger swath of white Americans as ever before, dissent is patriotic and productive. It moves ourselves and our culture forward.

> ROSE: I CAN'T BELIEVE PEOPLE ARE SAYING MR. ROGERS IS TOO WOKE!
>
> DOROTHY: IT'S NOT ABOUT ANY REAL MORALITY. PEOPLE ARE REJECTING DECENCY JUST TO GET ATTENTION. I DISAGREE.
>
> ROSE: I MEAN, SO DO I! WHO WANTS TO WATCH A SHOW WHERE THE HOST IS ASLEEP THE WHOLE TIME?

The year 2020 is over, and the world is remarkably changed in numerous ways. Many of us experienced the greatest losses of our lives, and many of us are still grappling with the magnitude of what we collectively have been through. Regardless of our individual circumstances, many of us will move forward in similar ways to how we persevered through one of the strangest and most difficult years in modern history—with lots of missteps, stress, and unknowns, but also with a sense of shared community in knowing that whether or not we like it, we are all in this together. If these fictional characters and imagined relationships can alleviate that burden in some way, even if it's just to make us laugh for approximately 22 minutes, then they are worth leaning on. There's a good chance that they're some of the same fictional characters others have been leaning on, too.

Whether we are dealing with a shelter-in-place order away from our families, fighting America's special breed of white nationalist fascism, or renegotiating what it means to live with discomfort for an extended period, a steady rudder of creativity and consolation for us will always be watching *The Golden Girls*. Consuming media, and reconsuming it, and reconsuming it again, to continue to measure our progress as the human beings we were, and the human beings we want to be. As Cristel Antonia Russell (2012) said, paraphrasing the Greek philosopher Heraclitus: "You never cross the same river twice—it's not the same river, and it's not the same you." Our ersatz relationships forged with these four fictional women not only helped to enhance our real relationships with our friends and family members, but also helped enhance ourselves. We continue to sift through words and actions shown on the screen—taking what qualities we admire from the characters, crafting podcast episodes and reconsumption analysis around them, and trying our damndest to live these values each day in our own lives. In that way, the comfort, guidance, and inspiration we and millions of others received, from Dorothy, Blanche, Rose, and Sophia will be part of our personalities and formative makeup for the rest of our lives.

How lucky we are to need naught but a device, network connection, and collaborative podcast to be able to find solace, guidance, and inspiration in *The Golden Girls*.

REFERENCES

Bennington-Castro, J. (2020, June 1). *How AIDS remained an unspoken-but-deadly-epidemic for years.* History.com. https://www.history.com/news/aids-epidemic-ronald-reagan.

Brown, J. B. (2013). *Sex and the City*, platinum edition: How *The Golden Girls* altered American situation comedy. (Electronic thesis). Retrieved from https://etd.ohiolink.edu/.

Browne, K. (2020). *The Golden Girls.* Wayne State University Press.

Burns-Ardolino, W. (2013). Female foursomes & their fans. Faculty scholarly dissemination grants. 1247. https://scholarworks.gvsu.edu/fsdg/1247.

Cherry, M. (Writer). Wooten, J. (Writer). Hughes, Terry (Director). Harris, S (Creator). (1990, March 3). Sisters and other strangers (Season 5, Episode 21) [TV series episode]. In T. Thomas, & J. Witt (Executive Producers). *The Golden Girls.* Witt/Thomas/Harris Productions. Hulu. https://www.hulu.com/.

Cohen, J. (2006). Audience identification with media characters. In J. Bryant & P. Vorderer (Eds.), *Psychology of Entertainment* (pp. 183–197). Lawrence Erlbaum Associates Publishers.

Colucci, J. (2020, September 13). Opinion: How *The Golden Girls* would handle Donald Trump. *CNN.* https://www.cnn.com/2020/09/13/opinions/golden-girls-35th-anniversary-trump-colucci/index.html.

Derrick, J. & Gabriel, S. & Tippin, B. (2008). Parasocial relationships and self□discrepancies: Faux relationships have benefits for low self□esteem individuals. *Personal Relationships, 15*(2), 261–280. https://doi.org/10.1111/j.1475-6811.2008.00197.x.

Gamble, T. (Writer). Vaczy, R. (Writer). Hughes, Terry (Director). (1989, April 15). Sophia's choice (Season 4, Episode 22) [TV series episode]. In S. Harris & T. Thomas (Executive Producers), *The Golden Girls.* Witt/Thomas/Harris Productions. Hulu. https://www.hulu.com/.

Gamble, T. (Writer). Vaczy, R. (Writer). Hughes, Terry (Director). (1990, February 17). 72 Hours (Season 5, Episode 19) [TV series episode]. In S. Harris & T. Thomas

(Executive Producers), *The Golden Girls.* Witt/Thomas/Harris Productions. Hulu. https://www.hulu.com/.

Goodwin, A., & Whannel, G. (2016). *Understanding television.* Routledge.

Harris, S. (Creator). (1985–1992). *The Golden Girls* [TV series]. Witt/Thomas/Harris Productions. Hulu. https://www.hulu.com/.

Hurwitz, M. (Writer). Perzigian, J. (Writer). Seigel, D. (Writer). Passaris, L. (Director). (1992, May 9). One flew out of the cuckoo's nest (Season 7, Episode 23) [TV series episode]. In S. Harris, T. Thomas & P. Witt (Executive Producers), *The Golden Girls*. Witt/Thomas/Harris Productions. Hulu. https://www.hulu.com/.

Horton, D., & Wohl, R. R. (1956). Mass communication and para-social interaction. *Psychiatry: Journal for the Study of Interpersonal Processes, 19,* 215–229.

Kaufman, G. F., & Libby, L. K. (2012). Changing beliefs and behavior through experience-taking. *Journal of Personality and Social Psychology, 103*(1), 1–19. https://doi.org/10.1037/a0027525.

Koblin, J. (2020, April 30). Lockdown TV: Netflix dominates, news surges and Bea Arthur is still golden. *New York Times.* https://www.nytimes.com/2020/04/30/business/media/coronavirus-television-netflix-ratings.html.

Leckey, J. (2011). The therapeutic effectiveness of creative activities on mental well-being: A systematic review of the literature. *Journal of Psychiatric and Mental Health Nursing, 18*: 501–509. https://doi.org/10.1111/j.1365-2850.2011.01693.x.

Lopez, G. (2016, December 1). The Reagan administration's unbelievable response to the HIV/AIDS epidemic. *Vox*. https://www.vox.com/2015/12/1/9828348/ronald-reagan-hiv-aids.

Lorenz, T. (2020, April 1). Stop trying to be productive. *New York Times.* https://www.nytimes.com/2020/04/01/style/productivity-coronavirus.html.

Macey, D.A. (2012). Ancient archetypes in modern media. In A. Ruggerio (Ed.), *Monster, mate, mommy: Media depictions of women as brides, wives, & mothers* (pp. 49–62). Lexington Books.

The Metropolitan Center. (2007). (rep.). *Thirty Year Retrospective: The Status of the Black Community in Miami-Dade County* (p. 8). Miami, FL.

Morreale, J. (2003). *Introduction. Critiquing the sitcom: A reader* (p. xi). Syracuse University Press.

"Nielsen ratings." *USA Today.* Gannett Company. 1990-02–21. p. D3.

Pear, R. (1981, December 20). Reagan officials seek to ease rules on nursing homes. *New York Times*. pp. 1–26. https://www.nytimes.com/1981/12/20/us/reagan-officials-seek-to-ease-rules-on-nursing-homes.html.

Podcast Stats: How many podcasts are there? (n.d.). https://www.listennotes.com/podcast-stats/.

Powell, E. H. (2018). 'Staying golden': The politics of gender, sexuality, and jazz in *The Golden Girls*. *Jazz Research Journal, 12*(1), 86–109.

Russell, C., & Levy, S. (2012). The temporal and focal dynamics of volitional reconsumption: A phenomenological investigation of repeated hedonic experiences. *Journal of Consumer Research, 39*(2), 341–359. doi:10.1086/662996.

Seigel, D. (Writer). Perzigian, J. (Writer). Passaris, L. (Director). Harris, S. (Creator). (1992, February 8). Questions and Answers (Season 7, Episode 17). [TV series episode]. In T. Gamble, T. Thomas, & P. Witt (Executive Producers), *The Golden Girls*. Witt/Thomas/Harris Productions. Hulu. https://www.hulu.com/.

Sörqvist, P., & Marsh, J. E. (2015). How concentration shields against distraction. *Current Directions in Psychological Science, 24*(4), 267–272. https://doi.org/10.1177/0963721415577356.

Thrasher, S. W. (2020, July 2). The real mud on *The Golden Girls. Vulture*. https://www.vulture.com/2020/07/the-real-mud-on-golden-girls.html.

Werner, R. M., Hoffman, A. K., & Coe, N. B. (2020). Long-term care policy after Covid-19—solving the nursing home crisis. *New England Journal of Medicine, 383*(10), 903–905. https://doi.org/10.1056/nejmp2014811.

NOTE

1. While we certainly wish that *The Golden Girls* could have covered these topics, these quotes are entirely the creation of the authors of this paper.

PART 3

Connection and Comfort

Chapter Twelve

Walking My Way to Community and Connection during the COVID-19 Pandemic

Theory and Practice

Theresa Conefrey

The March sun has long since set, and I am walking in my neighborhood, inhaling deeply the cool night air, listening to a podcast through my earbuds. After spending a long day in front of my computer, I welcome the signature tune of "Auf den Punkt (To the point)," a German news and current affairs podcast hosted by the affable Jean-Marie Magro. Speaking with Magro is his guest, fellow journalist, Matthias Drobinski, who is commenting on how the COVID lockdown restrictions in southern Germany will prevent the usual family get-togethers around Easter (Magro, 2020). Listening to German transports me back in time to Kirchheim-Teck, a town in Baden-Württemberg, where I lived and worked over twenty years ago. I mull over the impact of the ongoing restrictions on my German friends' lives, until the scent of Brugmansia wafting from a neighbor's front lawn jolts me back to my neighborhood. Following the scent trail of the fragrant, white blooms, I glance upwards, noticing a homemade rainbow poster in a bedroom window. I make a mental note to ask my students about similar posters thanking essential workers that they may have seen in their own neighborhoods. My gut tightens as I realize that some of them will have parents and other family members who are essential workers.

As I'm crossing the street, a neighbor, who is out walking his dog, waves and I smile back. Turning the corner, I spot Meyer lemons in a cardboard box near the sidewalk. Near their homes, neighbors have begun sharing garden produce and gently used items for anyone who wants them. I grab a lemon tossing it from hand to hand as I walk. The rhythmic thrum of my feet on the pavement is hypnotic and time appears to stand still until I spy a cat with a raised spine that appears startled. Distracted, I stumble when my toe stubs an uneven paving stone but promptly right myself. When the ending theme to "Auf den Punkt" begins, I start heading home, humming the melody silently and skipping along to the beat. Despite the uncertainty of the future, I am content in this moment.

CREATING A COMFORTING COVID-19 HABIT

Walks in my neighborhood listening to podcasts were what sustained me during the Santa Clara County lockdown of March 2020 and beyond. Curious to understand how this new and evolving habit supported my mental and physical wellbeing, I turned to the research in neuroscience, psychology, and communication. Soon, I discovered that there were limitations to what I could learn from quantitative scholarship to help me understand a habit which combined multiple activities and which was impacted by multiple social factors. Perpetuating Cartesian dualism, the view that the mind and body are separate, positivist research privileges the "objective," over the "subjective." Researchers generate hypotheses, collect data, create statistical models, and search for generalizable findings. As an empirical approach is reductionistic, it precludes measuring multiple overlapping and intersecting impacts of experiences that are partially generalizable and partially unique. It is ill-suited, for example, for interpreting the widely differing COVID-19 "R" numbers in my suburban neighborhood and in downtown San Jose, less than 5 miles from my home. This is because the "R" or reproduction number, the average number of people each person with the virus will infect, excludes social factors such as accommodation, occupation, socio-economic status, and ethnicity, which impact actual transmission rates.

Generalizable research findings on aspects of my experience such as walking and wellbeing, podcast use and multi-tasking, phatic communication and community, a tree-filled neighborhood, and so on, did not help me make sense of a habit whose benefit surely resulted from the synergy of these elements. To explore these complex interactions, I broadened my research to include qualitative approaches, poststructuralism, social constructivism, and feminist research on the messier, socio-historical embodied aspects of experience. I recognized that my unique experience was deeply interwoven with the experiences of others, the social, cultural, political, historical, and natural environment, as well as technological innovations such as earbuds and Bluetooth wireless technology. To unify these different approaches, I drew on critical embodiment theorizing, an approach which "illuminates the material elements of individuals' lives and the embodied nature of all sensory experience and sense making" (Ellingson & Borofka, 2020, p.2), and one which rejects binary oppositions between objectivity and subjectivity, self and others, and the personal and the political. This approach combined well with autoethnography, a research methodology, which aims to describe and analyze personal experience in order to understand cultural experience (Ellis, Adams, & Bochner, 2011).

Combining autoethnography with embodiment theorizing provided me with the tools I needed for reflecting on my experience of being a white, cisgender woman, listening to podcasts while walking in a middle-class neighborhood in northern California during the COVID-19 pandemic. As Barad notes, "Existence is not an individual affair. Individuals do not preexist their interactions; rather, individuals emerge through and as part of their entangled intra-relating" (2007, p. ix). In the following sections, I explore the interactions among different aspects of my newfound COVID-19 habit (podcasts, walking, neighbors, and the neighborhood), to make sense of how, although always in flux, they coalesced into a feeling of community and connection.

MOTIVATING OUTDOOR EXERCISE WITH PODCASTS

What I experienced as a beneficial habit emerged organically. Strolling in my neighborhood was not something I did before the COVID-19 pandemic. My social and fitness needs were met at work, the gym, or the yoga studio—places that were far from my neighborhood. However, when California issued its "shelter in place" order of March 16, 2020 (Office of Governor Gavin Newsom, 2020), mandating that all gyms, schools, offices, and non-essential businesses close and requiring everyone to "stay home," my habits had to change. Fortunately, socially distanced "outdoor activity" was permitted and even encouraged because of its anticipated (and later confirmed) impact on well-being during the pandemic (Dominski & Brandt, 2020; Matias et al., 2020).

Although running was my preferred choice for outdoor exercise, a flare-up of Achilles tendonitis led me to switch to walking. I tolerated walking if it was the fastest way to get from one place to another but did not view it as an efficient form of exercise and nor did my immediate family members. With restrictions on socializing outside the family, the prospect of solitary walks without even a pet for company was not enticing until I remembered the podcasts that I had planned to play during my commute to work. What if I wore earbuds and listened while I walked? Tedium turned to treat, and soon I began downloading additional podcasts and looking forward to walking.

With an increasing number of podcasts available to the approximately 80 million weekly listeners in the U.S., finding appealing content was easy (Edison Research, 2021). Once a niche market, focused mainly on music, the popularity of podcasts is growing with 37 percent (104 million) of Americans claiming to have listened to podcasts monthly and 24 percent (68 million) weekly in 2019 (Edison Research, 2020). I discovered I was also not alone in using podcasts to motivate exercise. Research on "temptation bundling" suggests that offering audiobooks increases gym visits (Kirgios et al., 2020; Milkman et al., 2014). Like me, exercisers often choose audio media over other forms of media because it affords multitasking, and podcasts are preferred over radio shows because of their flexibility (Perks & Turner, 2019). Recorded content can be played anytime, anywhere on a wide variety of devices, including smartphones, which are the most popular (65 percent) choice, and unlike live radio, the playback speed can be changed by the listeners, with about 26 percent of listeners like me choosing to alter processing speeds to personalize their listening experience (Edison Research and Triton Digital, 2020).

EXPLORING PODCASTS AND SOCIAL INTERACTION

Soon, I found that podcasts helped me meet not only my fitness needs but also my pandemic need for social interaction. In those early days, the topic was my guide for selecting what podcasts to play, but after becoming familiar with the hosts, I began choosing podcasts depending on with whom I wanted to spend time. Gabor Steingart, the host of the "der Achte Tag" and "Morning Briefing" soon became a favorite not just because of the informational and uplifting content of his shows but also because of the prosody of his warm opening greeting and the conversational tone of his interactions with his guests. Before introducing each guest on *The Eighth Day*, an inspirational podcast series that first aired on March 16, 2020, Steingart would remind listeners that the series was about how the pandemic would change us and what we could do to ensure that these changes benefited ourselves and society. His use of the plural pronoun as he introduced his guest and explained that we would be thinking through these questions together, facilitated the conceit that I was part of the conversation. This practice created a perception of authenticity and a sense of reciprocity, which research suggests that I was not alone in finding appealing (Perks & Turner, 2019). Choosing to listen to my preferred hosts also helped me avoid the "echo chamber" effect by introducing me to a wider range of thoughts and opinions than I might otherwise have been exposed to had I continued to select episodes based on prior interest.

As I twisted the cord-free earbuds so snugly into my ears that they afforded the intimacy of his voice in my head, the transcendent timbre of the theme music swelling at the beginning and end of the episode would send shivers down my spine. Apparently, I'm not alone in feeling a warm connection to certain podcast hosts. Research suggests that such feelings of connection to media personalities or parasocial relationships (Horton & Richard Wohl, 1956) are not uncommon and that many people use similar language to talk about media personalities and real friendships (Eyal & Dailey, 2012). Among podcast listeners, this figure is high, with about a quarter of respondents listing "companionship" as one of their main reasons for listening (Edison Research, 2020). Similarly, in their qualitative study on podcast listening, Perks and Turner discovered that "parasocial relationships were a driving force in many interviewees' decisions about what to listen to" (2019, p. 109).

Apart from enabling parasocial relationships, podcast-listening also facilitated actual interactions. Because the Bluetooth earbuds that I wore were unobtrusive, and not noise canceling, I could interact with other walkers and homeowners on my route by making eye contact and smiling or saying "hi." Over the course of the pandemic, opportunities for phatic communication waxed and waned as conversing from at least two meters apart and donning masks masked smiles and muffled conversation. Additionally, as spring progressed into summer, there were sunglasses and sun hats to contend with, which made reading faces even more challenging. Gradually, by closely reading body language (a slight shoulder turn in my direction, a slowed pace), I developed an intersubjective awareness of who was open to exchanging greetings (Merleau-Ponty, 2013). I knew that those who were taking calls as they walked were not; neither were walkers who were so preoccupied with their phone screens that their lack of awareness of others threatened to breach social-distancing rules. Gradually some nodding acquaintanceships progressed into brief exchanges about the weather or local happenings, and over time, I knew who to count on for a greeting or a longer micro-exchange and would plan my walks, accordingly, pondering on the health of those whom I did not see for a few days in a row.

While not claiming that phatic communication and parasocial relationships are comparable to meaningful face-to-face interactions, for me and others they fulfilled a valuable function in ameliorating loneliness during a time of forced isolation. When the opportunities for deeper interactions and everyday small talk were limited, this form of social interaction helped compensate for the loss of micro-exchanges with baristas, store clerks, colleagues, and so on that were common in pre-COVID times (Orbach, 2021). Unlike social interaction, which affirms our self-worth (Maslow, 1943), social isolation erodes our sense of being seen and heard and having a place in the community (Rokach, 2019). Studies of mental health during the COVID-19 pandemic are uncovering similar negative consequences (Czeisler et al., 2020; Ettman et al., 2020; McGinty et al., 2020; Torales et al., 2020) to the negative psychological effects reported with earlier quarantines (Brooks et al., 2020). An intriguing recent study using functional magnetic resonance imaging (fMRI) showed that social isolation and hunger led to similar patterns of craving in the midbrain (Tomova et al., 2020). However, as in my case, many people found creative ways to improve their resilience by staying connected virtually and interacting with others outdoors (Hwang et al., 2020; Luchetti et al., 2020).

WALKING AND THINKING

After coming home from a walk, I would often feel surprisingly eager to return to lesson planning, Zoom calls, and research. Sometimes, the podcast topic would have sparked new ways of approaching concepts I was grappling with and at other times, it would have provided fresh perspectives to weave into a class lecture. Remembering my days as the kind of student who struggled to stay focused in class, I was puzzled by how easy I found it to retain and integrate ideas from the podcasts. Was there something about an aural-only medium that fostered more focus? Some podcast hosts discussed with their guests how the reduction in visual distractions provided by the aural medium and its perceived intimacy could deepen focus and increase receptivity to new ideas (Fridman, 2021; Magnussen & Trautmann, 2019; Roll, 2020).

I also wondered if there was something about being in motion that facilitated learning. Was there just the right amount of haptic stimulation from the rhythmic treading of my left and right foot placements and visual and aural stimulation from the environment that it was easier for me to stay focused than when I was sitting at my desk? In his eponymous podcast, Huberman (2021) noted that movement can strengthen focus before learning and aid in its retention after learning (2021). Similarly, in a conversation between Shane O'Mara, a neuroscientist and avid walker, and Ragan Chatterjee, M.D. (2019), O'Mara explained that like a muscle, the volume of the hippocampal formation, the part of the brain that is involved in processing information, grows bigger as a result of exercise, resulting in improvements in memory. Likewise, in his recent book on walking, O'Mara (2019) explores research on how movement improves cognitive processing (Rosenbaum et al., 2017) and can lead to increases in both creativity and problem-solving or divergent thinking as well as focused thinking or convergent thinking (Oppezzo & Schwartz, 2014). O'Mara describes how walking improves his own thinking and includes accounts of celebrated writers and thinkers such as William

Wordsworth, Soren Kirkegaard, William Hamilton, and Bertrand Russell who also drew inspiration for their work from their walks.

Recent research also supports the benefit of movement and embodied approaches to maximizing pedagogical gains in formal education. Drawing on the field of embodied cognition Susan Hrach (2021) argues for an embodied approach to teaching making the case that we are "not brains on sticks, and neither are our students" (p. xiv). Based on her research, she advocates teaching outdoors, encouraging movement, and incorporating sensory activities into our classrooms as ways of acknowledging that our students bring their whole selves to their learning experience.

Learning in motion is innately human (Kirks et al., 2015). The current practice of sitting down at desks to acquire knowledge came much later in our history and paralleled the move from rural to urban living (Cregan-Reid, 2018). Before settled agriculture, when humans were hunters and gatherers, we spent a significant amount of time in motion. Today's modern hunter-gatherers still have an encyclopedic memory for edible plants, flora, and fauna, which they acquire while foraging on their territories (Wood et al., 2021). Daily walking also enabled me to create a cognitive map of my neighborhood (Tsanov & O'Mara, 2014). Soon, I learned where the trees were that would have grapefruits, figs, plums, and apples that neighbors would share with others during the pandemic. Despite teasing from my family about my "foraging behavior," I enjoyed participating in this sharing economy with my own fresh produce, which deepened my connection to my neighborhood and its seasonal rhythms.

FEELING CALM, CONNECTED, AND COMFORTED

Apart from helping me keep up with my workload, walking improved my mood. Combined with phatic communication and parasocial relationships, it fostered a feeling of well-being which surprised me given my overall anxiety due to all the uncertainty and change of the pandemic. I noticed the difference between the positive feedback loop, when my work was going well and I was feeling more relaxed, and the negative spiral, when I was feeling anxious and distracted and work was piling up, which generated more negative self-talk and a feeling of being overwhelmed. I also discovered that walking helped with more specific anxiety about the virus. For example, when I read that the number of COVID-19 deaths was increasing or learned that a family member or friend had become infected, walking could help me overcome amygdala hijacking (Goleman, 2006), an intense fight-or-flight response. Affirming the Latin aphorism, *solvitur ambulando*, "it is solved by walking," any worries that had been gnawing at me seemed less onerous when I could "walk" them out; the more I walked, the calmer I felt and within about twenty minutes my mood always lifted.

My experience is supported by research, which suggests that patterned rhythmic activity moves us from higher anxiety states to calmer, more cognitive ones (O'Mara, 2019; Perry & Hambrick, 2008) and that walking can reduce depression (Belvederi Murri et al., 2018; Laskowski, 2016; O'Mara, 2019'; Perry & Hambrick, 2008). I found walking in the park or in a neighborhood with numerous trees and green spaces was especially soothing as it triggered feelings of being connected to something more eternal. My experience aligns with Attention Restoration Theory, which suggests that nature has a restorative effect, promoting feelings of calm, relaxation, and improved focus (Kaplan, 1995). Awareness of the benefits of nature has also led to a renewed interest in the Japanese concept of shinrin-yoku or "forest bathing" (Hansen et al., 2017). The focus for participants is not on exercise but rather on the meditative and relaxing aspect of being immersed in nature, breathing in the forest air, hearing the birds chirping and tuning in to all one's senses. Researchers have found that feeling connected to the natural world, which is alive and enduring, can ease stress and bring a sense of comfort (Li, 2018).

During weeks when I was too busy to walk as much as I wanted to, I turned to meditation apps like "Balance" and mindful practices like breath control (Bostock, 2020; Hof, 2020; Nestor, 2020) to support my well-being. However, as usual, I struggled with consistency in my practice because I could not reign in my thoughts when I was sitting cross-legged on the floor. About to give up, I discovered that I could practice mindfulness techniques on the go. Moreover, I could amplify my understanding of breathwork by listening to podcasts on them while I walked. Mindful walking allowed me to feel tiny stones and seed pods under my feet and to delight in these different textures and feel connected to the earth below. When the rhythmic movement had performed its magic to move me into a calmer state of mind, by tipping my nervous system from sympathetic to parasympathetic mode, I'd sometimes walk with my arms slightly away from my body and my palms facing outwards. As I walked, I drew comfort in telling myself that right here, right now, I was safe in that moment. Of course, what I discovered is not new. Walking meditation is a part of many traditions and even my digital apps included meditations that were specially designed to be used while walking. In addition, several well-established practices such as mindfulness-based stress reduction program (MSRP) advocate meditative practices that involve walking (Kabat-Zinn, 2016; Kabat-Zinn & Kabat-Zinn, 2017).

A mind-body approach was also evident in media messaging during the pandemic, which acknowledged that catching COVID-19 was not the only possible health consequence but that extreme loneliness because of social isolation could also lead to a myriad of physical symptoms as well as mental health issues. This whole person approach has led to a practice of social prescribing, whereby doctors write prescriptions for patients to join community activities such as walking groups (Bertotti et al., 2018). More broadly, this is an example of more recent integrated health care approaches locally and globally (Drinkwater, Wildman & Moffatt, 2019; U.S. Department of Health and Human Services, 2015; WHO, 2016). Indeed, recent research suggests, that walking has been helpful in supporting resilience during COVID-19 (Seifert et al., 2020) and that it has been particularly beneficial for adolescents (Jackson, Stevenson, Larson, Peterson & Seekamp, 2021).

CONNECTING TO THE NEIGHBORHOOD

During the early days of the pandemic, it surprised me to realize that my feeling of connection to my childhood home in the UK was stronger than to the house in San Jose, where I had lived for almost two decades, after completing my graduate studies in the U.S. I also noticed my preference for German, British, and Irish hosts, and wondered if the uncertainty of the pandemic had led me to yearn for the familiar accents of countries where I had lived before emigrating to the United States. At the start of the pandemic, I barely knew my neighbors and treated my house as a place to rest and refuel rather than imbuing it with the emotional attachment of "home." Although I had sometimes waved at my street's long-term residents as I drove in and out of my garage, I could attach very few names. Over the course of the pandemic, however, my neighborhood became a place of engagement rather than estrangement (Sennett, 1991). As I started becoming acquainted with my neighbors, their dogs, and the layout of the streets, I became more attentive and attached to the rhythms and the specificity of my neighborhood as a community located in a particular time and place, spring 2020 to spring 2021, suburban, San Jose, California, USA, during the COVID-19 global pandemic. As Gieryn (2000) notes, a neighborhood is "not inherent in any arrangement of streets and houses but is rather an ongoing practical and discursive production/imagining of people" (p. 472).

The transition from house to home occurred as I came to know my neighbors and my neighborhood through a fluid array of both human and non-human interactions. Latour's (2005) actor-network theory (ANT), a methodological approach that explores actants (i.e. nonhuman agents) in networked systems helped illuminate for me the technological interplays that existed between my phone, my earbuds, my podcasts, my neighborhood, and my experience of listening to podcasts while strolling. His view of an individual in fluid and dynamic relations with actants aligns with Ash and Gallacher's (2015) post-humanism perspective and in particular with their concepts of "attunement," "vibration," and "tone" as ways to approach research from an embodied perspective that views the body as less determined by physiology or biology and "more an open and plastic boundary whose basic condition is change, porosity, and augmentation" (p. 69). I began feeling more connected to my neighbors and my neighborhood through multiple interactions in a specific place at a specific historical time.

In the early days of lockdown, the weather in northern California was chilly, but as the pandemic continued, winter gave way to spring, then summer, and fall, and winter and spring returned. As well as the natural rhythms, I observed the "Hallmark" rhythms of holiday decorations such as bunnies and eggs in spring, Fourth of July flags in summer, and Halloween and holiday decorations in fall and winter. Decorations for these cultural celebrations were more elaborate than ever during the pandemic possibly because the increased time spent at home led to more time being available to decorate and possibly because the festive spirit made being more confined more bearable. In addition, public displays appeared that were more specific to the times such as posters expressing appreciation for essential workers marking the early days of the pandemic, banners denouncing racial injustice and affirming solidarity with Black neighbors after the murder of George Floyd, graduation decorations when it became clear graduation ceremonies would be canceled, and political signage in the run-up to the 2020 presidential election. These natural and anthromade rhythms, the neighbors sharing seasonal garden produce or placing teddy bears in windows to cheer up children all contributed to my feeling of community and the sense that my neighbors and I were in this together, and that by supporting one another, we would all get through the pandemic (Lewis & Westlund, 2015).

CONNECTING MIND AND BODY

Daytime walking offered more opportunities for social interaction, but the busier, noisier streets could make listening to challenging content difficult. Night walking was relaxing because the streets were quiet except for occasional small gatherings of teenagers smoking on the street near their cars. Fewer pedestrians (mainly only couples or lone dog walkers) meant that less attention was required for maintaining social distance and more could be allocated to podcast listening. While lockdown's decrease in vehicular traffic reduced my fear of traffic accidents, I remained vigilant when walking at night and was conscious of needing to choose routes with adequate lighting and of avoiding shortcuts through green spaces. While men and women are equally likely to be injured by a car, women are more likely than men to be injured by men when walking alone at night (Miller, 2015).

Such fears notwithstanding, I recognized my privilege of living in a neighborhood that was considered safe and of appearing to fit in or belong there, that is "performing" my identity as a white, cisgender woman, (Butler, 1988). Explicit and implicit power relations are mutually constitutive of any specific socio-historical context so that discourses of power position the body in different ways. As Barad notes, "Existence is not an individual affair. Individuals do not preexist their interactions; rather, individuals emerge through and as part of their entangled intra-relating" (Barad, 2007, p. ix). Crenshaw's concept of "intersectionality" (1991) in a society structured on systemic racism helps to explain the complex interactions of gender and race that could, for example, embolden a white, female dog owner to call the police on a Black, male bird watcher as both walked in Central Park, New York (Hamad, 2020).

Similar calculations of intersectional identities come into play when determining who gives way to whom to maintain social distancing requirements. Although it seems obvious that younger, vigorous walkers might give way to frailer, older individuals, the outcome is harder to predict when a young mother pushing her stroller and holding a dog on a leash is walking toward an elderly couple, or when young women are walking toward persons of a similar or different age, ethnicity, or other social variables, with or without masks. Transgressions against another pedestrian's unwritten, informal rules are consequential and led to stressful walks. For example, early in the pandemic, if I had decided that I was going to walk on the grass in order that a parent with a toddler could continue walking on the pavement, I would often wait until I was within a car's length of them to move, reasoning that 15–16 feet was well in keeping with the guidance to maintain at least 6 feet distance. Angry glances from mothers, roughly pulling their kids toward them and stepping off the sidewalk led me to make similar moves much sooner next time.

More generally, Wacquant's concept of a "carnal sociology" (2009) and Pitts-Taylor's feminist version (2015) reminds us of the need to focus on the body as well as the mind. Similarly, Ellingson's concept of "intersubjectivity" denote how our bodies are always "intermingled, reciprocal and enmeshed" (2017, p. 21), that is, always in dynamic relationships to others, animals, non-humans, our surroundings, current social and cultural narratives, and so on. Not only are our bodies continually mediated by the relationships and interactions described earlier but every aspect of our embodied self is in a perpetual state of change. Added to the familiar flux of our cells continuously shedding and being replaced until our death, our body-selves are continually tweaking how we perform our bodies in a physical and social world that is constantly changing. The continually evolving COVID-19 pandemic with its sudden changes increased the speed and unpredictability of these changes, which led to drastic changes in how I viewed other walkers. For example, the same neighbors that I viewed in the early days of the pandemic as familiar faces taking themselves and their dogs for needed walks, I came to view later in the pandemic as potential virus transmitters.

FOSTERING COMMUNITY AND CONNECTION AFTER THE COVID-19 RESTRICTIONS ARE LIFTED

The purpose of this autoethnographic account was to make sense of how walking in my neighborhood listening to podcasts sustained me during the COVID-19 pandemic. Drawing on multiple research frameworks from a variety of disciplines, I came to reject dualist attempts to discover certainty in favor of messier embodied ways of creating knowledge. After researching broadly from qualitative and quantitative perspectives, I concluded that my new habit was comforting not just because of the health benefits of exercise but also because it deepened my sense of community. During a time of enforced isolation, it led me to feel more connected to my neighbors and my neighborhood, and to a virtual community of podcast hosts and their guests. I concluded that all the human and nonhuman elements interacted synergistically to strengthen my feeling of community and connection with others who were also living through the pandemic. Together these actual and parasocial relationships protected me from COVID-19 induced social isolation and strengthened my resilience. In addition, walking enabled me to begin blurring the mind-body divide in my own body-self to start viewing my body and brain as integrated and to trust more in my embodied knowing. Instead of continuing to subscribe, like many academics, to Thomas Edison's view that "the chief function of the body is to carry the brain around," I began paying attention to what I felt in my heart and gut to draw on multiple forms of knowing.

While the COVID-19 pandemic has challenged us all in numerous ways, it has also provided opportunities to take stock of who we are and to clarify who we want to become. In reflecting with Steingart and his guests on the opportunities inherent in the pandemic, I am optimistic about the changes to our societies and ourselves. Since discovering how walking can draw me out of my head and into to my body, inducing a comforting feeling of focused calm, I plan to change my sedentary work habits. I intend to put into use for myself and my students what I have learned from research and personal experience about how movement can strengthen learning. I plan also to support efforts to make neighborhoods safer and greener so that everyone can benefit from getting to know their neighbors and experiencing nature. I am grateful for newer technologies that enable us to stay connected to our global community as well as our local one. Perhaps my story is not unique; perhaps it is a version of the hero's journey, a tale of a crisis overcome, and a return home transformed.

I still twist my earbuds into place, change into clothes with phone pockets and go for walks when I can. I still see some of the same neighbors that I did before, and I am curious about whether they returned to their daily routines, or if they too made changes. While COVID travel restrictions remain in place, I still rely on virtual connections to maintain a sense of global community with friends and family overseas. With a podcast queued on my phone, I move forward in this pandemic, pondering my place in this neighborhood and this world.

REFERENCES

Ash, J., & Gallacher, L. A. (2015). *Becoming attuned: Methodologies of Embodiment* (1st ed., pp. 69–85). Routledge.

Barad, K. (2007). *Meeting the universe halfway*. Duke University Press.

Belvederi Murri, M., Ekkekakis, P., Magagnoli, M., Zampogna, D., Cattedra, S., Capobianco, L., Serafini, G., Calcagno, P., Zanetidou, S., & Amore, M. (2018). Physical exercise in major depression: Reducing the mortality gap while improving clinical outcomes. *Frontiers in Psychiatry, 9*, 762. https://10.3389/fpsyt.2018.00762.

Bostock, R. (2020). *Exhale*. Penguin Publishing Group.

Brooks, S. K., Webster, R. K., Smith, L. E., Woodland, L., Wessely, S., Greenberg, N., & Rubin, G. J. (2020). The psychological impact of quarantine and how to reduce it: Rapid review of the evidence. *The Lancet (British Edition), 395(*10227*)*, 912–920. https://10.1016/S0140-6736(20)30460-8.

Butler, J. (1988). Performative acts and gender constitution: An essay in phenomenology and feminist theory. *Theatre Journal (Washington, D.C.), 40*(4), 519–531. https://10.2307/3207893.

Chatterjee, R. (Host). (2019, November 20). Why walking in the superpower you didn't know you had with Professor Shane O'Mara (No. 84) [Audio podcast episode]. In *Feel Better Live More.*

Cregan-Reid, V. (2018). *Primate change: How the world we made is remaking us*. Octopus Publishing Group.

Crenshaw, K. (1991). Mapping the margins: Intersectionality, identity politics, and violence against women of color. *Stanford Law Review, 43*(6), 1241–1299. https://10.2307/1229039.

Czeisler, M. É, Lane, R. I., Petrosky, E., Wiley, J. F., Christensen, A., Njai, R., Weaver, M. D., Robbins, R., Facer-Childs, E. R., Barger, L. K., Czeisler, C. A., Howard, M. E., & Rajaratnam, S. M. W. (2020). Mental health, substance use, and suicidal ideation during the COVID-19 pandemic—United States, June 24–30, 2020. *MMWR. Morbidity and Mortality Weekly Report, 69*(32), 1049–1057. https://10.15585/mmwr.mm6932a1.

Dirks, Paul H G M, Berger, L. R., Roberts, E. M., Kramers, J. D., Hawks, J., Randolph-Quinney, P. S., Elliott, M., Musiba, C. M., Churchill, S. E., de Ruiter,

D. J., Schmid, P., Backwell, L. R., Belyanin, G. A., Boshoff, P., Hunter, K. L., Feuerriegel, E. M., Gurtov, A., Harrison, J. d. G., Hunter, R., . . . Tucker, S. (2015). Geological and taphonomic context for the new hominin species Homo naledi from the Dinaledi Chamber, South Africa.https://10.5167/uzh-120196.

Dominski, F. H., & Brandt, R. (2020). Do the benefits of exercise in indoor and outdoor environments during the COVID-19 pandemic outweigh the risks of infection? *Sport Sciences for Health, 16*(3), 583–588. https://10.1007/s11332-020-00673-z.

Drinkwater, C., Wildman, J., & Moffatt, S. (2019). Social prescribing. *BMJ*, 364, 1285. doi: https://doi.org/10.1136/bmj.l1285.

Edison Research and Triton (2021). *The Infinite Dial 2021.* Edison Research. https://www.edisonresearch.com/the-infinite-dial-2021-2/.

Edison Research and Triton Digital (2020). *The Infinite Dial 2020.* https://www.edisonresearch.com/wp-content/uploads/2020/03/The-Infinite-Dial-2020-from-Edison-Research-and-Triton-Digital.pdfport/.

Ellingson, L. L. (2017). *Embodiment in qualitative research* (1st ed.). Routledge.

Ellingson, L. L., & Borofka, K. G. E. (2020). Long-term cancer survivors' everyday embodiment. *Health Communication, 35*(2), 180–191. https://10.1080/10410236.2018.1550470.

Ellis, C., Adams, T. E., & Bochner, A. P. (2011). *Autoethnography: An overview.* University of Cologne Press.

Ettman, C. K., Abdalla, S. M., Cohen, G. H., Sampson, L., Vivier, P. M., & Galea, S. (2020). Prevalence of depression symptoms in US adults before and during the COVID-19 pandemic. *JAMA Network Open, 3*(9), e2019686. https://10.1001/jamanetworkopen.2020.19686.

Eyal, K., & Dailey, R. M. (2012). Examining relational maintenance in parasocial relationships. *Mass Communication & Society, 15*(5), 758–781. https://10.1080/15205436.2011.616276.

Field-Springer, K., & Margavio Striley, K. (2018). Managing meanings of embodied experiences theory: Toward a discursive understanding of becoming healthier. *Health Communication, 33*(6), 700–709.

Fridman, L. (Host). (2021, February 28). Andrew Huberman: Sleep, dreams, creativity and the limits of the human mind (No. 164) [Audio podcast episode]. In *Lex Fridman Podcast.*

Goleman, D. (2006). *Social intelligence*. Random House Publishing Group.

Hamad, R. (2020). A white damsel leveraged racial power and failed. *New York Times*. https://www.nytimes.com/2020/05/27/opinion/amy-cooper-central-park-racism.html.

Hansen, M. M., Jones, R., & Tocchini, K. (2017). Shinrin-Yoku (Forest Bathing) and nature therapy: A state-of-the-art review. *International Journal of Environmental Research and Public Health, 14*(8), 851. https://10.3390/ijerph14080851.

Hof, W. (2020). *The Wim Hof method: Activate your full human potential*. Sounds True.

Horton, D., & Richard Wohl, R. (1956). Mass communication and para-social interaction: Observations on intimacy at a distance. *Psychiatry (Washington, D.C.), 19*(3), 215–229. https://10.1080/00332747.1956.11023049.

Huberman, A. (Host). (2021, May 17). How to learn skills faster (No. 20) [Audio podcast episode]. In *Huberman Lab.* https://hubermanlab.com/how-to-learn-skills-faster/.

Hwang, T., Rabheru, K., Peisah, C., Reichman, W., & Ikeda, M. (2020). Loneliness and social isolation during the COVID-19 pandemic. *International Psychogeriatrics, 32*(10), 1217–1220. https://10.1017/S1041610220000988.

Jackson, S. B., Stevenson, K. T., Larson, L. R., Peterson, M. N., & Seekamp, E. (2021). Outdoor activity participation improves adolescents' mental health and well-being during the COVID-19 pandemic. *International Journal of Environmental Research and Public Health, 18*(5), 2506. MDPI AG. Retrieved from http://dx.doi.org/10.3390/ijerph18052506.

Kabat-Zinn, J. (2016). *Mindfulness for beginners: Reclaiming the present moment and your life*. Sounds True.

Kabat-Zinn, J., & Kabat-Zinn, J. (2017). Walking meditations. *Mindfulness, 8*(1), 249–250. https://10.1007/s12671-016-0638-1.

Kaplan, S. (1995). The restorative benefits of nature: Toward an integrative framework. *Journal of Environmental Psychology, 15*(3), 169–182. https://10.1016/0272-4944(95)90001-2.

Kirgios, E. L., Mandel, G. H., Park, Y., Milkman, K. L., Gromet, D. M., Kay, J. S., & Duckworth, A. L. (2020). Teaching temptation bundling to boost exercise: A field experiment. *Organizational Behavior and Human Decision Processes, 161*, 20–35. https://10.1016/j.obhdp.2020.09.003.

Laskowski, E. R., MD. (2016). Walking throughout your day keeps depression (and a host of other health problems) away. *Mayo Clinic Proceedings, 91*(8), 981–983. https://10.1016/j.mayocp.2016.06.005.

Lewis, S. C., & Westlund, O. (2015). Actors, actants, audiences, and activities in cross-media news work. *Digital Journalism, 3*(1), 19–37. https://10.1080/21670811.2014.927986.

Li, Q. (2018). *Forest bathing: How trees can help you find health and happiness.* Penguin Publishing Group.

Luchetti, M., Lee, J. H., Aschwanden, D., Sesker, A., Strickhouser, J. E., Terracciano, A., & Sutin, A. R. (2020). The trajectory of loneliness in response to COVID-19. *The American Psychologist, 75*(7), 897–908. https://10.1037/amp0000690.

Magnussen, C. & Trautmann, M.(Hosts). (2019 October, 19). Mit Gabor Steingart, Journalist und Buchautor mit unterneherischem Erhgeiz. (No. 166) [Audio podcast episode]. In on the way to new work-der Podcast über neue Arbeit.

Magro, J. (Host). (2020, April 9). Seltsame Ostern (No. 434). [Audio podcast episode]. In *Auf den Punkt.* Süddeutsche Zeitung.

Maslow, A. H. (1943). A theory of human motivation. *Psychological Review, 50*(4), 370–396. https://10.1037/h0054346.

Matias, T., Dominski, F. H., & Marks, D. F. (2020). Human needs in COVID-19 isolation. *Journal of Health Psychology, 25*(7), 871–882. https://10.1177/1359105320925149.

Merleau-Ponty, M. (2013). *Phenomenology of perception*. Taylor and Francis. https://10.4324/9780203720714.

McGinty, E. E., Presskreischer, R., Han, H., & Barry, C. L. (2020). Psychological distress and loneliness reported by US Adults in 2018 and April 2020. *JAMA: The Journal of the American Medical Association, 324*(1), 93–94. https://10.1001/jama.2020.9740.

Milkman, K. L., Minson, J. A., & Volpp, K. G. M. (2014). Holding the hunger games hostage at the gym: An evaluation of temptation bundling. *Management Science, 60*(2), 283–299. https://10.1287/mnsc.2013.1784.

Office of Governor Gavin Newsom (2020, March 16). *California issues directive to fight COVID-19*. CA.Gov. https://www.gov.ca.gov/2020/03/16/california-issues-directive-to-fight-covid-19/.

O'Mara, S. (2019). *In praise of walking: A new scientific exploration*. W. W. Norton & Company.

Oppezzo, M., & Schwartz, D. L. (2014). Give your ideas some legs: The positive effect of walking on creative thinking. *Journal of Experimental Psychology. Learning, Memory, and Cognition, 40*(4), 1142–1152. https://10.1037/a0036577.

Orbach, S. (Host). (2021, February 19). A sense of an opening. [Audio podcast episode]. In *A point of view*. BBC Radio 4.

Perks, L. G., & Turner, J. S. (2019). Podcasts and productivity: A qualitative uses and gratifications study. *Mass Communication & Society, 22*(1), 96–116. https://10.1080/15205436.2018.1490434.

Perry, B. D., & Hambrick, E. P. (2008). The neurosequential model of therapeutics. *Reclaiming Children and Youth, 17*(3), 38.

Pitts-Taylor, V. (2015). A Feminist carnal sociology?: Embodiment in sociology, feminism, and naturalized philosophy. *Qualitative Sociology, 38*(1), 19–25.

Rokach, A. (2019). *The psychological journey to and from loneliness*. Academic Press.

Roll, R. (Host). (2020, July 20). How to change your brain with Dr. Andrew Huberman. (No. 533) [Audio podcast episode]. In The Rich Roll Podcast.

Rosenbaum, D., Mama, Y., & Algom, D. (2017). Stand by your stroop: Standing up enhances selective attention and cognitive control. *Psychological Science, 28*(12), 1864–1867.

Seifert, G., Jeitler, M., Stange, R., Michalsen, A., Cramer, H., Brinkhaus, B., Esch, T., Kerckhoff, A., Paul, A., Teut, M., Ghadjar, P., Langhorst, J., Häupl, T., Murthy, V., & Kessler, C. S. (2020). The relevance of complementary and integrative medicine in the COVID-19 pandemic: A qualitative review of the literature. *Frontiers in Medicine, 7*, 587749.

Steingart, G. (Host). (2020, March 16). Der Achte Tag: Deutschland neu denken. In Mediapioneer. https://mediapioneer.com/der-achte-tag-2/.

Sennett, R. (1991). *The conscience of the eye: The design and social life of cities*. Faber & Faber.

Thomas F. Gieryn. (2000). A space for place in sociology. *Annual Review of Sociology, 26*(1), 463–496. https://10.1146/annurev.soc.26.1.463.

Tomova, L., Wang, K. L., Thompson, T., Matthews, G. A., Takahashi, A., Tye, K. M., & Saxe, R. (2020). Acute social isolation evokes midbrain craving responses similar to hunger. *Nature Neuroscience, 23*(12), 1597–1605. https://10.1038/s41593-020-00742-z.

Torales, J., O'Higgins, M., Castaldelli-Maia, J. M., & Ventriglio, A. (2020). *The outbreak of COVID-19 coronavirus and its impact on global mental health*. SAGE Publications. https://10.1177/0020764020915212.

Tsanov, M., & O'Mara, S. M. (2014). Decoding signal processing in thalamo-hippocampal circuitry: Implications for theories of memory and spatial processing. *Brain Research, 1621*, 368–379. https://10.1016/j.brainres.2014.12.003.

U.S. Department of Health and Human Services. (2015). *Step it up! The Surgeon General's call to action to promote walking and walkable communities*. U.S. Dept of Health and Human Services, Office of the Surgeon General.

Wacquant, L. (2009). *The body, the ghetto and the penal state*. Springer Science and Business Media.

Wood, B. M., Harris, J. A., Raichlen, D. A., Pontzer, H., Sayre, K., Sancilio, A., Berbesque, C., Crittenden, A. N., Mabulla, A., McElreath, R., Cashdan, E., & Jones, J. H. (2021). Gendered movement ecology and landscape use in Hadza hunter-gatherers. *Nature Human Behaviour, 5*(4), 436–446. https://10.1038/s41562-020-01002-.

World Health Organization. (2016). *Integrated care models: An overview*. World Health Organization. https://www.euro.who.int/__data/assets/pdf_file/0005/322475/Integrated-care-models-overview.pdf.

Chapter Thirteen

The Class of 2020

Parents' Perspectives of the Pomp and Terrible Circumstance

Michelle Napierski-Prancl

> I said "Kate, shhh. Come on." I said, "I got to use to the bathroom." So we snuck in the school . . . and we went down the hall, because every graduating class . . . the entire class is part of painting a mural, they design it, decide it, and everything. Well, their mural is unfinished. It's untouched from that moment that the school shut down. . . . I took some pictures of it, and her face, it was crushed, like "there's our mural, the unfinished one." It goes from floor to ceiling and probably 15 feet long and it'll stay there forever. . . . People will ask, "why does theirs' look that way? Why is it still an outline and not all painted?"
>
> Vicki, Class of 2020 Parent from Colorado

PARENTS OF THE CLASS OF 2020

High school seniors in the Class of 2020 were born only a few months before or after the terrorist attacks on September 11, 2001. As their parents grieved with a distraught nation, their new lives served as a symbolic sign of hope, resilience and a wonder for what good things the future may hold. As time went on this cohort seemed no more unique than any other, and they celebrated milestones and the mundane like those before them: the first day of Kindergarten, the tooth fairy, and driver's permits. However, before senior prom and graduation, this cohort and their parents would face another enormous and unexpected tragedy—the global pandemic caused by the coronavirus. Seniors were in final rehearsals for high school musicals, playing in championship basketball games, and shopping for prom dresses when it all came to a screeching halt. School—no, in fact, the world—would pause. At home, parents like Lydia[1] from Texas had an impossible task; "I couldn't fix it. I'm a fixer." Politicians, news sources, and others described it as an unprecedented time and for parents like Beth from Minnesota, "it was the worst of times and it was the best of times."

Twenty-two parents of the Class of 2020 shared their stories with me for this study. They represent 19 different states and Puerto Rico, from Alabama to Washington, New Jersey to Nebraska. They were sampled through social media using a combination of random and nonprobability sampling and are of different races, ethnicities, and marital statuses. Their children attended a variety of different types of schools: from a large public school in Texas, to a small magnet school in Delaware, to a Charter school in Minnesota, to homeschool in Maine.

Two themes from Reinharz's (1992) work on feminist research resonates especially well with this project; "Feminist research frequently includes the researcher as a person" (p. 240), and "Feminist research frequently attempts to develop special relations with the people studied . . . " (p. 240). As a parent of a Class of 2020 student, I understand the magnitude of all that was lost when schools closed and I understand the difficulty in explaining this loss to those who did not have a high school senior. Caroline from California explains, "I really feel like people are unable to embrace the gravity and reality of this unless you are directly connected." I also understand the frustration felt by parents like Celeste from Delaware who says, "I was so salty, I was so mad . . . it was rough . . . he's my only child, no graduation, nothing. . . . I was beyond frustrated, for both of us . . . " I was also familiar with remarks that Cara from Nebraska describes as "dismissive" from those who said other generations went to war and had it worse than the Class of 2020.

> Some people were so insensitive, "Oh they'll get over it." Yeah, they will but that's not really the point. You got to go to graduation and if somebody told you that you couldn't go, you would be upset too. These kids were 17 years old. These are big things that they look forward to and they worked hard.

As Reinharz (1992) suggests, by acknowledging my own experience, I earn "the trust of others in doing the research" (p. 259). Accordingly, I believe that I experienced a genuine connection with the participants. For instance, almost every parent stopped on their own accord at some point during the course of our interview to show me a photo of their child. Many parents also paused to ask me about my son. We shared tears and laughter because we are parents, not because we were a researcher or interviewee. I laughed when Celeste showed me a picture of herself holding a megaphone out of a car window in the surprise graduation parade she organized for her son. I also laughed when Scott from Illinois apologized for swearing too much as he recounted the terrible senior year his son experienced; it clearly conveyed his anger but he jokingly attributed it to his Chicago upbringing. I got teary-eyed when Dan from Alabama said, "I'm so sorry, I can't believe I'm so emotional," when talking about his twins. I assured him he was not the only parent to do so. In fact, Michaela from Michigan described herself as "a crying mess," but then we both laughed when she could not find a tissue to dry her eyes and she improvised by grabbing her husband's sock from the basket of folded laundry sitting next to her on the sofa. She jokingly insisted that she would return it to the dirty clothes hamper and with a similar sense of humor, I promised that I would make note of that in my write-up. This type of connection comes from our shared experiences as Class of 2020 parents who watched their children lose their senior year. Additionally, I was conscious of my unique status and at some points stopped to remind respondents of this when I thought they might have revealed sensitive information. I relate this to Hesse-Biber (2007) who writes,

> I am aware of the nature of my relationship to those whom I interview, careful to understand my particular personal and research standpoints and what role I play in the interview process in terms of my power and authority over the interview situation. (pp. 113–114)

The stories in this chapter are through the eyes of parents so that we can see what it was like to parent a Class of 2020 student. Take for example, a poignant scene described by Laura from Virginia. "I came home from work and Liam and his girlfriend were sitting in the driveway and literally they had a tape measure between them 6 feet apart and they both had masks on." Similarly, we can empathize with Scott, who describes his feelings of helplessness.

> I'm a spectator to my son's horror. It's like I'm in a movie theater, you know when you yell at the screen, 'Don't go in there, don't go into the basement 'and you know, they can't hear you on the screen, and that's what it's like being the parent of a 2020 kid. It's like you're watching a freaking horror movie . . . and you just hope to God that at the end of this your son is still standing.

The parents of the Class of 2020 had a lot to share about how they and their children persevered, sometimes positively and sometimes not, during the pandemic. Their insights validate the significance of the lost senior year and they offer examples of what brought them comfort during this time of grief. Caroline shared that like her son, her grandmother never had a high school graduation because of the U.S. entry into World War II. "She's 95 and she still brings up what they did wrong and what bothers her to this day." Thus, Caroline feels, " . . . you need to talk about loss in order to go through the grieving process and if we don't talk about what these kids have lost then they're stuck in their feelings and that will manifest mental health problems . . . " Other parents felt the same way, like Will from Massachusetts who said, "I'm scared about his mental health," even now with his son in college.

SENIOR YEAR, RITES OF PASSAGE, AND COLLECTIVE EFFERVESCENCE

Senior year is a highly anticipated and meaningful time for students and parents. Some look forward to and even plan their senior year long before 12th grade. Lydia, a teacher, began our interview with this very point.

> It was devastating. He and I spent three years of his high school career talking about his senior year. "Oh Mom, how are you going to act when I'm a senior?" They normally have a senior clap out day where the seniors wear their cap and gown and the faculty stand outside and clap for them. . . . It was sad to say, that day did not happen. Even he was like, "you didn't get to see me do that." "I know babe, I didn't get to see you do that." That was definitely a devastation for us because we had planned that for like three years.

The loss from senior year varied from one extreme to another. In Maine, Bridget who homeschools her daughter said that the COVID-19 restrictions had little impact on their school day. "We still did our normal routine which is obviously a bit different from public schools . . . we don't have the typical high school milestones, we don't have homecoming, we don't have prom, so we didn't miss out there." In Texas, Sherry felt fortunate, as her daughter was able to attend her debutante ball just days before schools closed. Yet in contrast, Scott's son had a difficult year even before schools went remote beginning with a teacher's strike that put an early end to his son's senior football season. That was followed by a student walk-out that ruined the National Letter of Intent signing day and a "coyote shutting down the city and closing school . . . " To put it bluntly, Scott says, "it was a shit show . . . a tire fire . . . we went straight from strike, to tire fire to COVID. Jake had a month of senior year." Anna from Puerto Rico shares another extreme case and reflects on her son's overall high school experience. "First, we had Hurricane Maria, then we had the earthquake, and then we had the pandemic. The kids that have survived catastrophic events are the kids in Puerto Rico."

When schools shut down it threatened students' opportunities to participate in rituals and rites of passage. Pascoe's (2012) ethnography of a high school found that school rituals are "talked about for months in advance, covered in the school newspaper, and talked about for years afterwards as the stories about assembly content, after-dance parties, and who drank how much grew larger and more outrageous with the passing of time" (p. 41). However, for the Class of 2020, much of this never occurred. Christine from Pennsylvania describes each loss her daughter felt as the events she waited for senior year were canceled one by one.

> She was supposed to go to France . . . and the first thing they did was they canceled the French trip . . . and they had this meeting at the school and everybody was crying and the French teacher was crying, it was just days and days of crying. . . . And then she finally got this big role in the spring play . . . and then the play got canceled. And then the music trip, she was supposed to go to Virginia, and then that got canceled. She just cried.

Sherry talks about it as "dominos falling." Her daughter's school unsuccessfully rescheduled graduation twice. "My daughter handled it really well until the day that they canceled the second graduation. And then she was just a hot mess for 24 hours." Vicki describes "devastating" losses for her daughter. "It was like someone slammed the door on her face. She had these huge plans and none of them occurred." Cindy from New York explains that the abrupt end to senior year meant that her son lost his "lasts."

> The biggest loss he felt was missing his last season of track. . . . He was the captain, that was his everything, and he didn't get it. They didn't know it was their last track meet. . . . He didn't get to run in his last races. He didn't get to see what times he would get in his last season.

It was a similar story for Wendy's daughter in Washington.

> Probably the most devastating thing, she was on the varsity fast pitch team. We had all these big plans for the season and all these cool things. . . . Luckily, another coach from a town just north of us called our coach . . . "Hey you want to just get together for a quick scrimmage . . . " Thank God . . . because the next day they gave them notice that the school was going to close and they canceled everything. That one scrimmage was all we got for fast pitch . . . and that was heartbreaking because that was her one sport; that was her love. So then we just muddled through.

Unfortunately, senior year is not designed for muddling through. It typically includes a series of special events to mark students' achievements before they move on to their next chapter. Social theorists and philosophers have been thinking about the importance of rituals and rites of passage for a long time. The writings of Arnold van Gennep and Émile Durkheim in particular, offer us valuable insight into why the loss of senior year experiences or even the shift to virtual celebrations is far from meaningless. Writing in 1908, van Gennep states, "The life of an individual in any society is a series of passages . . . " (1960, pp. 2–3). While van Gennep (1960) focused much of his attention on rites related to birth, marriage, and death his work provides valuable insight to senior year, graduation in particular, as embodying a rite of passage. Vicki explains, "For us, in the United States in our culture . . . this is how ending our childhood and moving into adulthood happens. It's a milestone for us. You're moving on." Bridget's daughter was anxious to move on from high school.

> Even though we were homeschooling, she's just not a book kinda kid and she doesn't really like school so she was really looking forward to graduating. . . . So, I promised her, "you will graduate, we will have your official graduation . . . we'll figure it out . . . " We ended up having to wait until July.

Fasick (1988) applies van Gennep's rites of passage to the high school experience and argues, "Whatever else the graduation ceremonies may mean, they have become a symbol of entrance into young adulthood for the vast majority of young people" (p. 467). Without a graduation ceremony, it is difficult to see the completion of a high school degree as a rite of passage. Sherry explains,

> I think . . . as humans we like things tied up with a nice little bow. We like things compartmentalized and packaged . . . so when you finished school doing Zoom, and then you have a couple . . . weeks of not doing anything and then you start Zoom online college courses, there was no period at the end of the sentence.

Thus, when van Gennep describes liminal rites as, "most of these rites should be understood as direct and physical rites of entrance, of waiting, and of departure—that is, as rites of passage" (1960, p. 25), we can see how not having a graduation ceremony makes a life transition from one stage to another virtually incomplete.

Scholars on the high school experience recognize prom and graduation serve as significant markers in one's high school life. In Hoffman's (2002) study students predicted these events would be the "most memorable aspects" of high school (p. 36). In fact, parents in my study, like Lydia, still held vivid memories of these events. "I remember my graduation, I remember standing in the mirror, undoing my rollers. I remember my grandmother coming over and we all rode to the stadium together." As a result, Lydia wanted to give her son "moments" to remember. "He was having a lot of woulda, coulda, shoulda . . . 'Oh, I wish we would've done this.' 'Oh I wish we could've done that,' . . . I just didn't want him to have . . . regrets." Her solution was to host a "Prom Shenanigans" party in her backyard. She insisted on two things; that his friends have a COVID-19 test prior to attending and that there was a prom king.

> I did go ahead and name him prom king. . . . I even had a sash that said "Quarantine King" and his friends just laughed. . . . They just thought it was the funniest thing. He even gave a speech because they were all like, "Speech! Speech! Speech!" So he was like, "Thank you all so much for coming and for voting for me." It was a nice little night for all the guys. . . . They just needed to go back to being kids. . . . It was the one time in, I guess you could say in 6 weeks where he had something to look forward to, he could hang out with his friends . . . he didn't have to worry about Covid . . . he had fun, for one night.

There are many reasons for us to take a critical look at proms. Scholars have conducted cultural analyses of proms (Best, 2000), challenged us to reconstruct the heteronormative components of proms (Smith, 2011), and called our attention to racism and racial segregation of proms (Harrison, 2007). The ACLU (n.d.) has even created a "Know Your Prom Night Rights" guide for LGBTQ+ youth in case they experience discrimination. In sum, proms "are key sites at which a politics of youth is formed, where identities are fashioned and cultural struggles waged" (Best, 2000, p. 17). Thus, proms deserve a critical eye, because as Best (2000) describes, "Proms are a big deal" (p. 18). In 2020, much of the big deal surrounding proms concerned their cancellation.

According to Chen (2012), proms highlight the role high schools play in students' transition from youth to adulthood. One specific way is in the planning of proms, which empowers students and gives them decision-making responsibilities on par with adults. However, in 2020 many parents took over planning so that their children would not miss out. Caroline acknowledges, " . . . my heart bled for these kids." Therefore, she hosted an unofficial prom for about 200 students. She contacted the Department of Parks and Recreation in her town, asked about the rules for social gatherings, got clearance from the city manager and hosted a prom using her own funds and community donations. It was not a traditional prom as couples arrived at socially distant scheduled times and there was no crowded dance floor. However, there was a DJ and different stations for students to promenade through combining photo-ops with carnival-like games. They received goody-bags and a take-out dinner. As a result, Caroline says students "got to dress up and they got to post on social media, 'Hey, going to prom!'"

Even during a pandemic, high school cliques affect prom. Dan explains, "just like any school . . . one of the popular groups had this big barn prom and they invited the select group of kids . . . and I was like, you know what? We can do it better, we can go to the beach . . . " He believed prom was important.

> It's one of those coming-of-age things you look forward to and dream about. . . . Did it turn out the way they expected? No. But, I think my wife and her best friend were like, "Well, we are going to do something for them . . . " The kids can dress up. We ordered a nice meal and let them have some last memories . . . of high school. It wasn't anything I'll say spectacular but it was just a way for them to be celebrated . . . an opportunity to have fun and be kids because they grow up too quick and what are you going to look back on and think about? I think that is why we chose to do it. They needed those memories . . .

Despite their best efforts, parents could not fully replicate the prom experience. Christine explains,

> All six of us dressed up, and we had my daughter pinning a boutonniere on my husband . . . everybody played along . . . and then they all looked at me and said, "Can we just take this stuff off and go?" It was really anti-climactic. . . . I pictured us: "Let's dance in the living room . . . " and they were like, "This is uncomfortable and can we not?" So, it was disappointing. . . . I did not want her to miss out and I guess I didn't realize that that experience in and of itself wasn't necessarily something that could be replaced.

While not all high school students attend prom, most students do attend graduation. Originally published in 1912, Durkheim's writing on religion, on the sacred and profane, helps us to better understand the importance of the graduation ritual. Specifically, Durkheim's notion of collective effervescence describes how a meaningful connection can emerge from shared ritual experiences (Durkheim, Cosman & Cladis, 2008). Graduations are not mundane, daily occurrences, but instead are ceremonious occasions that invite a student cohort to celebrate their achievements collectively. In 2020, commencement took on a multiplicity of different formats from virtual events to socially distant in-person affairs. Such celebrations did not necessarily provide an opportunity for classmates to bond and they varied in quality of experience. In Connecticut, Rachel's son graduated without his peers. Yet, Rachel describes the principal's delivery of diplomas via a school bus and police escort as "special" and "nicely done."

> She played the "Pomp and Circumstance" music. It was fast, she put her table out, put the diploma out and she said to Tim, "I want you to turn your tassel." . . . and then she said, "You can throw your cap . . . " We set up a tent in our driveway. . . . I said, "I have to do something spectacular . . . " So I had a banner made with his graduation picture. It was big and it was in the front yard. He was so embarrassed and I said "I don't care, you have to have something . . ." I asked all my neighbors, "would you help us celebrate Tim?" . . . It was awesome, everyone came out . . . and his girlfriend came and his hockey coach came . . . and it was really nice, even the principal was like, "Wow, this was awesome . . ." We lucked out, they had a plane fly over that had a "Congratulations 2020" banner and it happened right when Tim was getting his diploma.

In contrast, Cara and Scott described their schools' drive-through graduations as a "joke." Cara explains,

> When I tell you there was nothing put into it, I mean there was nothing put into it. It was four card tables set up in the parking lot. The kids drove through. They literally tossed their stuff through the window, "Bye . . . " There wasn't a balloon. I mean nothing. . . . I was appalled. They had plenty of time to put some sort of effort into it. They didn't give a shit.

There were other disappointments as well. Limits on social gatherings meant that some parents could not attend their child's graduation even if it was in-person. Jessica from New Jersey describes feeling left behind.

> You know Nick drove off by himself to his graduation and I was crying in the driveway. . . . that is not how it should be . . . we watched it on the computer . . . it was okay, I mean it was fine. It was a nice graduation. And we saw like two sets of ginormous empty bleachers where we could be sitting and it was just so frustrating. I don't know why we couldn't have been there as well. It seemed like there was enough room.

No matter the format of the ceremony, certain aspects of the graduation ritual were significant to both students and parents. In New York, Tom's daughter helped plan an outdoor ceremony and "she said one of the biggest things that everybody seemed to want was the bagpipes. There were certain things that they felt were ceremonious and necessary . . . " For Celeste, it was "Pomp and Circumstance." She waited in the parking lot while her son went into the school building to be recorded walking across the stage for their virtual graduation ceremony.

> I was like "Okay, fine, whatever. It's still graduation." I went with my megaphone and my balloons . . . and I recorded "Pomp and Circumstance" onto the

> megaphone so that when my kid came out, I had my megaphone playing so he got his little celebration.

Lydia felt the same way about music and made it an important part of her son's drive-through graduation.

> We all loaded up in the car. The line was an hour and a half long wait. I played graduation music the entire time. . . . I wanted him to have a graduation where he would remember, "No I didn't have this, but I had that . . . " At first . . . I was lame mom. For the first 30 minutes he was like, "Ugh" in the back seat, "Oh Mom." But, as we got closer and closer he just got excited. . . . I just saw his genuine smile. Not the fake one. The actual real Stephen smile. It meant a lot to me, but I know it meant a lot to him. . . . He truly was himself. And that's really what I wanted for him to have little moments.

For Beth, the cap and gown was essential. However, because of concerns about cleaning gowns during COVID-19, the school decided to forgo them. Parents thought this was a mistake.

> Well, we had some drama about the gowns . . . we ended up at the last minute, a group of us parents all donated a small fortune and we bought all the kids brand new gowns . . . we were like, my kid is graduating and my kid is wearing a gown and I will pay for my kid and five others . . . we needed the gowns. . . . It was the only thing that we could do that was tradition. We knew we couldn't go to prom, and we knew we had to have a weird graduation, we knew we couldn't do senior trip, we knew we couldn't do senior skip day, this was the one thing we knew that we could buy ourselves and it was only money, you know. . . . It was the only piece of tradition that we could get in place.

The graduation season of 2020 underscores the fact that graduation and other rituals are valued not only by students but also by parents. Tom's daughter asked, "'I wonder, do the parents need this more than we do?" His response was,

> There's something about this that needs to happen for parents because of all the time and effort we feel we put into getting you there . . . we feel like we want you to have that, so you can look back on it, saying, "there were rituals, there were traditions that happened despite the limits."

Laura would agree.

> I think some of it was more important to me than it was to him to be honest with you. . . . The graduation, the honor of having a kid graduate with a 3.75 . . . the academic pieces were more important to me. The ritual was more important to

> me and I missed it because I knew from my older two boys what I was missing. . . . Graduation was hard. They did a virtual graduation . . . and I made him wear his cap and gown . . . and he was like, "Why am I wearing this? Nobody's going to see me but you." And I said, "I know, but to me it's important, just wear it for five minutes until your name is flashed, turn your tassel and move on."

Parents also described other rites of passage that occurred outside of school that the pandemic affected as well. Laura was emotional when talking about her son withdrawing from Scouts before earning the rank of Eagle.

> He was a Boy Scout, he was on his way to Eagle . . . and he said, "You know what Mom? I'm not going to Eagle, I'm going to stop where I am." . . . and I'm begging him, "Please Eagle, you've done the work." And he's like, "This is a global pandemic and I know this is important to you but the reality is that I don't want to." . . . that was hard. . . . I'm still choked up about it. . . . It was harder for me truly, than it was for him.

While Durkheim challenges us to think about the significance of rituals because they mark that which we think is special and separate from the mundane aspects of everyday life, contemporary scholars in psychology argue that the mundane is meaningful too. The research of Gabriel, Naidu, Paravati, Morrison, & Gainey (2020) suggest that collective effervescence is a common occurrence that "happens regularly and it is psychologically important" (p. 151). This is illustrated by Cindy who says that her son did not miss "the big hoopla stuff" like prom as much as he missed being in school with his friends.

> It's more the smaller things with his friends. . . . I think what he missed . . . was the free time in school when they would all meet. . . . There was a desk in the hallway where they would all meet and have their silliness, that's what he missed . . . that unstructured time in school was huge for him and that's where he connected with his friends.

Gabriel et al. (2020) argue, "collective effervescence doesn't separate the sacred from the profane, it turns the everyday profane into the meaningful and sacred" (p.152). Research shows that during normal circumstances students' interactions in the hallways are "significant and distinct parts of students' school day" (Pierce, 2005, p. 6). Students in Hoffman's (2002) study, "repeatedly indicated that being with, interacting with, and seeing friends and acquaintances on a daily basis in and out of school were critical components of their high school experience" (p. 26). Even more, Pierce (2005) found that "hallway passings are vital moments with varying degrees of social function and weight" (p. 7). When schools closed in the spring of 2020, students lost months' worth of vital moments.

CONCERN FOR MENTAL HEALTH

Overwhelmingly, parents felt concern for their children's mental well-being when schools went remote because many, like Anna's son, missed "human contact with other students." Parents tried to talk to their children but were not always successful. Vicki felt "shut out."

> It was bizarre because you couldn't even get them to talk . . . you would try to bring it up and . . . they kept trying to act like, "I just don't want to talk about it." It was almost a revert back to when they're in 6th grade, you know when your kids are that age? "I don't want to talk to you about anything," that's kinda what it felt like. I was like, "Okay, you're obviously struggling with this, 'cause you're not able to talk about it and express how you really feel."

Christine describes it as trying to maintain a "constant balance."

> Sometimes we would do things and she would really appreciate it and other times we would do things and it would just make her cry because we were reminding her of the things she was missing. We couldn't really figure out with any real accuracy which was going to go which way. . . . It was just like we walked around on eggshells with her.

When talking about her daughter, Wendy says she "never gave her a chance to get depressed."

> I'm poking and prodding and picking. . . . "If you don't want to talk to me, talk to your sister. You got to talk to somebody. Do you want me to call one of your friends? I don't want anything to happen to you . . . " There were days when I was like, "if you're thinking anything" and she was like, "Mom, I'm not thinking anything." "I know, but I need to know and these are the questions I'm going to keep asking you because I don't know how this is effecting you unless you tell me."

In Florida, Andy was tragically aware that the risk of suicide ideation and attempts was higher for youth during some points of the pandemic than before the lockdown (Hill et al., 2021). Two students in his son's school took their own lives. Andy had many conversations with his son and classmates so that,

> . . . they were not basically slipping into a black hole and then feeling there is no purpose of living. . . . I think he and his friends kinda rallied around each

> other. . . . They were going to be by each other's side and pick each other up. . . . If something looked weird, or something looked off with somebody, it was a red flag so I would always make sure I would communicate that with my son and I always would communicate that with my son's friends, "Hey let me know if something is odd about Ben."

During the lockdown, students also felt the weight of the world's problems from the global pandemic, to social unrest, to a growing political divide. Andy explains, "It just gets so overwhelming . . . dealing with not just everything with society and politics, but everything else that builds on these young minds . . . " Michaela was surprised when she read a sonnet her son wrote for his English class that talked of grieving, an abyss, and a black hole.

> It didn't help to be in today's climate when you have the George Floyds going on and all the racial divide and there were marches all over the place. . . . He got accepted to multiple universities both HBCU and regular universities and I asked him, "Why are you going to go to the HBCU?" And he was like, "because I feel safe . . . " and I'm like, "you don't feel safe?" And he's like, "Mom, I don't know where I go from being a beloved drum major to becoming a threat and . . . I'm only 18 . . . " and at that moment I'm like . . . I don't know how to comfort you with Covid, with quarantine, with . . .

Michaela had difficulty finishing her thought, as we were both in tears. It was the most painful segment of all the interviews I conducted and it gives us only a glimpse into how her son was experiencing the effects of racism during the pandemic.

COMFORTING THE CLASS OF 2020

As time went on and the school calendar started to run out, many schools, parents, and communities looked for ways to comfort the Class of 2020. There were lawn signs, banners, and car parades. Some efforts, but not all, brought comfort. In special instances, collective effervescence occurred. Will describes such a time:

> You walked into the athletic facility; it was like a grand hallway of all these pictures of your kids and their names and graduation picture . . . and a collage picture of their friends . . . and it was this amazing very spiritual connection. . . . Then trying to meet the moment of just being with all our fellow families going through the same thing so there was that strange sociological connection that we're all in this together. And there was this really great expression of unity.

One successful idea that took off at both the local and national level was the "adopt-a-senior" concept. Mary Storey from New Mexico created "The Original Adopt a High School Senior" Facebook group. I asked Mary, who is not a parent of a Class of 2020 senior, to explain why she created the group:

> When I was watching the Governor give her address back in last March, I was like, "Oh man some of these seniors are really going to miss out . . . " I just thought I'd start a page to adopt a high school senior, no biggie. I really thought it was going to stay local. I had no idea in the world that it was going to blow up the way that it did. . . . Oh my gosh, it grew so fast. Within the first 48 hours I had 5,000 members and then it just continued to get bigger and bigger. By the end of it we had 63,000 members.

The premise was that members of the online group could symbolically adopt seniors from around the country. Parents nominated their child and wrote about their interests and even their favorite snacks. Adopters, usually complete strangers, sent a care package. Michaela was very touched by a local version of adopt-a-senior.

> I cried when she came. . . . She went online to his school to order him his Nike sweatshirt and a t-shirt and his school flag, and went and got a blanket and spent so much money and I never met that lady until she came, and I was so overwhelmed . . . and she was like "if he needs anything else, let me know."

As it turns out, the woman who adopted Michaela's son had watched him grow up through the music program and felt especially moved to make his care package special.

Many parents talked about the generosity and thoughtfulness of those who adopted their senior. Will describes his son's care package as "awesome" and "personalized to the T." Wendy's daughter received so many candles that she was still burning them when I interviewed her mother a year later. "Stuff would just show up in the mail. She got candles . . . and boxes of candy and just little notes wishing her well." Adopting a senior provided comfort to parents, not just in seeing their child celebrated but also by participating in adopting someone else's child. Celeste described herself as "crafty" and made several care packages. She showed me pictures. "She was just so thrilled . . . look at that picture. Her mom said she hadn't smiled for that long for a long time and that made me feel good."

The community came out in full force when a county in Texas canceled the rodeo due to COVID-19; students participating in Future Farmers of America were in a tough situation. Sherry's daughter was able to show her rabbits at the rodeo the day prior, but her daughter's boyfriend was not so lucky.

> . . . they're in the truck waiting to drop the animals off and they start walking down the line telling people, it's been canceled, don't even stop . . . and people are like, "What are we going to do with these cows?" . . . Some of these people have driven across the state to get here so there's no place to even stop with your cattle, you've got to get them out, you've got to let them eat.

Farmers from a nearby county without the same restrictions came to the rescue:

> A couple of farmers who were probably 20 miles north of us . . . they said, 'We have fields that have barbwire fences, bring your trailers, you can sleep at your trailers, there's a couple of motels in town, we have water in our barns, ya'll can come in our houses and take showers if you need to, just come get the cattle safe and we'll figure something out.' By the next morning they had . . . a mini cattle show and gave the kids the ribbons from the rodeo . . . the judges volunteered their time, then while they're sitting there watching this, people are like, "Well how are we going to sell them?" Two moms get online with an auction company, "Can we do an online auction with these cattle?" In 48 hours every cow was sold for at least $1,000 more than what they thought they would've gotten at the rodeo. It was just amazing . . . people went, "Okay this is what we need to do to support these kids."

Some communities planned to recreate important rituals later in the summer when they expected COVID-19 restrictions to change. However, there was an expiration date as to when things could be done. Anna describes it as a loss of momentum. "The momentum of the senior prom is gone. The momentum of the graduation was gone. . . . It's all about the momentum." Her son's school held a car parade with a symbolic turn of the tassel in case they could not hold a graduation, but then restrictions changed and they were able to have a traditional ceremony. Unfortunately, by that time her son had lost interest. "I said 'Listen the school is going to do a graduation,' he was like 'For what? We already symbolically graduated. Heck with it . . . We already graduated Mom. Chill. Relax. Done is done.'" Eventually, to Anna's delight, she was able to convince her son to attend the graduation ceremony. Meanwhile, Jessica found that the momentum for a post-graduation party was lost.

> Against all odds, they were going to have . . . this great fun day at the football stadium . . . and can you believe that not enough kids signed up because they were just done and they had to cancel it? That was another disappointment. Nick was one of the kids who wanted to go but couldn't find many of his friends who wanted to go. . . . I felt bad for the parents who put it all together. It sounded amazing after everything they had been through. . . . I was shocked that not enough kids wanted to go.

Many parents, including Andy, Rachel, and Cindy, said there came a point when their children were "just done." COVID-19 and school closings had taken their toll and it was time to move on to the next chapter with or without the traditional rituals.

LESSONS LEARNED

The perspectives of the parents of the Class of 2020 show that senior year rituals as well as mundane daily school attendance play an important role in the lives of adolescents. The rituals are also important to parents and in some instances, may hold even greater significance for them. They feel a sense of pride in their children's accomplishments that is likely coupled with a nostalgia for normalcy and even for their own high school days. Their stories illuminate how emotionally vested they are in their children's experiences. As I listened to them, I recalled my own experiences, my own grief, and my own sense of loss. I remember telling a friend that during the uncertain time of school closings it felt like I was sucker-punched on a daily basis. Every day, there was another loss, another reason to lose hope, and another day of worrying about my son. These stories tell me that I was not unique in my experience. The interviews also show that it makes a difference for those who, like me, lived in a community that recognized the loss and reacted in some way. To me, the most effective way my community responded was to decorate the village park in school colors with flowers, lights, banners, and individual signs with the students' senior pictures printed on them. At first, it seemed like a nice thing to do but surprisingly it was much more than nice, it was healing because it symbolized that others cared.

To be clear, the parents in this study do not diminish the gravity of the pandemic; some had been ill and more than one had lost a loved one. They do not believe in prioritizing prom over public health. However, they do feel that in addition to the trauma of the pandemic there was another layer of loss that was deeply significant and worthy of recognition. Thus, if and/or when stay-at-home orders occur again, we cannot be complacent; we cannot get lazy or desensitized to the magnitude of what may be lost. These stories tell us that when schools and communities attempt to recreate rituals and provide opportunities to experience collective effervescent, it makes a difference. We also see that these events must be done in a timely fashion and coincide with the school calendar as much as possible otherwise, students will likely feel it is too little, too late. In the end, when communities respond it validates students' feelings and provides comfort during a time of grief, ultimately enabling families to persevere during the pandemic.

REFERENCES

American Civil Liberties Union Foundation. (n.d.) "Know your prom night rights!" Retrieved September 3, 2021, from https://www.aclu.org/sites/default/files/field_document/Prom_Rights.pdf.

Best, A. L. (2000). *Prom night: Youth, schools and popular culture*. ProQuest Ebook Central https://ebookcentral.proquest.com.

Chen, C. S. (2012). *Prom: How a high school ritual brought youth closer to adulthood, 1890–1970*. (Dissertation, UC Berkeley). https://Escholarship.org/UC/item/96N4586k.

Durkheim, E., Cosman, C., & Cladis, M. S. (2008). *The elementary forms of religious life/Emile Durkheim; Translation by Carol Cosman; Abridged with an introduction and notes by Mark S. Cladis*. New York, NY: Oxford University Press.

Fasick, F. A. (1988). Patterns of formal education in high school as *Rites de Passage*. *Adolescence*. *23*(90), 457–468.

Gabriel, S., Naidu, E., Paravati, E., Morrison, C. D., & Gainey, K. (2020). Creating the sacred from the profane: Collective effervescence and everyday activities. *The Journal of Positive Psychology*. *15*(1), 129–154. dio:10.1080/17439760.2019.1689412.

Harrison, R. J. (2007). Black and white prom nights: The unconstitutionality of segregated high school proms in the 21st century. *Journal of Gender, Race and Justice*. *10*(3), 505–530.

Hesse-Biber, S. N. (2007). The practice of feminist in-depth interviewing. In Hesse-Biber, S. N. & Leavy, P. L. (Eds.), *Feminist research practice: A primer*. (pp. 111–148). Sage Publications, Inc.

Hill, R. M., Rufino, K., Kurian, S., Saxena, J., Saxena, K., & Williams, L. (2021). Suicide ideation and attempts in pediatric emergency department before and during COVID-19." *Pediatrics*. *147*(3), Online. doi: 10.1542/peds.2020–029280.

Hoffman, L. M. (2002) Why high schools don't change: What students and their yearbooks tell us. *High School Journal*. *86*(2), 22–37.

Pascoe, C. J. (2012). *Dude, you're a fag: Masculinity and sexuality in high school*. University of California Press.

Pierce, K.M. (2005). Posing, pretending, waiting for the bell: Life in high school classrooms. *High School Journal*. *89*(2), 1–15. doi:10.1353/hsj.2005.0023.

Reinharz, S. 1992. *Feminist methods in social research*. Oxford University Press.

Smith, P. K. (2011). The prom as a spectacle of heteronormativity. *Counterpoints*, *392*, 156–170.

van Gennep, A. (1960). *The rites of passage. Translated by Monika B. Vizedom and Gabrielle L. Caffee*. USA: University of Chicago Press.

NOTE

1. Names of parents and students have been changed to maintain confidentiality.

Chapter Fourteen

Bridging Social Distancing Boundaries

Food Consumption and Community during Quarantine

Edith Ritt-Coulter

The act of eating is a part of the everyday human experience both as a biological need to sustain life and the performance of communal identity through the sharing of culinary knowledge and practices. The COVID-19 pandemic changed how people engage with one another and their relationship with food. This change included consumers' access to communal eating spaces like restaurants or even having friends over for dinner. Grocery store shelves ran low on stock and financial unknowns perpetuated the fear of food insecurity. In response to the shift in the social norms people began looking for comfort and sustainability in their food selections (Flynn, 2020; Lusk & McCluskey, 2020). Staying at home created space for individuals to experiment with new cooking practices or reinvent old ones to stabilize the uncertainty of the COVID-19 pandemic.

When my aunt, Karen Insolia, passed away in November 2018, I began to crave food items that I associated with her. After a phone conversation with my father, I realized that he was also experiencing this phenomenon. As a culinary historian I became curious about the interconnection of memories and food during the grieving process. In the spring of 2020, I found myself turning to food once again to grieve not the loss of a person but the loss of my sense of community. I wanted to understand the relationship between eating practices and the COVID-19 pandemic, partially out of my own need to stimulate the intellectual and creative parts of my personality. This inspiration also came about because I became bored during quarantine. My kitchen was a space where I could curb the boredom I felt and deal with the underlying sense of longing I had for normal social behavior that usually included sharing food with my friends. Before the shutdown, I had been reading the work of Cruz Miguel Ortiz Cuadra (2013) and grappling with his theories on palate memory and communal identity through culinary knowledge. The idea that eating is an embodied experience that is tied to and contributes to our sense of self intrigued me (Wallach, 2019). After realizing that my relationship with food changed during the COVID-19 pandemic, I pondered, if food is the embodiment of nostalgia that links communal eating habits with an individual's sense of belonging, then how can food be used to reestablish a sense of belonging during a global pandemic where social distancing and quarantining are the new norms (Fischler, 1988; Cuadra, 2013; Abarca, 2017). Exploring the concepts of palate memory and sensory embodied experiences allowed me to answer this question. I adopted these concepts by reshaping my kitchen's culinary atmosphere by utilizing methods and practices that were both familiar and unfamiliar to me as a means to bridge the social distancing boundaries. For me finding comfort and a sense of belonging during the pandemic meant applying food history concepts to my own lived experience and partaking in the palate memories of my friends and family's generational food culture. At first, this curiosity manifested in a subconscious return to my great-grandmother's culinary knowledge from the Great Depression. I then revisited interviews I had conducted before the pandemic lockdowns on Oklahoman's culinary history. As the year progressed, I began recreating dishes that held significant value in my interpersonal relationships. Through the sensory experience of cooking and eating a meal, I found that I was able to briefly reconnect with my sense of community.

Jean Anthelme Brillat-Savarin's 1825 declaration," Tell me what you eat, and I shall tell you what you are," has been rearticulated and repeated since he uttered the phrase, but what does this mean when we are looking at the interconnection of food and communal identity during a pandemic (Brillat-Savarin, 1825/2009). Food is central to our sense of identity. The way any given human group eats helps it assert its diversity and hierarchy at the same time, both its oneness and its otherness with whoever eats differently (Fishler, 1988, p. 171). The identity formation associated with cultivating, preparing, and eating food items reveals a constructed system that connects and rejects individuals based on their consumption. The COVID-19 pandemic restrictions limited communal eating and challenged individual's sense of oneness by disrupting established eating practices. For example, a friend group's Wednesday night dinner at a local pub to grab burgers and beer would become part of an individual's culinary and communal identity because of the consistent nature of the behavior. COVID-19 restrictions prohibited these interactions in public and private eating spaces, which contributed to feelings of disconnect and isolation (Matias et al., 2020). When the initial COVID-19 pandemic shutdown occurred, food became a stabilizing factor because of its role in establishing communal and individual identities through eating practices. People turned to food to regain a sense of security and normalcy by investing in their home cooking experiences, stockpiling nonperishables, purchasing comfort food items, new kitchen gadgets, reinventing new recipes, and revamping old, while documenting their experiences on social media (Doering, 2021). Journalists and researchers noticed this shift in people's relationship with food and eating during the COVID-19 pandemic and began looking into the trends and changes in habits from several different points of view (Matias et al., 2020; Doering, 2021; Lusk & McCluskey, 2020; Creswell, 2020).

One of the first trends that researchers analyzed was consumer purchasing behaviors. During the early weeks of the stay-at-home orders across the United States, grocery stores began seeing shoppers stockpile nonperishable goods because of the fear of not knowing when the next time they were going to be able to resupply their pantries or, worse, have a paycheck to purchase pantry items. Grocery providers saw a 90 percent increase in sales during the early quarantine period, with consumers stocking up on paper products, frozen foods, packaged foods, and meat (Lusk & McCluskey, 2020, p.11). This increase in panic buying can be attributed in part to the disruption of everyday eating practices. Before the COVID-19 pandemic, 54 percent of consumer food spending went towards meals purchased outside the home (Lusk & McCluskey, 2020). Consumers turned to home-cooked meals because of stay-at-home orders, and restaurants no longer provided full-service dining experiences. At the beginning of the lockdown, consumers turned to quick and comforting food items. In the year leading up to the pandemic, processed items such as Kraft Macaroni and Cheese and Hamburger Helper saw a decline in consumer purchases due to health-based trends towards fresh and organic food items (Creswell, 2020). After the CDC released their social distancing guidelines, comfort and convenience food brands saw a significant rise in demand. For example, Campbell's soup saw a 59 percent increase in sales compared to 2019 (Creswell, 2020).

Faced with uncertainty, consumers turned toward nonperishable products that provided them with a sense of comfort and nostalgia. Many of the items being purchased held emotional value rooted in childhood memories. Julie Creswell wrote an article for the *New York Times* over the shift in consumer diets. One respondent said, "One of the first things I grabbed was Kraft Easy Cheese, the disgusting orange stuff in a can. But it was one of the foods I ate growing up; it is a nostalgia thing" (Creswell, 2020). Another interviewee claimed, "I am eating ice cream, ice cream bars. Tonight, I am eating a spinach-artichoke lasagna, there is so much dairy in it, but I just need the comfort that I get from that food right now" (Creswell, 2020). Google data showed that from March 11, 2020, to August 20, 2020, there was more interest in cookies, ice cream, and burgers than interest in salads and veggies (Moreno, 2020). Overall, the trends in COVID-19 consumer habits reflected a need for comfort through food.

REVISITING CULINARY PRACTICES FROM THE GREAT DEPRESSION

Many people turned to classic recipes that originated in the Great Depression to save money, cook with limited ingredients, or even just enjoy the nostalgia factor of dishes cooked by their grandparents (Flynn, 2020). The trend toward restrictive and resourceful diets emerged during the early twentieth century (Viet, 2013). Research in nutritional science, progressive ideals, and the U.S. involvement in World War I came together to fundamentally change American thinking on food by developing a culture of self-control (Viet, 2013, p. 2). The modernization of the U.S. food culture solidified during the Great Depression when rationing and making do with whatever was on hand became crucial to survival. During this era, on the radio and in women's magazines, home economists taught women how to stretch their food budget with casseroles and meals like creamed chipped beef on toast or waffles, chili, macaroni and cheese, soups, and creamed chicken on a biscuit (Reinhardt & Ganzel, 2003). Home cooks had to become creative with their dishes because of the scarcity of staple pantry items like eggs, flour, and meat products. Depression recipes substituted rice and beans for meat as a way to integrate protein into diets. The dishes from this period were often simple fare that was easy to prepare, using canned and dried foods that did not require an icebox, let alone a refrigerator (Huffstetler, 2021). People who lived during the Great Depression internalized the eating habits needed to survive and created culinary knowledge transmitted to future generations through subtle culinary rituals. Paul Crenshaw's 2007 article "The Giving of Food" best describes the small ways that the children of the Great Depression manifested their relationship to food. The memory of not having enough to go around as a child lingered in Crenshaw's grandmother's memory and influenced her culinary practices (Crenshaw, 2007). The meals she prepared for her family as an adult were simple yet plentiful dishes that ensured everyone had enough to eat (Crenshaw, 2007). The subtle mannerism and use of food as a language of security was transmitted to the generation that followed the children of the 1930s and has reemerged as a stabilizing force in the eating practices present during the COVID-19 pandemic (Flynn, 2020).

PALATE MEMORY EATING AS AN EMBODIED AND SENSORY EXPERIENCE

The physical act of eating is an embodied experience rooted in sensory knowledge and a vital component in forming socio-political identities. The interconnection of food and identity that is passed down through generational eating practice is called palate memory. Palate memories are formed by the intimate bonds that individuals have during food preparation, such as a mother's cooking or frequently consuming various dishes and meals (Cuadra, 2013). This bond created with food speaks to and evokes memories and emotions, good and bad, fixations on flavors, taste, and at times sensations of estrangement (Cuadra, 2013, p. 2). Palate memories are often associated with an individual's ethnic background and the food consumed by their ancestors. When a child consumes dishes that hold cultural value, this culinary knowledge is transferred to the child and stored within their memory. This practice creates generational eating habits that contribute to the formation of identity through cultural capital that includes cuisine. Food is historical knowledge that is transmitted through the act of eating and inherently connects groups of people through a collective palate memory (Abarca, 2017). Food preferences, or in the case of the COVID-19 pandemic, what we chose to consume during times of crisis reflects a broader connection to our past that provided us with a sense of belonging and security. This desire for normalcy triggers a neurological response, which manifest as an individual's need to consume food items associated with their childhood (Creswell, 2020; Matias et al., 2020).

Palate memory is a system of knowledge stored in the body and reproduced through embodied sensory experiences. Through the habitual bodily movements in the act of watching, dicing, kneading, baking, serving, offering, and sharing food, culinary subjectivities are performed and displayed: embodied memory (Abarca, 2017, p. 7). Therefore, the act of preparing and eating a meal is not just a visceral act of nourishment but also a sub-cognitive representation of how we identify with members of our cultural and ethnic communities. Through the senses, the reproduction of unwritten recipes takes place with the sensory memory (Abarca, 2017, p. 34). The connection between smell and taste with emotions and memories lies within the amygdala (Shepard, 2012). When the senses encounter a familiar smell or taste, it will activate the amygdala and associated inferotemporal regions to evoke the emotions and memories tied to them (Shepard, 2012, p. 170). In this neurological process, sensory-based food memories become a depository of culinary knowledge, stored and reenacted through our generational eating habits (Abarca, 2017).

Although palate memory is a theory that connected modern eating practices to previous generations, it can also be used to alleviate feelings of isolation from one's community. Different dishes evoke sensory-based memories in this concept, and in the context of quarantine, partaking in these recipes can elicit feelings of togetherness while remaining within social distancing guidelines. The embodied and sensory experience tied to food creation and consumption can be a powerful mechanism rooted in communal identities both past and present.

NEW CULINARY QUARANTINE EXPERIMENTS: BRIDGING THE SOCIAL DISTANCE WITH FOOD

Memories of Betty Jean Miller's Potato Soup

Like many others, when the COVID-19 pandemic quarantine began, I became concerned about my family's access to food and purchasing enough sustainable items so we could stay at home for an extended period. I found myself referring back to my great-grandmother's culinary culture that she handed down to me, along with a beautiful set of cast-iron skillets. Betty Jean Miller was a child of the Depression and World War II, which contributed to her repertoire of resourceful meals that did not waste any food items she had at her disposal. I lived with my great-grandmother from my birth in 1992 until her death in 2011. Every homemade meal I ate as a child was provided to me by her. Most of my early childhood memories are with her in the kitchen, learning how to bake, cook, and preserve items from our garden. I learned how to stretch my food budget by having a pantry full of staple items that could be transformed into multiple dishes. I watched as my great-grandmother repurposed leftovers and created new meals for our family. This culinary knowledge is what I turned to when the shelves at my local grocery store ran low on stock. I walked down the aisles looking for items that could make hearty soups, stews, or casseroles that could be reheated and served until the dish was gone. This system of culinary knowledge from my great-grandmother's experience during the Great Depression was ingrained in her relationship with food, which she transmitted to me through her subtle practices and meal preparations (Crenshaw, 2007).

The food my great-grandmother prepared for me as a child provided me with a sense of comfort, and in the face of uncertainty, I turned to her dishes to find familiarity. One evening, as I scoured my pantry, figuring out what to feed my family, I remembered my favorite comfort food that my great-grandmother made for me as a child, potato soup. I gathered the potatoes, bacon, white onion, chicken broth, and cream from my pantry. I recalled the smell of black pepper dominating the air in the kitchen and how the steam coming from soup gave off an almost buttery aroma. Unlike most potato soups, my great-grandmother's soup was very thin in texture, almost brothy. Visually it was a plain dish, but what it lacked in visual appeal it made up with flavor. After reflecting on my great-grandma's cooking, I began working on dinner that night. As I chopped, sauteed, and boiled, a feeling of nostalgia came over me as I remembered how Grandma Betty used to make that very soup while I sat at her feet in the kitchen, usually getting in the way. When the soup was done, my father, Richard Ritt Sr., and I sat together at our kitchen table and savored the flavors of my grandmother's soup and the memory of her. At that moment, our household's isolation cohort did not feel so disconnected from the outside world as we reminisced on our family's culinary history.

The experience that my father I shared at our kitchen table was rooted in our neurological wiring. This is an example of how our brains respond to the taste and smell of familiar cuisine (Maslow, 1943). After my father and I shared potato soup and memories, I was inspired to create a quarantine experiment that combined my two passions, history and cooking. My kitchen during lockdown became an outlet for me to grapple with the underlying emotions I had associated with the COVID-19 pandemic. For other people their kitchens also represented a similar space of creative expression and searching for a sense of normalcy (Doering, 2021).

If, as palate memory suggests, cooking and eating can be used as a tool to connect the past to the present, food could also be used to reestablish a sense of communal identity during a global pandemic where isolation is the new norm. I hypothesized that adopting the kitchen practices of my socially distanced friends and family could be one creative way I could combat the feeling of isolation and bridge social distancing boundaries that challenged my sense of self during the COVID-19 pandemic. I asked the members of my household if they would assist me in this academic culinary adventure. My father, husband, and three children knew that it would involve eating and graciously agreed.

THE CULINARY HISTORY OF OKLAHOMANS

Before the COVID-19 social distancing restrictions, I worked on an oral history project that explored the culinary histories of Oklahomans. Interviewees detailed the culinary practices passed down from their ancestors and then invited me into their kitchens to teach me one of their favorite family recipes. These interviews were conducted with my friends and family. With the stay-at-home orders, I found these interviews to be an essential resource that allowed me to theoretically enter someone else's kitchen. Through eating cuisine associated with my friends and family, I engaged with their palate memories, which alleviated my psychological response to isolation and reestablished a sense of communal identity that helped me persevere through the COVID-19 pandemic.

Remembering James O. Lawson's Onion Burgers and Fries

I stumbled upon the resourcefulness of these oral histories through a conversation I had with my father. We began talking about how much we enjoyed my grandmother's soup which led to him reminiscing about the individuals in his life who had passed away. My father's best friend, Bishop James O. Lawson, Sr., became the focus of this conversation. Specifically, their Monday morning meetings at Panera and going out for lunch after church on Sundays, which was a consistent part of their routine since 2008. When Lawson passed away on September 19, 2019, this culinary and social practice in my father's life ceased to continue. Shortly after the death of Lawson, the COVID-19 pandemic reached the United States and caused churches, including my father and Lawson's congregation, to shut their doors. This period marked a significant time of upheaval and uncertainty in my father's life. In our conversation, he expressed that he had begun questioning his identity and wondering where he would fit within the new norms of society or even his own group. As I sat listening to my father, I searched for something to comfort him. I remembered that I had conducted an oral history interview with Lawson, and I offered this piece of history to my father to hear his friend's voice again. My father was surprised that I had not shared this information with him earlier and we proceeded to listen to the oral history of James O. Lawson Sr.

On March 14, 2019, I interviewed Lawson in Oklahoma City, Oklahoma. He described the community he grew up in and the food culture of Lawson Temple, his family's church in Stillwater, Oklahoma. Lawson was born on October 25, 1952, and grew-up in Stillwater. His father, Bishop Fred D. Lawson, Sr., operated the local Church of God in Christ congregation in the Southern Woods neighborhood, the African American section of the city. Segregation created an atmosphere where African Americans in Stillwater, and throughout the United States, had to rely on their ethnic enclave for support. Specifically, Black churches became religious, social, and political spaces for members of the African American community. Lawson believed the food ministry at his father's church was an essential tool in bringing people of diverse backgrounds together in Stillwater. Lawson described how onion burgers and hand-cut fries were served at the church as a fundraiser. The burgers, fries, and the different varieties of soda available at the church became a treat for members of the congregation and the surrounding community. Lawson remembered:

> Mother Abington she was superb with onions; she had those original onion burgers that stank up the whole town. She cooked so many hamburgers that people in the community would come out [to the church], and the hamburgers would cost a quarter. (J. Lawson, Interview, March 14, 2019)

Lawson further explained the process of making Mother Abington's burgers:

> Back in those days the way they cooked them; see they didn't have a fancy grill. They had an original old-style grill, and I don't remember what sauce she put on it, but I remember they would stick onions inside the meat, and the buns didn't come in until later. A lot of times, it was flat bread. You put the bread on [the grill] and toasted the bread, and then they would have some cheese in there. (J. Lawson, Interview, March 14, 2019)

As the interview progressed, Lawson's notorious sweet tooth began speaking when he said:

> Peach cobbler was off the charts; I will tell you one that really got me was rhubarb pie, the best pie I've ever eaten in my life. I don't know how they sweetened it, but it was the most! I've been trying to figure out who made that pie. (J. Lawson, Interview, March 14, 2019)

As Lawson described the food of his childhood, the sensory memories took over. He detailed the taste and smells as if he had just eaten those items making the interview a sensory experience in itself.

As my father and I finished listening to the oral history interview, we hungrily realized that we had to make onion burgers and hand-cut fries. I set up my laptop in the kitchen and turned-on Lawson's interview for the second time that evening and proceeded to engage in his culinary history. The smell of caramelized onions filled my kitchen as Lawson's voice described all of his favorite dishes growing up and how he envisioned his family's role in the community. My father rejoined my palate memory experience and reflected on his friend's food choices and the ministry they both loved. He expressed that my experiment helped him feel closer to his departed friend and his congregation that he missed due to social distancing restrictions.

Re-creating Graduation Gumbo and the Emotional Meaning of Beignets

The next interview I decided to work with was my longtime friend and godfather to my eldest child, Robert Harland. He grew up in Opelousas, Louisiana, and inherited creole cooking culture from his parents and grandparents. When asked what his favorite food was growing up, he responded:

> Whew, it is a list! My favorite then and now is still jambalaya. That is when you take chicken and sausage, and you know to mix it with rice, some people put shrimp in there, but I grew up on the chicken and sausage jambalaya (R. Harland, Interview, March 3, 2020).

Harland described how both men and women in his family cooked and took the time to teach him their culinary knowledge. His grandparents and father cooked Creole-style dishes while his mother leaned towards a more southern style. Harland recalled, "My dad made the best jambalaya. Oh, my lord, my grandmother made beignets, that is a French doughnut. She made things like collard greens and did a lot of different gumbos" (R. Harland, Interview, March 3, 2020). When asked about his mother, he stated, "she did a lot of the meatloaf, brisket, macaroni and cheese, and lasagna. That was her side of cooking; she was more like home cooking" (R. Harland, Interview, March 3, 2020). At the age of fourteen, Harland moved from Louisiana to Oklahoma. I asked him what the difference was between Oklahoma and Louisiana cooks. Harland chuckled and said, "We cook with more flavor, we have more heart in our cooking, we have different seasonings" (R. Harland, Interview, March 3, 2020). Curious, I asked what is this heart thing, what does it feel like? He responded:

> It is when you are in the kitchen, and you feel everything that you are doing. Like some people like to dance, like a ballet dancer who loves to dance, you are going to see the passion in the way she dances, and you are going to realize she is not just up there dancing, like a musician playing a piano or blowing a trumpet, it is the same as cooking. You will taste someone's food and be like yeah, they put some love in that pot. You know we don't rush things (R. Harland, Interview, March 3, 2020).

Harland's description of heart is an example of how cooking is an embodied experience. Throughout Harland's interview, his love of creole cooking culture resounded in his recollections and represented how culinary knowledge can create generational identities through food (Abarca, 2017). His personal style of cooking is the culmination of his ancestor's culinary practices that were taught to him by his family members. Currently, Harland is teaching his two daughters how to cook the dishes from his youth. This is an example of Abarca's concept of generational culinary knowledge and how it is passed down.

Harland's passion for cooking is one that he shares with anyone who enters his home. Growing up, Harland's flavor-packed dishes always ended up on my plate either at church potlucks or private dinners. For my high school graduation party, he cooked a pot of gumbo that I enjoyed and crave to this day. One evening I decided to recreate his gumbo using chicken and sausage but my attempt at making a roux failed. I added butter and flour to my cast-iron skillet and took my time. After thirty minutes, as Harland suggested in his interview, my roux looked and tasted unappealing. I gave up and decided to cook a frozen pizza. After dinner, my inner amateur chef would not let me surrender, and I remembered that I had a box of beignet mix from Café De Monde in my pantry that I purchased during a trip to New Orleans. After our interview on March 3, 2020, Harland took over my kitchen to make beignets and instructed me not to follow the directions on the box; instead of water, he added milk and little vanilla. He did not measure the ingredients with cups or tablespoons but by his senses. After failing to make a decent roux, I attempted to make beignets with my children as an apology for delaying dinner that evening. I mixed all the ingredients until the batter became an airy dough. I dropped a few beignets into a pot halfway full of hot cooking oil, baked them until they were golden brown, and dusted them with powdered sugar. My youngest daughter, Evelyn, made a mess with powdered sugar, and her older sister Jocelyn commented on how our kitchen smelled like the fair. The smell reminded me of walking around Jackson Square near Café De Monde with my husband in 2019, a time before travel restrictions. I recalled for my children the sights that I witnessed and played them jazz music like what I heard on the streets of New Orleans. I attempted to give the kids a pseudo cultural history lesson, but they were more interested in eating and talking about going back to the fair after the COVID-19 pandemic. We laughed and enjoyed eating beignets, which was also a part of Uncle Robert's culinary history. Harland's culinary knowledge was linked to his family's history but also a place. Louisiana is signified by its culture and food practices. Harland's interview and sharing his knowledge with me allowed me to bring the outside world into my own kitchen by utilizing distinct smells and sounds that evoked sensory memories of the fair or Jackson Square (Shepard, 2012).

What occurred that evening was rooted in my children's and my sensory memories and revealed how smells, sounds, and taste could elicit emotions associated with those places and expand our sense of space within confinement. My children associate the fair with interesting smells, sweet treats, and the feeling of happiness. This experience with food trigged those memories (Shepard, 2012). For me, I associate the taste and smells of beignets to a meaningful trip with my husband, which was something that we had put on our bucket list as teenagers. Memories associated with food and place can have powerful emotional connections that can be a source of comfort during periods of instability. My kitchen became a space that allowed me to transcend the lockdown by reliving culinary experiences through the tactile process of preparing and consuming food items that invoked palate memories of a time before social distancing.

Coulter Family Culinary Traditions

Leading up to Thanksgiving, my husband mentioned how he missed his family's holiday cooking that included greens, macaroni and cheese, and his favorite, neck bones. Collard greens and macaroni and cheese were two of my husband's favorite dishes that I had perfected, but neck-bones were a dish that I had always entrusted my mother-in-law to provide. Since we couldn't gather together this Thanksgiving, I decided to try to recreate my mother-in-law's neck bones as a part of my culinary experiment. Her list of ingredients included pork neck bones, red potatoes, onion, garlic powder, Cajun seasoning, salt, and pepper. No measurements, just the advice to make sure my water was well seasoned. In my kitchen, I repeated the mantra "what would mom do" as I searched my memory to recover how her neck bones tasted and smelled. My mother-in-law's dish contained a mixture of sweetness from the onions and a hint of spice from the Cajun seasoning that created a savory yet buttery feeling in my mouth.

From this memory of eating my mother-in-law's neck-bones, I seasoned until the flavor matched the one in my thoughts, but the real critic would be my husband. As we gathered around the dining room table for Thanksgiving dinner, I anticipated his first bite hoping that my attempt at recreating one of his mother's dishes would help him feel connected to his family, if only through the act of eating a food item from his childhood. To my surprise, the flavors were spot on, and the dish's similarities to what he remembered at his family's holiday dinners allowed for a discussion about our families' culinary history. Later that evening, I called my mother-in-law excited that I had successfully recreated one of her dishes. We talked about how she learned how to cook from her mother and that she was happy that someone in the next generation wanted to learn the family recipes. As my mother-in-law ended our conversation, she mentioned that my children always asked for sugar rice when they visited. She explained that this dish containing rice, butter, salt, and sugar was one of my husband's favorite breakfast items as a child. I could not help but laugh because that is the one dish my husband knows how to cook. Our children always request sugar rice on Saturday mornings when he is off work, and he gladly serves it to them. Sugar rice is a simple dish, yet it has become the childhood favorite of three generations in my husband's family. This event is an example of how palate memories are transmitted through everyday actions—no recipes but a sensory memory that guides the cooking process (Abarca, 2017).

Goulash, Good Wine, and Lifelong Girl Friends

As my experiment in testing the theories of palate memory and embodied food experiences evolved, I continued to search for recipes that held significant meaning for my family. For me, the one person I missed the most during quarantine was my best friend, Cheyenne. During our early teen years, we spent the majority of our time after school in the kitchen and frequently cooked dinner together. We sat around the dining room table to do homework as we waited for our parents to return home from work. The kitchen became a space where we developed our friendship dynamic and cultivated our sense of self as young adolescent girls. Cheyenne and I continued this tradition of cooking a savory meal and spending time with each other into our adulthood. When the CDC implemented stay-at-home guidelines, we stayed in our family bubbles to protect our immune-compromised parents. The absence of our shared meals together did not shake my identity but inherently made me feel disconnected from someone vital to my sense of community.

One dish that has become a staple in our meals together is goulash. As we came of age, we added a bottle, or two, of wine to accompany our meal depending on our collective level of stress. Cheyenne's rendition of goulash is her grandmother's recipe that called for crushed tomatoes, diced onions, hamburger meat, macaroni, and ranch-style beans instead of kidney beans because we are from Oklahoma.[1] Goulash was a simple dish that filled our stomachs growing up but I always associated it with one of my closest friends. Like my previous attempts to engage with palate memory theory, I entered my kitchen to transform staple pantry items into a meal that represented more than just something to eat. I put on my friend group's playlist and danced around my kitchen, listening to songs from our teenage years, prom, our twenty-first birthdays, baby showers, and weddings. I started by browning the ground beef with the onions, added the seasonings and then the remaining components. That evening I was heavy-handed on the garlic. The smell lingered in the air while the sauce simmered, and I knew it did not have the same fragrance as Cheyenne's goulash. I have never prepared it right in the fifteen years that Cheyenne and I have been friends; it just tastes better when she makes it. Although my attempt at goulash did not have to same umami as my friend's dish, the memories associated with goulash did provide me with comfort rooted in Cheyenne and my shared culinary history. Food based comfort is rooted in the memories associated with dishes that hold significant emotional capital in an individual's life (Shepard, 2012; Abarca, 2017; Cuadra, 2013). When preparing and consuming food items the brain responds to the familiar sensations and recalls the emotions linked to that food memory. In the case of goulash, I associate that dish with comfort because of the sentiments subconsciously tied to eating it with Cheyenne over the years. Food has become a significant component of my relationship with Cheyenne, much like my father and his late friend James O. Lawson. Eating practices within friend groups contribute to the development of communal identities and thus becomes a defining factor in one's sense of self (Fischler, 1988).

CULINARY KNOWLEDGE BEYOND THE QUARANTINE

The culinary knowledge stored within our bodies directly correlates to feelings of nostalgia. This biological response does not solely manifest during periods of uncertainty and isolation but also in every aspect of our culinary memory. The kitchen is a place to link past experiences with the present moment in a creative endeavor. Cooking enables us to recall sensory memories through the preparation process. The almost ritualistic dance between the panty, stove, and the kitchen table engages the subconscious in ways that unlocks not just feelings of comfort, but of joy and sadness as well. After the passing of my aunt, Karen Insolia, I craved chicken and dumplings, which was one of my favorite dishes that she made. I entered my kitchen a started cooking as way to cope with the grief I felt. Kneading the dough for the dumplings became tactile way to grappling with the emotions I was processing. Food nostalgia is also linked to feelings of joy. Every year at Christmas I attempt to re-create Portillo's Italian beef sandwich recipe because it makes my dad happy and helps him recall his childhood in Chicago.[2] My father is proud of being from Chicago, much like Harland is proud of being from Louisiana. Both of these men claim cultural capital in the culinary heritage from the places they grew up and use it as signifiers of their identity. Understanding culinary knowledge as an embodied experience rooted in our neurological formation of memories allows for broader conversations regarding the role of food in the development of communal and individual identities.

The COVID-19 pandemic disrupted the everyday flow of society and created social voids in people's lives. A significant aspect of an individual's sense of community revolves around the food practices that defines their identity. The risk of food insecurity and restrictions on communal eating challenged people to find new methods of supplementing their culinary norms by revisiting old practices and trying new ones within their homes. Kitchens during lockdown represented a transformative space for creative culinary exploration and grappling with new social structures. Early researchers found that consumers turned to food as a source of comfort during the COVID-19 pandemic. In my own attempt to acclimate to the new social distancing protocols, I explored the interconnections of food and identity within the concept of palate memory in the hope to reestablishment my sense of community. Through the adoption of culinary knowledge shared with me by my friends and family, I found that the sensory act of preparing and eating a meal alleviated the feeling of disconnection through memories linked to emotions (Shepard, 2007). Scientists and food historians suggest that eating is an embodied experience that links ancestorial food habits to present practices, but I suggest that understanding the importance of communal food practices will allow us to better understand our current interpersonal relationships and the identities that form within these dynamics. As I reflect on the shift in consumer's relationship with food during COVID-19 pandemic and my own culinary journey, I am curious how this event will impact food practices going forward. I believe that much like our grandparents and great-grandparents, who lived through the Great Depression, we will continue to view food as a source of stability and comfort. I also look forward to teaching my children, and grandchildren, how sharing a meal can be a meaningful tool in developing bonds with the people around them.

REFERENCES

Abarca, M.E. (2017). Afro-Latina/os culinary subjectivities: Rooting ethnicities through root vegetables. In M. Garcia, E. Melanie Dupuis, & D. Mitchell (Eds.), *Food across border* (pp. 24–43). Rutgers University Press.

Brillat-Savarin, J. A. (2009). *The physiology of taste: For meditations of transcendental Gastronomy*. (F. Robinson, Trans.). Everyman's Library. (Original work published in 1825).

Crenshaw, P. (2007). The giving food. *Southwest Review*, *92(2)*,262–270. http://www.jstor.org/stable/43472811.

Creswell, J. (2020, April 7). I just need comfort: Processes foods make a pandemic comeback *New York Times*. https://www.nytimes.com/2020/04/07/business/coronavirus-processed-foods.html.

Cuadra, C. M. O. (2013). *Eating Puerto Rico: A history of food, culture, and identity*. University of North Carolina Press.

Doering, C. (2021, April 6). Many at-home trends adopted during COVID-19 to remain after pandemic, Nestle says. *Food Dive*. https://www.fooddive.com/news/many-at-home-trends-adopted-during-covid-19-to-remain-after-pandemic-nestl/597825/.

Fischler, C. (1988). Food self and identity. *Social Science Information*, *27*, 275–92. https://doi.org/10.1177/053901888027002005.

Flynn, C. (2020, May 29). 15 depression-era foods you won't believe are making a comeback. *Eat This Not That*. https://www.eatthis.com/depression-erafoods.

Gunderson, C., Hake, M., & Dewey, A. (2021). Food insecurity during COVID-19. *Applied Economic Perspective and Policy. 1(43*), 153–61. https://doi.org/10.1002/aepp.13100.

Huffstetler, P. (2021, May 17). The great depression era recipes. *The Spruce Eats*. https://www.thespruceeats.com/depression-era-recipes-1388459.

Gunderson, C., Hake, M., & Dewey, A. (2021). Food insecurity during COVID-19. *Applied Economic Perspective and Policy. 1(43*), 153–61. https://doi.org/10.1002/aepp.13100.

Lusk, J. & McCluskey, J.J. (2020). Consumer behavior during the pandemic. *CAST Commentary Economic Impacts of COVID-19 on Food and Agricultural Markets*, 11–13. https://www.cast-science.org/wp-content/uploads/2020/06/QTA2020-3-COVID-Impacts.pdf.

Maslow A.H. (1943). A theory of human motivation. *Psychological Review. (50)4*, 376–396.

Matias, T., Domoniski, F.H.,& Marks, D.F. (2020). Human needs in COVID-19 isolation. *Journal of Health Psychology*. 25(7), 871–882. https://doi.org/10.1177/1359105320925149.

Moreno, J. (2020, August 31). Google trends show comfort food has dominated COVID-19 diets. *Forbes*. https://www.forbes.com/sites/johanmoreno/2020/08/31/google-trends-show-comfort-food-has-dominated-covid-19-diets/?sh=480ea07232c7.

Reinhardt, C., & Ganzel, B. (2003). Feeding the family, *Wessels Living History Farm*. https://livinghistoryfarm.org/farminginthe30s/life_04.html.

Shepard, G. (2012). *Neurogastronomy: How the brain creates flavor and why it matters*. Columbia University Press.

Viet, H. Z. (2013). *Modern food, moral food: Self-control, science, and the rise of modern American eating in the early twentieth century.* University of North Carolina Press.

Wallach, J. J. (2019). *Every nation has its dish: Black bodies and black food in twentieth century America.* University of North Carolina Press.

NOTES

1. Ranch-style bean are pinto beans in a spicy sauce. The brand that Cheyenne and I use is called "Ranch Style Beans" with the catchphrase "real western flavor."

2. Portillo's is a restaurant chain founded in Villa Park, Illinois, in 1963. One of their specialties is the Chicago-style Italian beef sandwich. This dish is thinly sliced beef served on Italian bread and dipped in au jus. This sandwich is often served with sweet peppers.

Chapter Fifteen

The Escapism and Social Bond of Pandemic Binge Watching

Gwendelyn S. Nisbett, Stephanie Schartel Dunn, and Newly Paul

There's a certain cozy comfort in sitting down for a long TV binge session. You grab your favorite seat on the sofa, wrap up in a fuzzy blanket, and settle in for hours of escape into another world and another reality. Maybe you pick a show you know by heart; maybe it's the latest season of a new favorite. Occasionally, you get sucked into watching something completely outrageous. Your friends beckon over social media: *You HAVE to watch it . . . you're not gonna believe this stuff!* They send video clips of a colorful character singing to tigers—"I saw a tiger, and the tiger saw a man," he bellows. The show is a bit like a train wreck that you cannot look away from, leaving you a little bit disquieted and completely enraptured.

Tuning into Netflix's *Tiger King,* audiences were introduced to a cast of wacky characters and their outrageous antics. The show was a slow burn hit, with audience social media buzz creating the eventual avalanche of viewers for what *Vulture* dubbed a "WTF-filled docuseries" (Adalian, 2020). Within ten days of being released on Netflix, 34 million viewers had watched the docu-series (Clark, 2020).

Tiger King landed in our binge lists at the height of the pandemic lockdown, when many found themselves oscillating between the terror of the situation and the boredom of idleness. We knew little about COVID-19 spreading across the globe, other than it was deadly and we needed to stay socially distant from the people around us. It was a bit like a weeks-long snow day, with a morbid edge. Not surprisingly, many opted to binge endless hours of television (Feldman, 2020), from news conferences to reality television and from old favorites, like *Golden Girls,* to feel-good newcomers like *Ted Lasso*.

Vorderer et al. (2004) argue that people seek out entertainment for many reasons, including stimulation, as a form of escape, and to feel better about one's current situation. Bingeing meets many of the needs.

This chapter explores viewer reactions to one of the break-out hits of the pandemic binge season—Netflix's *Tiger King* (Hersko, 2020). Using viewer response data during the spring 2020 lockdown, we examine bingeing motivations, the potential for watching as an escape from pandemic stresses, and possible reasons for the show's popularity. Of particular interest was whether the buzz generated by the show, and the subsequent social sharing of clips and memes, was a product of a desire to connect and share during the early days of the pandemic.

Research suggests that binge watching surged during the pandemic (Dixit et al., 2020) and people sought out bingeing as a coping mechanism (Boursier et al., 2021). A marketing survey among U.S. adults found that about 71 percent had subscribed to a new streaming service during the pandemic, and nearly 50 percent got a new television set (2021 Streaming Habits Survey, n.d.). Americans spent an average of nine more hours watching TV per week in May 2020 than they did in early March the same year (Pevos, 2020). Media reports indicated that people were choosing to binge on reality shows (Syfret, 2021) and past seasons of popular shows such as *The Office* or *Game of Thrones* (Giorgis, 2020). Media streaming platform Netflix experienced a rise in viewership during the COVID-19 pandemic, with documentaries and reality programming frequently being binge watched by audiences (Feldman, 2020).

Binge watching is defined by Castro et al. (2021) as "the self-determined consumption of multiple episodes of a serialized show consecutively" (p. 5). Binge behaviors are associated with time-consuming, extremely repetitive activities (Sung et al., 2018). The idea of multiple episodes depends on the source of the definition. For example, while Netflix defines binge watching as consuming two to six episodes of a given show in one go, others have defined it as watching more than one episode of a show "in a single sitting at one's own time and pace" (Merikivi et al., 2020, p. 6). Audience control over the specific programs viewed and the timing of such media consumption is relatively new and rose in popularity along with the rise of content streaming services (Terfertiller & Conlin Maxwell, 2018). As such, there is limited research about binge watching (Vaterlaus et al., 2018; Starosta & Izydorczyk, 2020). The study of how binge watching is used to cope with stress and escape from stressors, especially in response to the COVID-19 pandemic is particularly novel. Though the situation itself is unique, understanding audiences' use of binge watching to escape from everyday stress allows media creators and researchers valuable insights on behavioral motivation.

Uses and Gratifications (U&G) and the concept of narrative transportation give us a lens to explore motivations for binge watching during the pandemic. U&G suggests audience members select media for a specific purpose depending on their individual needs (Katz et al., 1973). The phenomenon of narrative transportation, an audience's ability to become enthralled with a narrative, is a mechanism for maintaining feelings of escape.

UNDERSTANDING BINGE WATCHING USES AND GRATIFICATIONS AND NARRATIVE TRANSPORTATION

Binge watching can be driven by emotional needs such as the need to feel excitement or the need to control one's emotions (Rubenking & Bracken, 2018). Binge watching is also known to influence a person's affective state. For example, comedy, sci-fi, and drama genres are known to increase positive affect (Castro et al., 2021). While some consider binge watching to be a waste of time, others see it as a restorative experience that helps people recharge their minds (Pang, 2014). According to Pang (2014), shows that have intricate plots whose details get revealed throughout the season, and those that feature strong characters inhabiting a fascinating world are likely to encourage binge watching. People may choose to binge watch alone to get rid of loneliness or watch shows in the company of other people (Pittman & Tefertiller, 2015), but overall, they attribute positive feelings toward binge watching and perceive it as a kind of reward for their struggles (Feeney, 2014). Watching shows together helps couples share a social identity. This strengthens the relationship and makes couples feel closer to each other (Gomillion et al., 2017). The few studies that have examined binge watching in the context of COVID-19 in particular have found that certain emotional states are likely to trigger binge-watching behavior. For example, Boursier et al. (2021) conducted a survey among Italian respondents during the pandemic and found that women who reported feeling more anxious and stressed than men were more likely to watch television, and their binge-watching behavior was motivated by a need for escapism. The motivations of binge watching differ depending on unique individual qualities. Shim & Kim (2018) found that people tend to binge watch shows that are recommended by others, and high sensation seekers are more likely to indulge in binge-watching behaviors.

Loneliness and depression, both feelings commonly experienced during the pandemic, are predictors of binge behaviors (LaRose & Eastin, 2004; Sung et al., 2018). Studies suggest escapism via binge watching is more likely when individuals are facing stressful situations (Leppink et al., 2016). Indeed, some argued during the pandemic, that bingeing a show was a positive experience

(Pierce-Grove, 2020). In 2020, the pandemic presented many with the perfect opportunity to tackle their binge to-do list, catching up on past seasons that they had missed (Giorgis, 2020). One British show, BBC's *Staged*, embraced the awkward detachment of the social distancing and teleconferencing to work. The show allowed the audience to commiserate with the boredom of being stuck at home and feeling uninspired to get much done. Other shows, like Netflix's *Tiger King*, were so unique they tapped into the audience's desire to escape.

While binge watching as a cultural phenomenon had developed in pre-pandemic times, it took on a special importance during the pandemic. Media outlets reported on plenty of examples of binge watching during the pandemic, and many of these exemplify U&G theory in context. According to a *Forbes* article by Feldman (2020), the pandemic inspired people to binge watch foreign language shows, documentaries, reality TV, and romance shows. Feldman argued that as a result of being asked to isolate at home, people chose to watch foreign language shows that depicted faraway lands and allowed them to travel through their screens. She wrote viewing numbers for such shows rose by more than 50 percent as compared to 2019. In addition to shows depicting faraway lands, documentaries, including *Tiger King* and *Killer Inside: The Mind of Aaron Hernandez,* were among the most-watched media categories on Netflix. Feldman theorized that people watched these types of shows, about faraway places or lives most audiences cannot imagine living, to escape the "hardship and sadness" (Feldman, 2020) brought on by the pandemic. People opted for comedies, especially during the election season in October and November, to escape the politics of the presidential elections.

Interestingly, when Netflix rolled out its new lineup of movies to stream on March 1, 2020, *Outbreak*, a 1995 movie about a virus causing havoc in a small town in California, quickly became one of the top 10 most-watched movies in the country. Another movie called *Contagion*, which was based on a similar topic, also ranked among the top 10 movies in the country in March. Pandemic-related movies were popular because though they created a sense of terror and fear among viewers, these emotions could be controlled—the shows could be paused or fast-forwarded, which viewers found reassuring. Pandemic-related shows also helped audiences visualize the pandemic and prepare for it, while reminding them about the resilience of humans (Kelly, 2020).

Others wrote about pandemic viewing choices being guided by a yearning for escaping into simpler times; the shows acted as a "balm for the unrelenting sameness of daily life" and as an "anchor" (Giorgis, 2020) that prevented people from being swept away. Burbank (2020) theorized that audiences who were escaping into binge watching reruns of their favorite television shows were having a "natural response to COVID-19." According to Burbank, the option to binge watch was brought on by a combination of an endless choice of streaming titles provided by media platforms and the need to escape from decision-making and risk-taking. In such cases, an escape into familiar shows and genres was a way of escaping into friendly territory and exerting control over the unknown because people tended to remember the ins and outs of the shows they had already watched. *Tiger King* is an example of this friendly territory viewing in that it follows the formulaic pattern of the ever-popular true crime genre.

Uses and gratifications suggests that audiences seek out media to fulfill specific needs (Katz et al., 1973). Katz argued that U&G theory was related to the social and psychological origins of needs, which generate expectations of the mass media or other sources, which lead to differential patterns of media exposure (or engagement in other activities), resulting in need gratifications and other consequences, perhaps mostly unintended ones. (p. 510). U&G theory posits that audiences achieve gratification or satisfaction when they access media services and offerings that match their expectations. Thus, the theory highlights the role of individuals' motivations in media choice, with the end goal of satisfying their needs (Rubin, 2009).

Over time, researchers have adapted U&G theory to include changes in entertainment media and audience behaviors. For example, Sundar & Limperos (2013) posited that new media platforms offer alternatives to the traditional model of television viewing and this can affect viewership patterns. These new media affordances include second screening, and features that improve the interactivity and navigability of the media viewing platforms, which could encourage binge watching.

Scholarly research using U&G theory shows that people have several different motivations for watching television, online media, and binge watching in particular. Television viewing is motivated by the need to relax and escape, work through real-life struggles, pass time, inform oneself, watch out of habit, and to feel socially connected (Papacharissi & Mendelson, 2007). Online viewing is fueled by convenience and ease of access to entertainment (Haridakis & Hanson, 2009). Binge watching behavior is fueled by a need to catch up, relax, feel a sense of completion and cultural inclusion, feel excitement, and enjoy the narrative immersion provided by the availability of full seasons of a show instead of the week-by-week release common to broadcast television (Steiner & Xu, 2020; Zuckerman, 2014).

Regardless of the motivations for media consumption, an audience member can become transported by the narrative. Getting caught up in a great story is narrative transportation (Green et al., 2004). Narrative transportation begins with engagement in the narrative or media source. Engagement refers to the amount of focused attention an audience member expends on a particular media source (Green et al., 2004). Narrative engagement has been studied in a variety of contexts including reading (Gerrig, 1993), television and film (Riddle, 2013), and even social media posts (Nisbett & Schartel Dunn, 2019).

Depending on the level of engagement with the narrative depicted, an audience may even lose full perception of reality (Van Laer et al., 2014). Even if reality is not fully blurred, focusing on non-real-world events can offer audiences a desired escape. Audiences may become so engrossed in the story they focus more on the fictional world than the real world (Green et al., 2004). As discussed above, escaping from reality is one motivator audiences have for media use: therefore, audiences are likely to select engaging narratives in stressful times. The early weeks of the COVID-19 pandemic were particularly stressful for most people, so audiences were more likely to select narratives that could mentally transport them from the pressures of their current situation.

Part of the appeal of binge watching a show involves escaping reality for a period of time via narrative transportation. Because narrative transportation occurs when an audience member becomes absorbed in a narrative, prolonged viewing may increase the likelihood that an audience member will become transported by the narrative. Binge watching audiences have reported feelings of being engrossed in the storyline (Petersen, 2016). Being enthralled in a narrative allows for escapism, even momentarily, from reality. When this desired escapism is achieved, audiences learn they are able to "get away" from reality by engaging in narrative. Escapism, especially during the COVID-19 pandemic, is a goal for many media audiences. Once audience members identify stories or programs that enabled them to transport into the narrative, this frequently leads to increased television watching. Warren (2020) looked specifically at the relationship between narrative transportation and binge television watching. In this longitudinal study, findings suggest both frequency of viewing and length of time spent viewing a program both contributed to likelihood of narrative transportation.

CASE STUDY: BINGE WATCHING NETFLIX'S *TIGER KING*

Tiger King was a relatively short (just seven episodes released simultaneously and a later-added "Tell All") docu-series released March 20, 2020 on Netflix. The first episode follows the show's central character, Joe Exotic, and gives viewers a glimpse of his life and the history of the Greater Wynnewood Exotic Animal Park, where big cats, primarily tigers, are raised. Subsequent episodes introduce owners of similar animal facilities and details of their out-of-the-ordinary lifestyles. The show focuses on one of these owners,

Carole Baskin, who is in a long-term feud with Joe Exotic about their competing zoos and their styles of working with animals. Most of the remaining episodes explore the possibility of criminal actions taken by the pair, culminating in the accusation (and prosecution) of Joe Exotic for hiring a hitman to kill Carole Baskin. Throughout the seven episodes situations become increasingly bizarre (suspicious circumstances around deaths of Carole's multiple husbands and Joe's campaign for political office) and distant from the average person's lifestyle (staff consuming truckloads of expired meat from local grocery stores and zoo owners with harems of women). Oddly enough, much of the buzz about the show centered on the cast's outlandish behavior, rather eclipsing the animal rights issues brought up by the filmmakers.

Inspired by the popularity of *Tiger King*, we recruited feedback from viewers across the country to share about binge watching. Using a snowball-sample survey (using Qualtrics survey software) shared through social media networks, 312 respondents answered questions about how they were feeling during the pandemic, their bingeing habits, and reactions to *Tiger King*. Data was collected between April 6 and May 7 while the show was enjoying viral popularity.

The participant sample was composed of 73.4 percent individuals identifying as females, 26 percent identifying as males, and .6 percent identifying as non-binary. The mean age among respondents was 33.86 years (SD= 14.84). Ethnicities represented included 74.8 percent White, 7.1 percent Black/African American, 3.5 percent Asian, 8.1 percent Hispanic/Latinx, 2.3 percent Native American, and 4.2 percent mixed/other. Of the participants, 12.5 percent self-reported as Hispanic/Latinx (regardless of race).

In the survey, respondents answered a series of questions concerning their media-inspired transportation, escapism, views on the pandemic, and their reaction to watching *Tiger King*. Data included both quantitative and qualitative responses. Descriptive quantitative responses as well as a thematic analysis of the qualitative responses fell into two main themes: distraction/escapism and staying connected with others. These themes are in line with existing research related to binge watching—entertainment, social connection, and escapism have all been previously linked to binge watching behaviors (Sung et al., 2018; Laor, 2020).

Theme: Distraction and Escapism

One major theme to emerge in the data was watching the show as a distraction from the pandemic and escape from pandemic stress. When asked if they viewed the show to escape news about COVID-19, a majority somewhat agreed (42.3 percent) or strongly agreed (31.8 percent). Participants also reported that the show allowed them to think about something other than the dire pandemic news. A majority of participants reported thinking less about the news while watching the show (39.3 percent somewhat agreed and 28.9 percent strongly agreed).

One respondent reported wanting "non-Coronavirus entertainment" while another suggested watching *Tiger King* would "help take people's minds off the global pandemic." While people sat home, they watched a strange new world unfold where a set of oddball tiger zoo owners became the rulers of their tiny fiefdoms of true believers and desperate hangers on. This theme falls in line with narrative transportation research that finds when people get sucked into a show there is a link with feelings of escapism (Irimiás, Mitev, & Michalkó, 2021). Narrative transportation was also present in this theme as people cited getting sucked into the "train wreck" world present in the show. A respondent noted, "The people are characters so removed from most people's own experiences that it is as if it were fiction." As if running big cat zoos wasn't strange enough, the show eventually revolved around an outrageous feud between Joe and Carole resulting in a murder-for-hire plot. Another shared, "it is hard to believe they exist in my reality." A respondent summed up watching the show as "a mix of sensationalism, because the people in the show are soap opera levels of over the top, but I also think it's an escapism from all of the garbage going on in the world right now."

Above and beyond escapism and distraction, watching for entertainment value was a major sub-theme which falls in line with U&G research. As one respondent stated, *Tiger King* was interesting because of the "twist of stories, the complex and unique characters, the fantasy of it all." Another noted, "all of the characters seem like they're from a wild fiction novel." For instance, the primary narrative of the show involves Joe and Carole harassing each other all the while he was allegedly plotting to have her killed off. At the periphery, Carole's husband loyally did her bidding, and Joe's two husbands led a ragtag band of tiger wranglers. Many noted that the show was fascinating because it was such a departure from their everyday lives. One respondent called it "a window into an unknown world."

Theme: Staying Connected with Others

Another prevalent theme to emerge from the data suggests people participated in pandemic binge watching as a way to connect with others. Sharing memes was a major component of the *Tiger King* bingeing experience. An example of the memes referenced how wild both the show and the pandemic were, saying "If 2020 were a person" pasted over a photo of Joe and his tiger. Another example showed Joe in a crown, sitting on a throne, with a tiger nearby with "me when I get my government stimulus check" written at the bottom.

People cited wanting to distract others and bring levity to a dark time. As one respondent noted, they wanted to "help take people's minds off the global pandemic." Similarly, others wanted to laugh and help others laugh, as one respondent stated, "it's just a good laugh in a time we all need to laugh." Viewers particularly liked laughing at Joe's music videos, especially the one alluding to the rumor that Carole chopped up her ex-husband and fed him to tigers. Another respondent offered:

> My motivation has mostly been to get friends to laugh, to make fun of our nearby wild safari, and to get more friends to watch the show so we can talk about it and have some social interaction so I don't go stir crazy from social isolation.

Some spoke as though they wanted to suck people into the show so they could have something to chat about that did not revolve around COVID-19. One respondent explained they wanted to "make people smile and laugh, but more so to continue the social bond people who have watched the show share." Moreover, people seemed to enjoy getting caught up in a show that everyone was caught up in. One respondent noted that "we need a positive shared experience. People miss shared experiences."

People also cited the viral popularity of the show as a major reason for watching and a bonding point with other people. One respondent noted, "I'm bored in the house and everyone was talking about it" taking note of the isolation and boredom that came along with pandemic stay-at-home orders. People shared meme after meme quoting Joe complaining about "that b*tch Carole Baskin" and the audience even started jokingly blaming the pandemic on Carole as well. Another stated they "couldn't escape it—everyone was talking about it all the time." Others loved that the show was so popular, as one said they were "continually enjoying the phenomenon." Other respondents noted having "a bit of FOMO" and "I guess it's fun to have inside jokes with people who have watched it."

Tiger King & Pandemic Bingeing Reflections

The pandemic presented a unique opportunity to study bingeing and the need for escapism that made shows such as *Tiger King* so popular. The content of the show combined with the timing of its release, along with the buzz surrounding the show, made it a binge-worthy watch. U&G suggests media consumption allows consumers to satisfy both social and psychological needs (Ruggiero, 2000), and individuals are generally aware of their needs and select media in accordance with their needs (Lin, 1999; Laor, 2020). Studies suggest television viewing is frequently selected for relaxation, escapism, entertainment, and social need fulfillment (Rubin, 1983). *Tiger King* entertained audiences and helped people deal with boredom and anxiety during the quarantine. The characters were engrossing with their true-crime lifestyles and invited strong opinions (about everything from animal rights to Carole's social media videos to Joe's many husbands) which provided fodder for discussion on social media and interpersonal communication with family and friends.

Though some studies have suggested individuals use binge watching simply to pass time (Sung et al., 2018) or alleviate boredom (Vaterlaus et al., 2018), other studies suggest there may be deeper motivations or uses of binge watching (Flayelle et al., 2019; Panda & Pandey, 2017). Our data suggests people focused on the COVID-19 pandemic as a source of stress and sought out binge watching shows to escape. This is in line with previous research by Panda and Pandey (2017) who found respondents to be motivated to binge watch for social reasons and to escape reality.

A psychological exploration of binge motivations by Flayelle et al. (2019), found many factors including emotion, pleasure seeking, social aspects, and escapism. Binge watching, especially when motivated by escapism, allows audience members to distract themselves from elements of the real world (West, 2014). Our findings suggest escapism was a primary motivator for watching *Tiger King*. Respondents reported being deeply transported into the bizarre plotlines of the characters' petty crimes and animal exploits to the point they were able to forget about the pandemic (at least for a few hours). As an audience member becomes more absorbed in the narrative they are watching, especially during periods of prolonged viewership, their ability to escape into the narrative becomes stronger. Our data also suggests that the show not only worked as a form of narrative transportation during viewing, but also lead to recalling the narrative later and using is as a source of interpersonal bonding.

During the COVID-19 pandemic, nearly everyone found themselves in a more isolated, stressful situation, leading to different needs to fulfill. Media consumers are aware of their needs and select those media options that best suit their needs—including binge watching (Vaterlaus et al., 2018). Our case study found that people were bingeing to escape, but also bingeing to partake in a shared experience. Many found the characters and storylines in *Tiger King* to be way outside their everyday lives, so the show transported them to a weird and wacky world. Not only did the show profile big cat owners, it also profiled odd characters that found their way into the big cat lifestyle (either out of curiosity or desperation). The outlandish quality of the show also inspired interpersonal and social media sharing as a way to bond. People quoted the show and created memes to share with friends. Indeed, ratings data found that the show was not an instant hit, rather it began to take off when people starting sharing about it and generating buzz (Adalian, 2020).

We argue that *Tiger King* was a unique bingeing phenomenon and question whether the show would have had the same impact during a non-pandemic period. Study participants seemed to really enjoy the interactivity and buzz around the show because it allowed them to feel a part of something bigger than themselves. In a sense, they were craving human bonding that the pandemic stripped away and *Tiger King* was a great excuse to reach out, laugh about a meme, and share your "did you see that" moments. One such moment focused on a scene when Joe dressed up as a large stuffed animal to protest outside of Carole's zoo, further exacerbating their feud. Another moment included one of Joe's music videos that showed a Carole lookalike feeding chunks of meat to tigers, prompting the audience to wonder about the rumors surrounding her ex-husband's death. Some people even found Joe's music videos kind of catchy and started sharing them on social media.

CONCLUSIONS AND FUTURE RESEARCH

This chapter focused on how people sought comfort during the pandemic through engaging with pop culture content. Specifically, we looked at how people used binge watching as a coping mechanism, to seek comfort, and to bond with other people (especially those who were socially distant). Even though binge watching is often thought about in pejorative terms, bingeing during the pandemic was an important coping mechanism. People needed to take their minds off a virus that they did not understand and could not control. Study data suggests that one of the possible motivations and outcomes of bingeing is that it allowed people to transport to another world and become engrossed in fascinating stories. Many study respondents reported both being transported in the narrative and appreciating not thinking about the pandemic for a while.

Perhaps the most interesting finding focused on bingeing in order to bond with others. In a very viral sense, people heard about the show from friends and wanted to share in the collective experience. Bingeing helped many stay connected with friends and family and allowed us to take our minds off the stress of the pandemic. Even though the show was a silly and salacious way to pass the time, in a very real way it provided comfort during a very dark period. The implications of this study are not limited to pandemic television viewing; everyone has seasons in life that are more difficult than others. Understanding the role binge watching plays in coping with stressful situations allows for media creators to assess audience needs and allows individuals to recognize binge watching as a potential tool to cope.

As with any study, there were a few limitations. The study used snowball convenience sampling, so the participant pool ended up being slightly more homogenous than is ideal. Though a lab setting was not possible, especially during the early part of the pandemic, having a more immediate reaction to the show from respondents might provide more robust findings as people may have forgotten elements of their viewing motivations and how they responded initially to the show. Similarly, a longitudinal study such as was used by Warren (2020), tracking audience behavior and response, would be most ideal for future binge-watching studies. Future research should explore how binge watching is used by audiences to distract from a variety of stressful situations.

REFERENCES

Adalian, J. (2020, April 9). Tiger King is a gigantic hit for Netflix. *Vulture*. Retrieved from https://www.vulture.com/2020/04/tiger-king-ratings-netflix.html.

Boursier, V., Musetti, A., Gioia, F., Flayelle, M. V., Billieux, J. L., & Schimmenti, A. (2021). Is watching TV series an adaptive coping strategy during the COVID-19 pandemic? Insights from an Italian community sample. *Frontiers in Psychiatry*, NA. https://link.gale.com/apps/doc/A659204666/HRCA?u=txshracd2679&sid=HRCA&xid=0b52042e.

Burbank, M. (2020, September 1). Are you binge-watching reruns of your old favorite TV shows? You're having a natural response to COVID-19. *The Seattle Times*. Retrieved from https://www.chicagotribune.com/entertainment/tv/ct-ent-tv-show-reruns-coronavirus-20200901-tuuvm44fhzgl5k2tgrzssufxue-story.html.

Castro, D., Rigby, J. M., Cabral, D., & Nisi, V. (2021). The binge-watcher's journey: Investigating motivations, contexts, and affective states surrounding Netflix viewing. *Convergence, 27*(1), 3–20. https://doi.org/10.1177/1354856519890856.

Clark, T. (2020, April 8). Netflix's *Tiger King* was watched by 34 million viewers in the US in 10 days, according to Nielsen. *Business Insider.* https://www.businessinsider.com/netflixs-tiger-king-watched-by-34-million-viewers-2020-4#:~:text=Netflix's%20'Tiger%20King'%20watched%20by,in%20US%3A%20Nielsen%20%2D%20Business%20Insider.

Dixit, A., Marthoenis, M., Arafat, S.M.Y., Sharma, P., & Kar, S. K. (2020). Binge watching behavior during COVID 19 pandemic: A cross-sectional, cross-national online survey.*Psychiatry Research*, 289, 113089. https://doi.org/10.1016/j.psychres.2020.113089.

Feeney, N. (February, 18, 2014). When, exactly, does watching a lot of Netflix become a 'binge'? *Atlantic*. Retrieved from http://www.theatlantic.com/entertainment/archive/ 2014/02/ when-exactly-does-watching-a-lot-of-netflix-become-a-binge/283844/.

Feldman, D. (2020). Here's what we watched on Netflix in 2020 to escape the pandemic. *Forbes.* Retrieved from https://www.forbes.com/sites/danafeldman/2020/12/10/netflix-allowed-us-to-escape-2020-at-home-in-lockdown-heres-what-the-streamer-says-we-watched/?sh=15ac87811d2d.

Flayelle, M., Canale, N., Vögele, C., Karila, L., Maurage, P., & Billieux, J. (2019). Assessing binge-watching behaviors: Development and validation of the "Watching TV Series Motives" and "Binge-watching Engagement and Symptoms" questionnaires. *Computers in Human Behavior*, 90, 26–36. https://doi.org/10.1016/j.chb.2018.08.022.

Gerrig, R. J. (1993). *Experiencing narrative worlds: On the psychological activities of reading*. Yale University Press.

Giorgis, H. (2020, December 17). The year of ambitious TV watching. *The Atlantic.* Retrieved from https://www.theatlantic.com/culture/archive/2020/12/year-ambitious-tv-watching/617417/.

Gomillion, S., Gabriel, S., Kawakami, K., & Young, A. F. (2017). Let's stay home and watch TV: The benefits of shared media use for close relationships. *Journal of Social and Personal Relationships*, *34*(6), 855–874. https://doi.org/10.1177/0265407516660388.

Green, M. C., Brock, T. C., & Kaufman, G. E. (2004). Understanding media enjoyment: The role of transportation into narrative worlds. *Communication Theory, 14*, 311–327. https://doi.org/10.1111/j.1468-2885.2004.tb00317.x.

Haridakis, P., & Hanson, G. (2009). Social interaction and co-viewing with YouTube: Blending mass communication reception and social connection. *Journal of Broadcasting & Electronic Media 53*, 317–335. https://doi.org/10.1080/08838150902908270.

Hersko, T. (2020, April 8). *Tiger King* had 34 million viewers within 10 days of launch, Fox to air special. *Indie Wire*. https://www.indiewire.com/2020/04/tiger-king-netflix-viewership-fox-special-1202223808/.

Irimiás, A., Mitev, A. Z., & Michalkó, G. (2021). Narrative transportation and travel: The mediating role of escapism and immersion, *Tourism Management Perspectives*, 38, https://doi.org/10.1016/j.tmp.2021.100793.

Katz, E., Blumler, J. G., & Gurevitch, M. (1973). Uses and gratifications research. *The Public Opinion Quarterly, 37*(4), 509–523. https://doi.org/10.1086/268109.

Kelly, H. (2020, March 6). People have found a way to cope with pandemic fears: Watching *Contagion*. *The Washington Post*. Retrieved from https://www.washingtonpost.com/technology/2020/03/06/contagion-streaming/.

Laor, T. (2020). The race to escape: Location-based escapism and physical activity as a motivator in the consumption of the AR game Pokemon Go. *Cyberpsychology: Journal of Psychosocial Research on Cyberspace, 14*(2), Article 6. https://doi.org/10.5817/CP2020-2-6.

LaRose, R., & Eastin, M. S. (2004). A social cognitive theory of Internet uses and gratifications: Toward a new model of media attendance. *Journal of Broadcasting and Electronic Media, 48* (3), 358–377. https://doi.org/10.1207/s15506878jobem4803_2.

Lin, C. A. (1999). Uses and gratifications. In G. Stone, M. Singletary, & V. P. Richmond (Eds.), *Clarifying communication theories: A hands-on approach* (pp. 199–208). Iowa State University Press.

Merikivi, J., Bragge, J., Scornavacca, E., & Verhagen, T. (2020). Binge-watching serialized video content: A transdisciplinary review. *Television & New Media, 21*(7), 697–711. https://doi.org/10.1177/1527476419848578.

Pang, A. (February 19, 2014). Binge-watching *House of Cards* and *Breaking Bad* is 'good for you.' *Independent*. Retrieved from http://www.independent.co.uk/.

Papacharissi, Z., & Mendelson, A.L. (2007) An exploratory study of reality appeal: Uses and gratifications of reality TV shows. *Journal of Broadcasting & Electronic Media 51*, 355–370. https://doi.org/10.1080/08838150701307152.

Petersen, T. G. (2016). To binge or not to binge: A qualitative analysis of college students' binge watching habits. *Florida Communication Journal*, 44(1), 77–88.

Pevos, E. (2020, May 9). COVID-19 TV habits show a staggering change in viewing hours and what we're watching. *MLive.com*. Retrieved from https://www.mlive.com/coronavirus/ 2020/05/covid-19-tv-habits-show-a-staggering-change-in-viewing-hours-and-what-were-watching.html.

Pierce-Grove, R. (2020). Binge-watching can soothe the coronavirus quarantine blues, and no need for guilt. *USA Today*. Retrieved August 15, 2021, from https://www.usatoday.com/story/opinion/2020/05/02/coronavirus-quarantine-binge-watching-healthy-escape-column/3060846001/.

Pittman, M. & Tefertiller, A. (2015). With or without you: Connected viewing and co-viewing Twitter activity for traditional appointment and asynchronous broadcast television models. *First Monday, 20*(7). http://dx.doi.org/10.5210/fm.v20i7.5935.

Rubenking, B., & Bracken, C. C. (2018). Binge-watching: A suspenseful, emotional, habit. *Communication Research Reports, 35*(5), 381–391. https://doi.org/10.1080/08824096.2018.1525346.

Rubin, A. M. (1983). Television uses and gratifications: The interactions of viewing patterns and motivations. *Journal of Broadcasting, 27*, 37–51. https://doi.org/10.1080/08838158309386471.

Rubin, A. (2009). Uses-and-gratifications perspective on media effect. In J. Bryant, & M.B. Oliver, (Eds.), *Media effects: Advances in theory and research*, pp. 165–184. Routledge.

Ruggiero, T. E. (2000). Uses and gratifications theory in the 21st century. *Mass Communication and Society, 3*(1), 3–37. https://doi.org/10.1207/S15327825MCS0301_02.

Shim, H., & Kim, K. J. (2018). An exploration of the motivations for binge-watching and the role of individual differences. *Computers in Human Behavior, 82*, 94–100. https://doi.org/10.1016/j.chb.2017.12.032.

Steiner, E., & Xu, K. (2020). Binge-watching motivates change: Uses and gratifications of streaming video viewers challenge traditional TV research. C*onvergence: The International Journal of Research into New Media Technologies, 26*, 1, 82–101. https://doi.org/10.1177/1354856517750365.

Sundar, S., & Limperos, A. (2013). Uses and grats 2.0: New gratifications for new media. *Journal of Broadcasting & Electronic Media 57*(4), 504–525. https://doi.org/10.1080/08838151.2013.845827.

Sung, Y. H., Kang, E. Y., & Lee, W. (2018). Why do we indulge? Exploring motivations for binge watching. *Journal of Broadcasting and Electronic Media, 62* (3), 403–426. https://doi.org/10.1080/08838151.2018.1451851.

Syfret, W. (2021, April 13). I turned to reality TV to escape during the pandemic—until reality caught up. *The Guardian.* Retrieved from https://www.theguardian.com/tv-and-radio/2021/apr/14/i-turned-to-reality-tv-to-escape-during-the-pandemic-until-reality-caught-up.

Terfertiller, A. C., & Conlin Maxwell, L. (2018). Depression, emotional states, and the experience of binge-watching narrative television. *Atlantic Journal of Communication, 226*(5), 278–290. https://doi.org/10.1080/1546870.2018.1517765.

van Laer, T., de Ruyter, K., Visconti, L., & Wetzels, M. (2014). The extended transportation-imagery model. *Journal of Consumer Research*, *40*(5), 797–817. https://doi.org/10.1086/673383.

Vaterlaus, J. M., Spruance, L. A., Frantz, K., & Kruger, J. S. (2018). College student television binge watching: Conceptualization, gratifications, and perceived consequences. *The Social Science Journal, 56*(4), 470–479. https://doi.org/10.1016/j.soscij.2018.10.004.

Vorderer, P., Klimmt, C., & Ritterfeld, U. (2004). Enjoyment: At the heart of media entertainment. *Communication Theory*, *14*, 388–408. https://doi-org.libproxy.library.unt.edu/10.1111/j.1468-2885.2004.tb00321.x.

Warren, S. (2020). Binge-watching as a predictor of narrative transportation using HLM. *Journal of Broadcasting & Electronic Media*, 64:2, 89–110, https://doi.org/10.1080/08838151.2020.1718985.

West, K. (2014). Unsurprising: Netflix survey indicates people like to binge-watch TV. *Cinema Blend, Television*. Retrieved from http://www.cinemablend.com/television/Unsurprising-Netflix-Survey-Indicates-People-Like-Binge-Watch-TV-61045.html.

Zuckerman, M. (2014). *Sensation seeking (psychology revivals): Beyond the optimal level of arousal*. Psychology Press.

Chapter Sixteen

Ted Lasso

A Feel-Good Show in a Not-Feel-Good Time

Deborah A. Macey and Mary P. Erickson

It is obvious *Ted Lasso* has struck a chord with audiences and critics alike. With 20 Emmy nominations and seven wins, including Outstanding Comedy Series in 2021, *Ted Lasso* is more than a fish-out-of-water underdog up against a woman scorned. The series brings together a talented cast and excellent writers, creating characters with depth and heart, which allows them to move beyond typical tropes and stereotypes. Even some of the best cast and well-written series do not achieve this type of success so quickly. In an *Entertainment Weekly* YouTube interview, Brett Goldstein, who plays Roy Kent, attributes some of the show's success to "an element of magic." Part of the magic stems from the "just grimly perfect" timing (Spiegel, 2020) of the series. This magical timing coincides with changes in the television landscape, a mid-pandemic release date, and a need for a feel-good show in a not-feel-good time.

As the television landscape embraced a multitude of streaming platforms in the 2010s, programmatic offerings on Netflix, Amazon Prime Video, Hulu, and others enticed viewers to pay subscription fees and spend their time bingeing shows with marquee actors and large budgets. This new era of television programming, known as "quality TV" or "peak TV" occurred away from conventional network television structures, allowing for longer episodes, complex plotlines, and characters with depth (Lotz, 2014; Mittell, 2015). Apple TV+ is no exception, and *Ted Lasso* in particular follows this pattern of change in the industry.

Apple TV+, launched in November 2019, lined up high-profile talent, such as Reese Witherspoon and Jennifer Aniston starring in and producing *The Morning Show,* and Hailee Steinfeld and Jane Krakwoski in *Dickinson*, to compete with established streaming platforms. The company commissioned a *Ted Lasso* pilot, co-written by Jason Sudeikis and *Scrubs* showrunner Bill Lawrence and produced by Lawrence's company, Doozer Productions, and Warner Bros. Television.

Ted Lasso draws on a number of writers to shape the story and characters; Sudeikis and Lawrence developed the first two episodes with Brendan Hunt (who plays *Ted Lasso*'s Coach Beard) and Joe Kelly, a former writer on *Saturday Night Live*. As the season continued, other seasoned television writers and comedians took the helm for different episodes, including Brett Goldstein, Jane Becker, Leann Bowen, Phoebe Walsh, and Jamie Lee, among others.

The character of Ted Lasso first appeared on NBC Sports in 2013 in ads promoting England's Premier League televised football matches. Created and played by Sudeikis, previously a regular cast member of *SNL* and various comedy films, Lasso is an American college football coach recruited as manager for a Premier League team, despite having no experience or understanding of the sport. In the series, club owner of the fictional AFC Richmond, Rebecca Welton (played by Hannah Waddingham), is recently divorced from its previous owner, and bringing the supremely unknowledgeable Lasso onboard is her strategy to ruin one of her ex's favorite things. Apple TV+ ordered ten episodes, which premiered in August 2020. The show was quickly renewed for a second season, and soon, a third.

This chapter explores how Season One of *Ted Lasso* charmed audiences and critics, particularly two gender and media scholars. We engaged in a long soak (Hall, 1975) with the series as both critics and fans. We discovered that what makes *Ted Lasso* such a feel-good show is not only its well-written humor, but also its developed characters that allow for challenges to hegemonic gender norms and expectations. The series provides a stark contrast to the prevailing toxic masculinity of politics, particularly in the age of Donald Trump (Bellstrom & Hinchliffe, 2020) and presents more inclusive, varied, and even vulnerable, masculine representations. The female characters are developed with this same care. They have depth; they are strong, interesting, and funny. They support one another and are not interested in the typical catfight, which is ubiquitous throughout media (Reinke, 2010). Of course, much of *Ted Lasso*'s charm comes from its humor, which is often silly and sweet, but never trite, and at times, offers biting commentary.

More Than Midwestern Schtick

Many were surprised that the creators were able to take two NBC Premier League advertisements and transform them into a series with such heart (Surrey, 2020; Butler, 2021; Framke, 2020) and sustained comedy. We too were skeptical. While Erickson is not a sports fan, Macey is a super fan of soccer and admits the only reason she started watching the series was because it was about her favorite sport. Mostly she thought Sudeikis's faux Midwestern schtick would be tiresome. It is. But because it is not meant to ridicule and the series is otherwise brilliant, we were hooked with Marcus Mumford and Tom Howe's theme music establishing the tone. Yeeeaaaah!

There's lots to love about *Ted Lasso*. Its gentle humor is one of them (Spiegel, 2020). In times of crisis and uncertainty, humor can mitigate those feelings of discomfort, helping us to escape and manage those challenges (Achter, 2008). There are dozens of fish-out-of-water jokes for the audience to enjoy, ranging from Ted's dislike of tea to his inability to understand the game he is coaching to differences in language and culture. When asked how he takes his tea, Ted responds that he "take[s] it right back to the counter because someone has made a horrible mistake" (Sudeikis et al, 2020, 10:36). He plainly describes it as tasting "like hot brown water" and even doubts others' love of the beverage. "Be honest with me. It's a prank, right? The tea? Like when us tourist folks aren't around, y'all know it tastes like garbage?" (Walsh, 2020, 27:20)

At his first press conference Ted admits that you can "fill two internets with what I don't know about football" (Sudeikis et al, 2020, 13:13) When asked if he knows any footballers, he recounts, "Well, yeah, you got Ronaldo, and the fellow that bends it like himself" (Sudeikis et al, 2020, 14:38).

It is the humor that points to the absurdity of U.S. culture that is the most interesting. Sam Obisanya (played by Toheeb Jimoh), a young Nigerian player, asks, "Coach, is it true in America, you have so many beautiful dogs in pounds that some get put down for no reason?" Ted responds matter-of-factly, "That is true, Sam, it's also something a lot of female singer/songwriters are trying to change" (Wrubel, 2020, 16:06). When recognizing that the players are from all over the globe, Lasso mistakes a Welsh player for an English player and then questions, "How many countries are in this country?" Nate Shelley (played by Nick Mohammed), the kitman, and Coach Beard respond in unison, "Four." Lasso pauses and nods, "Kinda like America these days" (Sudeikis et al., 2020, 19:42). This line was especially resonant for us as we watched this episode in the lead-up to the supremely divisive 2020 U.S. presidential election. It is these quick-witted one-liners that make critical cultural scholars like us smile and remind us that there is more depth here than meets the eye. And our favorite cultural and political critique happens when

Lasso tries to share a little green army man (a gift from his son) with Sam. Sam's innocence plays well here as he politely rejects the offering. "Is it okay if I don't keep this? I don't really have the same fondness for the American military that you do." They agree: "Imperialism" (Hunt et al., 2020, 21:25).

Of course, *Ted Lasso* is more than just a much-needed comedy and a mirror to gently point out inanities of U.S. culture (and, as in the example above, American military aggression). It is more than a distraction during a global pandemic. At the end of episode one, sad music swells, and you see Ted exhausted in the shower. He calls his wife and Ted is presented as the loving father and heartbroken husband. He starts to grow on us as we realize he, and the other characters, are written—and brought to life by the actors—to be very real in their humanness. *Ted Lasso* is much more than a football comedy—much more than Midwestern schtick.

CONCEPTUALIZING GENDER IN THE 21ST CENTURY

The understanding of gender has seen dramatic cultural and social shifts in the first two decades of the 21st century, as the binary understanding of gender with masculinity and femininity as opposites has been unraveling. Examining gender representations in contemporary popular media necessitates more nuanced frameworks of how gender operates. As we are introduced to the main characters in the first episode, we begin to think perhaps these characters will take on an expected one-dimensional and stereotypical form. Very quickly, though, we find each character defying expectations and demonstrating thoughtful and (much-needed) more nuanced representations of gender.

Transcending Traditional Masculinity

Much of our viewing expectation has been shaped by the way that sports are televised as well as by narrative television. Televised sports have historically tended to prioritize "the specific form of manhood that is characterized by athleticism, muscularity, strength, power, and fearless domination . . . these men are said to disconnect their physical power from 'emotional understanding and the skills of emotional maintenance'" (Feasey, 2008, p. 101). There have been high-profile and influential exceptions to this presentation that open the range of characteristics that can define masculinity and athletes. Footballer David Beckham is one such example. According to Feasey, Beckham's public image transcends the boys' club, "violat[ing] every known norm associated with testosterone-pumped, homophobic, macho footballers," and has moreover been celebrated for doing so in media and by his fans (Cashmore, 2004; quoted in Feasey, pp. 102–103).

In narrative television, some of the most dominant depictions of masculinity have continued to emphasize "older and more traditional masculinities that are often characterized by anti-feminism, emotional stoicism, and misogyny" (Haywood et al., 2018, p. 5). Over the last two decades, the TV industry has courted male viewers with shows featuring male anti-heroes lovingly heralded by critics; these characters (among them, Tony Soprano, *The Sopranos*; Don Draper, *Mad Men*; and Walter White, *Breaking Bad*) lack conventional qualities that would otherwise position them as upstanding (Nygaard and Lagerway, 2017). The dark, shadowy corners of hegemonic (or orthodox) masculinity are explored in these shows, with little resolution or rectification; the characters' moral ambiguities reflect the political and cultural ambiguities of the first two decades of the 21st century, and further serve to reinforce traditional hegemonic masculinity (Albrecht, 2016).

As we think about where *Ted Lasso* sits, we see movement away from its television contemporaries in terms of masculine representations. We also see movement away from the orthodox masculinity of male athletes, as we come to know the show's various characters. Jamie Tartt (played by Phil Dunster), the cocky young football star, grows beyond the stereotyped footballer; his trajectory involves his struggle to come to terms with his absent and abusive father, the very real feelings he has for his former partner Keeley Jones (played by Juno Temple), and his relationship with his rival Roy Kent. Leslie Higgins (played by Jeremy Swift), named after his mother—"a feminine junior," is stereotypically the eunuch emasculated by Welton's dominance yet develops when he stands up to Welton late in season one, earning her respect. The stoic Coach Beard, the perfect antidote to Lasso's loquaciousness and inanity, is smart, sensible, and fair. While all the male leads deserve discussion, this section will focus on how Lasso, Tartt, and Roy Kent portray a more inclusive masculinity.[1]

Inclusive masculinity theory proposes that heterosexual men have increasingly grown to accept and practice a range of masculinities; this includes rejecting homophobia and violence, sharing emotional intimacy with friends, and practicing more feminine-coded behaviors and activities (Anderson & McCormack, 2016). As generational shifts broaden socially acceptable masculinities, many of these practices extend to male-dominated areas, such as sports. *Ted Lasso* is a place where these tenets can shine. Ted Lasso is the eternal optimist, which translates into warm and nurturing interactions with others. Jamie's self-centeredness is peeled back to reveal insecurity and desire for acceptance. Roy Kent is a surprising exemplar of inclusive and warm masculinity. While his gruffness and affection for the F-word point toward a closed-off, tough, angry presentation of masculinity, he continually surprises us with his compassion, his sensitivity, and his growing attention to personal accountability.

Ted Lasso is attuned to others' feelings. In episode one he drops his optimistic schtick as he asks Rebecca how she is doing with her divorce. It is their first real moment. He checks in on Rebecca again after Ernie Lounds from *The Sun* questions her about the newest revelation in her ex-husband's cheating scandal. In episode two, Lasso recognizes that Sam is a "little down in the dumps" (Hunt et al., 2020, 5:50). Lasso believes he is homesick and plans a birthday celebration for him.

Ted also works hard to foster a caring sense among the team; in his view, the collective is more important than the individual. In the second episode, he disarms Jamie, trying to win his favor and influence.

> I haven't known you that long, but I can honestly say that you are the best athlete I have ever coached . . . you are truly great at everything you do out there, except for one thing. . . . You might be so sure you are one in a million that sometimes you forget that out there you are just one of 11. If you could just figure out some way to turn that me into us. Sky's the limit for you. That was a heck of a goal out there. (Hunt et al., 2020, 23:39)

It is a poignant scene. Lasso does not try to strongarm or threaten Jamie into doing what he needs, but gently makes Jamie aware of his own influence and encourages him to wield it appropriately. It takes Jamie a while to learn this lesson (likely because Jamie is accustomed to being threatened and ridiculed by his own father), but he eventually comes around after Keeley breaks up with him and Lasso benches him for his arrogance.

Lasso employs this same gentle touch while trying to influence Roy Kent to use his role as captain to foster better teamwork and more care in the locker room. Roy, disgusted with the bullying of Nate, the kitman, complains to Lasso to "take care of it." Lasso responds,

> Roy, I learned two pretty big lessons on the rough-and-tumble playgrounds of Brookridge Elementary School. One, if little Ronnie Fauch offers you a candy bar, you immediately say no and you get the hell out of there because there's a good chance that little son-of-a-gun has just pooped inside a Butterfinger wrapper. No one ever saw him do it, but a couple people ate it. Number two, a teacher tells a bully not to pick on someone just makes it worse. (Becker, 2020, 10:48)

Coach Beard watches this exchange and, after Kent leaves, questions, "Why are you winding him up?" Lasso responds, "He's the one, coach. If we're going to make an impact here—First domino that needs to fall. Right inside that man's heart" (Becker, 2020, 11:20). And it turns out that Lasso's approach strikes a chord for Roy, who realizes that caring for another's dignity, rather than taking an every-man-for-himself approach, supports everyone's well-being.

Lasso cares about everyone. His constant refrain, no matter the insults thrown at him, is, "Hey, I appreciate you." And Ted cares deeply for Rebecca, as he recognizes a kindred spirit who is in as much pain over a marriage breakup as he is. During a fundraising event, Rebecca's ex-husband, Rupert (played by Anthony Head) shows up unexpectedly to assert his superiority over Rebecca and popularity among the event's attendees. Rupert's smugness upsets Rebecca. Ted later calls out Rupert in the most subtle way for crashing the party and canceling the musical guest. He tells Rebecca not everyone is fooled by Rupert's façade. "What a charmer . . . you know you may think you are the only one who can see who he really is, but you're not" (Lee, 2020, 30:54). Rebecca is surprised at Ted's astuteness. She knows she didn't really see who Ted was until that moment.

In Ted's next encounter with Rupert, Ted's depth is again revealed. In episode eight, Ted and Rebecca believe they are meeting with the Milk sisters, two minority owners of the club. To their surprise, Rupert and his new fiancé, Rebecca (played by Keeley Hazell), show up at the pub meeting and reveal that "New Rebecca" purchased the sisters' stake in AFC Richmond. Our Rebecca is distressed as Rupert threatens to sit in the owner's box and talk trash to the press. Ted tempts Rupert into challenging him to a game of darts. Rupert's initial wager of £10,000 is too high for Ted, so Ted counters, "If you win, I'll let you pick the starting lineup of the last two games of the season. But if I win, you can't go anywhere near the owner's box." (Bowen, 2020, 22:01). As the game wears on, Ted needs two triple 20s and a bullseye to win. No one thinks Ted can win, especially Rupert. Ted begins his monologue.

> Guys have underestimated me my entire life. And for years, I never understood why. It used to really bother me. But then one day, I was driving my little boy to school, and I saw this quote by Walt Whitman, and it was painted on the wall there. It said, "Be curious, not judgmental." I like that. (Bowen, 2020, 24:58)

Ted hits his first triple 20 and continues.

> . . . all them fellas that used to belittle me, not a single one of them were curious, you know. They thought they had everything all figured out, so they judged everything and they judged everyone. And I realized their underestimating me, who I was had nothing to do with it. 'Cause if they were curious, they would've asked questions. Questions like, "Have you played a lot of darts, Ted?" (Bowen, 2020, 25:23)

Ted hits his second triple 20. The crowd at the pub cheers in disbelief. Ted continues, "To which I would have answered, 'Yes, sir. Every Sunday afternoon at a sports bar with my father, from age 10 'til I was 16, when he passed away'" (Bowen, 2020, 25:58). Ted hits the bulls-eye. The crowd erupts; Rupert sulks away, and Rebecca is grateful for Ted's intervention on her behalf. This scene speaks to not only Ted's depth, but also Ted's ability to unmask the "tough guise" (Katz et al., 2016)—the bravado required of the performance of traditional masculinity.

It becomes clear in this scene that Ted is a complicated character; he is rescuing the damsel in distress, as it were, by defending Rebecca and fighting her fight for her, a traditionally masculine role. But he does so with a sense of deep and unselfish care for her emotional wellbeing.

Throughout the series, Ted's interactions evoke the emotional and care labor traditionally attributed to women's roles in relationships (Fixmer-Oraiz & Wood, 2019). On the other hand, Ted may also be dealing with his inadequacy in being able to care for his family. His wife has requested emotional distance (and eventual divorce), which Ted has conceded by physically distancing himself from his family. The care labor that Ted performs for his football family is his assertion of his role as provider, which has been amputated from his role in his own family.

As referenced earlier, television portrayals of male athletes' masculinity may shape viewers' expectations of what these athletes should be like (Feasey, 2008), which extends to what we might expect of fictionalized versions of male athletes. While *Ted Lasso* initially sets up a number of its male characters as conventionally masculine, the show repeatedly works to reveal the fragility of the characters' "tough guises." When we first meet Jamie Tartt, we see a cocky footballer whose athletic skill dominates the field. In his first dialogue with Lasso, Jamie is dressed in a floral-print warmup suit and a shoulder bag (a "man purse"), and is leaving to get a body wax. His comfortability with fashion and body image, a traditionally feminine domain (and reminiscent of Beckham's metrosexual pose [Cashmore & Parker, 2003]), is paired with his penchant for attention, and we recognize that Jamie is flashy and projects confidence in order to command the spotlight. In the next episode, Lasso asks him, "Which would you rather be, a lion or a panda?" Jamie responds, "Coach, I'm me. Why would I want to be anythin' else?" (Hunt et al., 2020, 9:48). While Lasso attributes this statement to being "psychologically healthy," we can also read it as masculine confidence in needing no improvement.

And yet, as we understand Jamie more, we find that he is indeed well aware of the "tough guise" he puts on. In episode six, Lasso benches Tartt for his arrogance after he shouted "Me! Me!" on the field in celebration of his two unassisted goals. After being substituted, Jamie walks off the field, leaves his uniform in the locker room, and skips the next practice. After some reflection, Jamie returns willing to contribute to the team-building exercise of exorcising the ghosts from the treatment room. The players are required to sacrifice something meaningful to them. Jamie brings his boots (cleats) to burn in order to "reverse the curse."

> My mum gave 'em to me. She was the one who got me into football in the first place . . . She's the reason I work so hard. Just wanted to make her proud. She doesn't even care if I'm any good. Just wants me to be happy. Be a good lad. Once I got good though, me old man started showing up, didn't he? You know bragging to all of his mates when I scored a goal. Calling me "soft" if I didn't dominate, you know. And I hated that. I actually fucking hated that. So, I made a vow to be so tough, so that he could never call me "soft" again. I wonder if sometimes I forget about making her proud. I don't think that she would be lately. (Wrubel, 2020, 26:05)

In this scene viewers see Jamie struggle with his performance of masculinity. He has embraced this hardened masculinity, so no one, especially his father, would see him as soft or in any way feminine. Julia T. Wood (1997) describes this as the main directive for young males—"don't be female." (p. 131). In later editions of her text *Gendered Lives: Communication, Gender, and Culture*, Wood and her co-author Natalie Fixmer-Oraiz acknowledge the changing nature of masculinity by adding to that theme that males must also "embody and transcend traditional views of masculinity" (Fixmer-Oraiz & Wood, 2019, p. 146). The male characters of Ted Lasso embody and transcend traditional masculinity and no character does that better than Roy Kent.

We are first introduced to aging footballer Roy Kent in the locker room as he walks in, shirtless, glaring in disbelief at the presence of Ted and Beard as the new coaching team. In the next episode, he is again shirtless in the locker room, post-practice, already questioning Ted's coaching method. His generally pissed-off demeanor continues in his interactions with Ted and the teammates, and we are genuinely surprised when Roy, Ted, and Trent Crimm (on assignment for *The Independent*) go to the grade school of Roy's niece, Phoebe, who softens Roy quite nicely. In his gruff fashion, Roy tells Phoebe's class he isn't much into public speaking or school and suggests, "Why don't we get out of this stuffy auditorium and go out on the pitch and have a proper fuck-about?" (Becker, 2020, 22:21). To this, the children sit stunned for a moment and then scream. Ted admires Roy for coming to the school, but Roy says he only does it for his niece, flashes her the biggest smile and waves as Phoebe runs over to him, pleading with him to do headers. He lifts her over his shoulders and viewers are treated to this sweet side of Roy Kent as he and Ted do headers with the kids until Phoebe kicks the ball right into Ted's nose; Roy praises her with "Good job, Phoebe" (Becker, 2020, 23:31). Every subsequent scene with Phoebe reinforces Roy's adoration of his niece; even though he is grumpy, he loves her dearly.

Roy Kent, the brooding and brusque footballer, reveals a depth that leaves us awestruck, especially in his relationship with Keeley. In episode eight, there is some miscommunication in their budding relationship. He doesn't want another empty one-night stand, which makes Keeley think he is not interested in her. Roy realizes he should have told Keeley that and apologizes as he is "trying to be more honest" (Bowen, 2020, 12:26). In the spirit of honesty, Keeley reveals she slept with her ex, Jamie Tartt, the night before because she was confused about their relationship. As Roy fumes, Keeley apologizes, but lets him know that he needs "to be okay with this" (Bowen, 2020, 13:06).

Roy seeks out Ted's advice who brings in the Diamond Dogs. Lasso, Beard, Nate, and Higgins make up the Diamond Dogs and convene to discuss relationship problems. The sheer existence of the Diamond Dogs challenges traditional aspects of masculinity; the informal grouping provides a sensitive and supportive way for these men to share their problems with and solicit advice from one another. After a series of Ted's silly comments that point out the inequitable treatment of male and female sexuality, Diamond Dogs come to an agreement. Ted says, "Don't let her past muck around with y'all's future" (Bowen, 2020, 15:47). To which Roy explains that Keeley slept with her ex last night. This information changes no one's opinion. To be sure Nate questions, "Are you two officially dating?" (Bowen, 2020, 15:54). And Higgins asks if Keeley and Roy have already slept together, two questions that might have changed the opinion of the group. The answers to both questions—no. Ted turns to Beard, who regularly provides sage wisdom to Ted, and says, "Coach, you want to bring this home?" Beard states, "Grow up and get over it" (Bowen, 2020, 15:59–16:05). Roy knows they are right and tells Keeley he is "done being mad about Jamie" because he is "a grown man . . . not a baby child" and he is "over it" (Bowen, 2020, 18:40–18:48).

In a hilarious faux press conference, Keeley questions Roy's change of heart. Roy repeats, "I'm over it." and explains, "I like you more than I hate him" (Bowen, 2020, 19:08–19:29). Later, on their first date, Keeley questions Roy, "Are you dating other people?" (Bowen, 2020, 23:02) because earlier she had asked him to coffee and he said he was busy and didn't offer an explanation. Roy explained:

> . . . It was private. . . . It was yoga. I do yoga with a group of women in their 60s. They have no idea who I am. It's twice a week and it is really good for my core. Normally it only takes an hour, but Maureen's just been going through a divorce and she needed to talk about it and blow off some steam. We all ended up at

G-A-Y 'til 2 a.m. and then we had crepes in Balham with some drag queens. (Bowen, 2020, 23:00–23:23)

The scene reveals how Roy transcends traditional masculinity. Traditional masculinity would find no use for women in their 60s, but Roy not only enjoys their company, he also is invested in their wellbeing. In addition, Roy is participating in yoga and sharing crepes with the women and drag queens—all things outside of the realm of traditional heterosexual masculinity. *Ted Lasso* is a kinder, gentler series, and its representation of masculinity reflects that transcendence from traditional masculinity, especially compared to the political machismo of the moment.

Formidable, Fallible, and Fully Human, Not Sidekicks and Catfights

As media scholars account for the changing representations of masculinity, others turn toward the examination of female character counterparts to assess how femininity and feminism are expressed. Females are still underrepresented in media about 2-to-1, and women over 30 rarely exist on screen (Fixmer-Oraiz & Wood, 2019). And still when women are represented, they are often in auxiliary roles, portrayed as weak, passive, and/or hyper-sexualized (Kilbourne, 2002), although television is slightly better given its historical designation as a feminine medium. Turner and Dunn (2018) observe that there are few television series that depict positive and realistic friendships between female coworkers. In addition, women are often pitted against one another (Reinke, 2010), even in series that are progressive (Macey, 2012). In television portrayals, relationships among teen girls often stereotypically depict relational aggression such as bullying, exclusion, and manipulation; the perpetrators of this aggression are "mean girls" or "queen bees" (Gonick, 2004). Media representations often continue these tropes in adult contexts, the workplace, and within friendships. Rarely do we see female relationships that provide mutual support or representations of females helping each other advance personally and professionally. Scholars suggest that comedies are less equipped to present these positive relationships (Turner & Dunn, 2018), however, perhaps driven by the perceived need to rely on tired stereotypes for jokes, particularly in network television (Macey, 2012; Turner & Dunn, 2018). But *Ted Lasso* exists outside of the broadcast networks.

The women of *Ted Lasso* shatter these stereotypes. The first scene of the pilot episode begins with a training session on the pitch, panning to a close-up of new owner, Rebecca Welton, while Sex Pistols' "No Future (God Save the Queen)" plays in the background. Welton is gorgeous and statuesque—powerful in her physical presence. She summons Head Coach George Cartrick (played by Bill Fellows), and viewers experience the fierce and formidable Welton for the first time. George walks in, grabs Higgins by the balls, makes a homophobic comment, followed by a sexist one, before Welton fires him. Shocked, he aggressively asks, "What the fuck for?" And we watch as Rebecca explains,

> For any number of reasons really. Your casual misogyny for one. I know it's a big word. Ask one of your daughters what it means. Or perhaps it's your performance, having led this team through yet another remarkably average season. . . . Still if I'm being completely honest, George, you're fired because I'm the owner now and I don't like you. Now do piss off, you fat twat. (Sudeikis et al., 2020, 2:27–3:17)

We watch as Rebecca exerts a power we only wish we had to tell off the powers that be as they continued to botch the COVID-19 response.

On his way out, George tries to humiliate Welton, but she is not having it. She has a plan—to take down AFC Richmond, the only thing her ex-husband loves. We worry for a moment that Welton will be the disposable, villainous, older-woman stereotype, who is just there as a foil to Lasso's optimism. That is not to be because this is Apple TV+ and these characters have depth and complexity. This is just a ploy to provide "some explanation . . . for why an American football coach with no soccer experience would be hired for the role" (Surrey, 2020).

Keeley Jones's entrance is equally formidable. Keeley, a model/influencer who is "sort of famous for being almost famous" (Goldstein, 2020, 7:03) walks into the men's locker room full of confidence with her hands pretending to cover her eyes. "Knock. Knock. Is everyone here decent? Oh! Boys, that is disappointing" (Sudeikis et al., 2020, 21:07). The character of Keeley could so easily become the vapid influencer stereotype, but the writers and Temple make her so much more than that. She is smart and driven, thoughtful and caring, and fully in charge of her sexuality. She speaks her mind and challenges people to be their best selves.

In episode three, we see Keeley assert and insert herself into Rebecca's office and life. It is their first scene together and sets the stage for Keeley and Rebecca's solidarity. Keeley brings Rebecca a cactus to thank her for preventing the publication of photos of her and Ted, the very same photos that Rebecca secretly commissioned to create chaos for the new coach. Keeley describes the gift, "Made me think of you. It's strong and a bit prickly" (Becker et al., 2020, 19:24). Keeley throws her bag on the couch, kicks off her shoes, and lies down. She states, "You know I've decided not to be scared of you anymore" (Becker et al., 2020, 19:31). Unselfconsciously, Keeley prattles on about how her then-partner Jamie would have been so mad had the press meddled in their private life. She reminds Rebecca about how the press did that to her and expresses her anger at how the press went after Rebecca instead of her cheating ex-husband. Rebecca responds, "Well, the press are never awful to men. No one ever pays a fortune for a photo of a naked man on a yacht in Mallorca a week after his divorce" (Becker et al., 2020, 19:59). Keeley realizes this is too specific of a comment and begs to see the picture of Rebecca sunbathing topless. Keeley squeals, "Holy shit, Rebecca. Are those your real tits? I feel like a teenage boy. I can't stop staring at them . . . I can't believe you stopped this from running. I would've shown everyone" (Becker et al., 2020, 20:24–20:37). While Rebecca acts unamused with Keeley's antics, Keeley's admiration makes Rebecca feel good.

In episode four, Keeley helps Rebecca feel less insecure at the red-carpet charity event. If these women were stereotypically competitive, the scene would play out much differently, foregrounding a catfight between the two. Keeley would feel jealous of the attention Rebecca receives and would want to one-up Rebecca by sabotaging her with suggestions for unflattering poses. Not these women. They want the other to succeed. Keeley sees Rebecca struggle to hide her discomfort and desire to present a front of confidence and strength in her newfound singlehood. Keeley winks at Rebecca as Rebecca mumbles that she "hate[s] this part" (Lee, 2020, 8:09). Keeley walks over to her, leans in and tells her exactly how to stand for the most flattering photos. Rebecca instantly feels more confident. Keeley wanders behind the photographers and shouts, "Ahh! Look guys. She's fucking fierce!" (Lee, 2020, 8:25). Rebecca laughs and Keeley blows her kisses. Rebecca twirls with confidence.

Later in the episode Keeley and Rebecca meet in the bathroom. Rebecca thanks her for the red-carpet confidence and then decides to reveal to Keeley that her then-partner Jamie had a second plus one. Keeley accepts, "Cheeky little prick" and asks, "Have you ever dated a footballer . . . When I was 18, I dated a footballer that was 23. Now I'm close to thirty and I am dating a 23-year-old footballer. I'm Leonardo DiCaprio. They are pretty fun though. Simple, rich, fit" (Lee, 2020, 24:43–25:30). Rebecca interrupts, "What about accountable? . . . I was married to a man for 12 years, who never once took responsibility for any single one of them" (Lee, 2020, 25:30–25:47). This scene hints at Keeley's sexual prowess and foreshadows the developing accountability theme of the series.

The following week, Keeley shows up to the stadium to coach Jamie at his branding event, Rebecca asks, "No judgment but are you back with that twat?" Keeley responds, "No. We're done. God, I love that you care though . . . You know, I put this whole thing [the branding event] together. I get 10 percent." Rebecca offers, "Keeley, if any of the other players needed some branding work done, is that something you would be interested in?" Keeley says, "I don't want you to offer me a job just 'cause I was nice to you in the loo the other night." And Rebecca questions, "Why not? Men give each other jobs in the toilets all the time." They laugh in cheeky solidarity (Goldstein, 2020, 6:02–6:45).

In episode seven, Rebecca is still the villain trying to destroy the team as they head to Liverpool to play Everton. Rebecca maliciously tells Higgins he is not welcome on the trip and Keeley will go in his place. However, when they arrive at the hotel in Liverpool, Rebecca confesses that it is her and Rupert's anniversary weekend. As she tears up, Keeley hugs her and lets her know it will be all right.

After a triumphant win over Everton, the team heads to a karaoke bar to celebrate. Rebecca stuns the crowd belting the lyrics to "Let It Go" while Ted has his first panic attack. It is Rebecca who consoles Ted outside of the karaoke bar and tells him it is okay as she knows the trauma of divorce. She is no longer the villain who sees Ted as a pawn in her plan. She is a human and sees another human struggling and seeks to help.

At the end of episode eight, Higgins finally stands up to Rebecca. She chides him for his role in hiding Rupert's infidelity. He apologizes and takes responsibility while urging Rebecca to stop her sabotaging antics. Higgins quits and storms out. Keeley storms in, and despite her girl crush and genuine affection for Rebecca, confronts her with evidence that she hired a photographer to take salacious-appearing photos of Ted and Keeley. Keeley states matter-of-factly, "You arranged for the photographer to take this . . . Don't deny it or pretend you don't know. Either you come clean to Ted, or I'll do it for you" (Bowen, 2020, 29:28).

Rebecca finally holds herself accountable in episode nine.

> Ted, I lied to you. I hired you because I wanted this team to lose. I wanted you to fail and I have sabotaged you every chance I had. It was me who hired that photographer to take the photo of you and Keeley. I set up the interview with Trent Crimm, hoping that he would humiliate you. . . . This club is all that Rupert has ever cared about and I wanted to destroy it. To cause him as much pain and suffering as he has caused me. And I didn't care who I used or who I hurt. All you good people just trying to make a difference. Ted, I'm so sorry. (Walsh, 2020, 11:19–12:14)

Ted simply and quickly forgives her because he knows "divorce is hard" (Walsh, 2020, 12:36). He holds out his hand. Rebecca refuses and hugs him tightly instead, and then Ted gently reminds her to make amends with Higgins, which she does. This series, on this streaming service, offers viewers depictions of females and friendships that are deep and complex. It shows female characters as powerful and prominent. *Ted Lasso* feels good because these female leads defy stereotypes and make each other better.

FÚTBOL IS LIFE

For the football (soccer) fan, the final match of season one doesn't disappoint. It is everything you want in a make-or-break game, including storied rivals, trick plays, a career-ending tackle, and an equalizing goal in stoppage time, complete with a beautiful scissor kick. It brings fans of the sport and the series the feeling of sheer exhilaration. But alas, it was not meant to be. Former Richmond player Jamie Tartt assists the winning goal for Man City, the rival team, and AFC Richmond is relegated. In soccer, and as in life, we are brought to our knees. The pandemic has taken a social, emotional, and physical toll on so many of us, yet we found small and large ways to persevere. And for two media scholars terribly weary from the ongoing pandemic, the less clichéd ending feels more fitting and sets up the struggle for the next season. Coach Lasso's speech to his defeated team speaks to how we all persevered through the pandemic. It is quiet in the locker room.

> You all played a heck of a game out there. We might not have won, but y'all definitely succeeded. . . . Now look, this is a sad moment right here. For all of us. There ain't nothing I can say standing here right now that can take that away. But please do me this favor, will you? Lift your heads up and look around this locker room. . . . And I want you to be grateful that you are going through this sad moment with all these other folks. Because I promise you, there is something worse out there than being sad, and that is being alone and being sad. Ain't nobody in this room alone. . . . Let's be sad now. Let's be sad together. . . . Onward. Forward. (Kelly et al., 2020A, 29:24–31:04)

As Marcus Mumford sings "You'll Never Walk Alone," Ted says they can be sad together and then forget the loss, "like a goldfish." We don't think we should forget the lessons the pandemic has taught. We learned that finding ways to connect and create have been the most important survival tools of the pandemic. We found new ways to connect with our students, our colleagues, and our leaders. We enjoyed our passions for the arts in new and unexpected ways. We connected to community through walking, through food, and yes, through scripted and reality programming that helped us escape, however briefly, from the traumas of the pandemic, the racial injustice, the political machismo and divisiveness of this time. In the end *Ted Lasso* made us laugh, showed us gentler representations of masculinities and more powerful visions of femininity. The series shows us that we are complex, conflicted, and imperfect individuals. It makes us want to be empowered, kind, and better humans by reminding us that we will be okay as long as we stay connected with and accountable to others. Ultimately, *Ted Lasso* made us feel good during a totally un-feel-good time. "Yeah, it might be all that you get."

REFERENCES

Achter, P. (2008). Comedy in unfunny times: News parody and carnival after 9/11. *Critical Studies in Media Communication, 25*(3), 274–303. https://doi-org.ezproxy-eres.up.edu/10.1080/15295030802192038.

Albrecht, M.M. (2016). *Masculinity in contemporary quality television*. Routledge.

Alexander, S. & Woods, K. (2019). Reality television and the doing of hyperauthentic masculinities. *Journal of Men's Studies* 27(2), pp. 149–168.

Anderson, E., & McCormack, M. (2016). Inclusive masculinity theory: Overview, reflection and refinement. *Journal of Gender Studies 27*(5), pp. 547–561.

Becker, J. (Writer), & Marshall, T. (Director). (2020, August 14), Trent Crimm: The Independent (Season 1, Episode 3) [TV series episode]. In B. Lawrence, J. Sudeikis, B. Hunt, J. Kelly, J. Ingold, B. Wrubel (Executive Producers), *Ted Lasso*. Ruby's Tuna Inc.; Doozer; Universal Television; Warner Bros. Television Studios.

Bellstrom, K., & Hinchliffe, E. (2020, October 30). President Trump and the rise of toxic masculinity politics. *Fortune*. https://fortune.com/2020/10/30/president-trump-and-the-rise-of-toxic-masculinity-politics/.

Bowen, L. (Writer), & Lowney, D. (Director). (2020, September 18), The Diamond Dogs (Season 1, Episode 8) [TV series episode]. In B. Lawrence, J. Sudeikis, B. Hunt, J. Kelly, J. Ingold, B. Wrubel (Executive Producers), *Ted Lasso*. Ruby's Tuna Inc.; Doozer; Universal Television; Warner Bros. Television Studios.

Butler, B. (2021, September 20). How *Ted Lasso* went from a viral NBC Sports promo to everyone's feel-good favorite to Emmy darling. *Washington Post*. https://www.washingtonpost.com/arts-entertainment/2021/09/20/ted-lasso-emmys/.

Cashmore, E., & Parker, A. (2003). One David Beckham? Celebrity, masculinity, and the soccerati. *Sociology of Sport Journal, 20*(3), 214–231. https://doi.org/10.1123/ssj.20.3.214.

Entertainment Weekly. (2021). *Meet 'Ted Lasso' stars Brett Goldenstein and Brendan Hunt* [video film] YouTube. https://www.youtube.com/watch?v=2nFsXwE3jCA.

Feasey, R. (2008). *Masculinity and popular television*. Edinburgh: Edinburgh University Press.

Fixmer-Oraiz, N. & Wood, J.T. (2019). *Gendered lives: Communication, gender, and culture*. Cengage.

Framke, C. (2020, September 19). For your reconsideration: *Ted Lasso*. *Variety*. https://variety.com/2020/tv/columns/ted-lasso-season-1-jason-sudeikis-1234772230/.

Goldstein, B. (Writer), & Hegarty, E. (Director). (2020, August 28), Tan Lines (Season 1, Episode 5) [TV series episode]. In B. Lawrence, J. Sudeikis, B. Hunt, J. Kelly, J. Ingold, B. Wrubel (Executive Producers), *Ted Lasso*. Ruby's Tuna Inc.; Doozer; Universal Television; Warner Bros. Television Studios.

Gonick, M. (2004). The 'mean girl' crisis: Problematizing representations of girls' friendships. *Feminism and Psychology 14*(3), pp. 395–400.

Hall, S. (1975). Introduction. In A.C.H. Smith. Paper Voices. (pp.11–24). Chatto & Windus.

Haywood, C. et al. (2018). *The conundrum of masculinity: Hegemony, homosociality, homophobia, and heteronormativity*. Routledge.

Hunt, B. (Writer), Sudeikis, J. (Writer), Kelly, J. (Writer), & Braff, Z. (Director). (2020, August 14), Biscuits (Season 1, Episode 2) [TV series episode]. In B. Lawrence, J. Sudeikis, B. Hunt, J. Kelly, J. Ingold, B. Wrubel (Executive Producers), *Ted Lasso*. Ruby's Tuna Inc.; Doozer; Universal Television; Warner Bros. Television Studios.

Katz, J., Young, J. T., Earp, J., Jhally, S., & Media Education Foundation, distributor. (2016). *Tough guise: Violence, media and the crisis in masculinity*. Kanopy Streaming.

Kelly, J. (Writer), Hunt, B. (Writer), Sudeikis, J. (Writer), & Lowney, D. (Director). (2020, September 11), Make Rebecca Great Again (Season 1, Episode 7) [TV series episode]. In B. Lawrence, J. Sudeikis, B. Hunt, J. Kelly, J. Ingold, B. Wrubel (Executive Producers), *Ted Lasso*. Ruby's Tuna Inc.; Doozer; Universal Television; Warner Bros. Television Studios.

Kelly, J. (Writer), Sudeikis, J. (Writer), Hunt, B. (Writer), & Delaney, M.J. (Director). (2020A, October 2), The Hope that Kills You (Season 1, Episode 10) [TV series episode]. In B. Lawrence, J. Sudeikis, B. Hunt, J. Kelly, J. Ingold, B. Wrubel (Executive Producers), *Ted Lasso*. Ruby's Tuna Inc.; Doozer; Universal Television; Warner Bros. Television Studios.

Kilbourne, J. (creator). (2002). *Killing us softly 3: Advertising's image of women*. Media Education Foundation.

Lee, J. (Writer), & Marshall, T. (Director). (2020, August 21), For the Children (Season 1, Episode 4) [TV series episode]. In B. Lawrence, J. Sudeikis, B. Hunt, J. Kelly, J. Ingold, B. Wrubel (Executive Producers), *Ted Lasso*. Ruby's Tuna Inc.; Doozer; Universal Television; Warner Bros. Television Studios.

Lotz, A. (2014). *The television will be revolutionized. (2nd ed.) second edition*. NYU Press.

Macey, D.A. (2012). Ancient archetypes in modern media. In A. Ruggerio (Ed.), *Monster, mate, mommy: Media depictions of women as brides, wives, & mothers* (pp 49–62). Lexington Books.

Mittell, J. (2015). *Complex TV: The poetics of contemporary television storytelling*. NYU Press.

Nygaard, T., & Lagerwey, J. (2017). Broadcasting quality: Re-centering feminist discourse with *The Good Wife*. *Television & New Media, 18*(2), 105–113. https://doi.org/10.1177/1527476416652485.

Reinke, R. (2010) Catfight: A feminist analysis. *Chrestomathy, 9*, 162–185.

Spiegel, J. (2020, December 31). *Ted Lasso* provided the warmest, kindest escape from the horrors of 2020. *Film*. https://www.slashfilm.com/578588/ted-lasso-and-2020/.

Sudeikis, J. (Writer), Lawrence, B. (Writer), Hunt, B. (Writer), & Kelly, J. (Writer), & Marshall, T. (Director). (2020, August 14), Pilot (Season 1, Episode 1) [TV series episode]. In B. Lawrence, J. Sudeikis, B. Hunt, J. Kelly, J. Ingold, B. Wrubel (Executive Producers), *Ted Lasso*. Ruby's Tuna Inc.; Doozer; Universal Television; Warner Bros. Television Studios.

Surrey, M. (2020, August 14). How on Earth Is 'Ted Lasso' Actually Good? *The Ringer*. https://www.theringer.com/tv/2020/8/14/21367994/ted-lasso-apple-tv-jason-sudeikis.

Turner, K. & Dunn, J. (2018). 'I'm your person': Television narrates female friendships in the workplace from *Cagney and Lacey* to *Grey's Anatomy*. In J. Dunn & J. Manning (Eds.), *Transgressing Feminist Theory and Discourse* (pp. 165–178). Routledge.

Walsh, P. (Writer), & Delaney, M.J. (Director). (2020, September 25), All Apologies (Season 1, Episode 9) [TV series episode]. In B. Lawrence, J. Sudeikis, B. Hunt, J. Kelly, J. Ingold, B. Wrubel (Executive Producers), *Ted Lasso*. Ruby's Tuna Inc.; Doozer; Universal Television; Warner Bros. Television Studios.

Wood, J. T. (1997). *Gendered lives" Communication, gender, and culture.* Wadsworth Publishing Company.

Wrubel, B. (Writer), & Hegarty, E. (Director). (2020, September 4), Two Aces (Season 1, Episode 6) [TV series episode]. In B. Lawrence, J. Sudeikis, B. Hunt, J. Kelly, J. Ingold, B. Wrubel (Executive Producers), *Ted Lasso*. Ruby's Tuna Inc.; Doozer; Universal Television; Warner Bros. Television Studios.

NOTE

1. It is important to note that, despite the expanded portrayal of masculinity in *Ted Lasso*, it remains a very heterosexual, cisgender portrayal; moreover, while there are some nonwhite characters, they are secondary. Sam and Nate are the only two who get character development, which happens in Season Two.

Index

About the Contributors

Lauren E. Burrow, Ph.D. is an Associate Professor of Education Studies at Stephen F. Austin State University. She is the co-founder and co-instructor of the Community Responsiveness and Engaged Advocacy in Teacher Education (CREATE) program track which focuses on encouraging service engagement in the community and partnerships with local families to increase social injustice awareness and improve the skills needed for pre-service teachers to take advocacy actions. She is a MotherScholar of three children who drive her to learn/UNlearn more every day. Her scholarship intersects her teaching and service with a focus on Service-Learning pedagogy in teacher education.

Theresa Conefrey, Ph.D. is the director of the Peer Educator program and teaches writing and communication courses at Santa Clara University. Her research interests focus on improving undergraduate learning and promoting the academic achievement of underrepresented learners.

Alicia Corts, Ph.D. is the director of the theatre program at Saint Leo University. Her research focuses on the intersection of virtual spaces and performance. She is the author of several chapters in edited volumes, and her articles can be seen in *Rebus*, *Theatre Journal*, *Theatre Symposium*, and *notches*. She is the assistant editor of *Ecumenica: A Journal of Religion and Performance.*

Chrissy Cross, Ph.D. is an Associate Professor in the Department of Education Studies at Stephen F. Austin State University. She teaches graduate and undergraduate courses in general and STEM pre-service teacher education. Her research areas include STEM pre-service teacher preparation and retention, STEM curriculum and instruction, academic motherscholarhood, and qualitative research methodologies. In 2016, she co-authored the NSF Robert Noyce Scholarship Grant, Talented Teachers in Training for

Texas (T4), and again in 2020 in the Talented Teacher in Training for Texas Expanded (T4X), which provide grants for STEM teachers in Texas.

Izabela Derda, Ph.D. is a researcher, lecturer, speaker, and industry professional. Currently she holds a position in the Media & Communication Department at the Erasmus School of History, Culture and Communication of Erasmus University in Rotterdam. She graduated from the Polish National Film School with a master's degree in film and TV producing and received her PhD in Media Studies from the University of Social Sciences and Humanities in Warsaw, Poland. In 2014 she was a visiting scholar at the Annenberg School for Communication and Journalism at the University of Southern California in Los Angeles. Her research interests lie in the investigation of the media as a practice. She is highly interested in how new technologies influence the storytelling design and shift creative processes.

Jan DeWaters is an Associate Professor at Clarkson University, with a joint position in the Institute for STEM Education and the School of Engineering. Her research interests focus on the factors that affect students' learning, competencies, and attitudes toward environmental and STEM studies and careers. Her work has been published in a range of education and sustainability venues, such as *Sustainability*, *Journal of Geoscience Education*, *Journal of Environmental Education*, and proceedings of the annual conferences of IEEE Frontiers in Education and the American Society for Engineering Education.

Mary P. Erickson teaches media studies at Western Washington University. Her research focuses on regional and independent screen media, distribution and marketing, gender, and technology. She co-edited *Independent Filmmaking Around the Globe* (University of Toronto Press, 2015). She has also worked in independent film as a publicist, researcher, and distribution consultant.

Heather J. Hether, Ph.D. is an Associate Professor of Teaching in the Department of Communication at the University of California, Davis. Dr. Hether's research focuses on public interest communication campaigns and innovative pedagogy. As an instructional researcher, Dr. Hether studies active learning, peer collaboration, and creative thinking. Dr. Hether teaches courses in health communication and communication campaigns. Prior to returning to academia, Dr. Hether worked for more than a decade in the private sector in marketing and public relations positions. She has held previous academic and research positions at the University of the Pacific in Stockton, California, and the Center for Healthcare Policy and Research (UC, Davis) in Sacramento, California.

Lauren Kelly is the co-host of *Enough Wicker: Intellectualizing The Golden Girls*, a scholarly podcast and website analyzing everyone and their grandmother's favorite 1980s television show. Based in Brooklyn, Lauren's professional background is in nonprofit strategy and fundraising, but she is very much looking forward to living life as a professional *Golden Girls* expert. In case that doesn't work out, she is also currently a graduate student studying public and social policy.

Sarah S. LeBlanc, Ph.D. is an Assistant Professor of Communication at Purdue University Fort Wayne. She teaches graduate and undergraduate courses in family, health, and relational communication. Her research focuses within two areas of maternal communication; communica-tion during the postpartum stage and how mothers communicate about taboo topics, like menstruation. Sarah is in the process of bridging her research with teaching to bring awareness to the issues she studies. Her publications include articles in *Health Communication*, *Journal of Motherhood Initiative*, *The Journal of Autoethnography*, *Death Studies*, *Journal of Loss & Trauma* to mention a few, as well as book chapters on mental illness and a few case studies. She has edited a case study book for family communication.

Deborah A. Macey earned her **Ph.D.** in communication and society from the University of Oregon. She has taught a variety of courses in human communication and media studies. Her research focuses on the intersections of gender, race, and class in popular culture, particularly television. As a lifetime member of the Organization for the Study of Communication, Language, and Gender, she frequently presents at its annual conference. Her work has appeared in *Media Depictions of Brides, Wives, and Mothers* (Lexington) and *Human Studies: A Journal for Philosophy and the Social Sciences.*

Matthew J. Manierre is an Assistant Professor of Sociology in the Department of Humanities and Social Sciences at Clarkson University. His research examines the relationships between social inequality and health, as well as methodological challenges therein. His work has been published in journals such as *Research on Aging*, *Gerontologist*, *Social Science and Medicine*, and *Health Communication.*

Derek Moscato is an associate professor in the department of journalism at Western Washington University in Bellingham, Washington. Moscato's research and teaching focuses on persuasion, global media, environmental communication, and political economy of media. Moscato is also affiliated with WWU's Border Policy Research Institute, Salish Sea Institute, and Canadian-American Studies program. His book *Dirt Persuasion,* focused on the populist appeals of heartland environmentalism, was published by the University of Nebraska Press in 2022.

Michelle Napierski-Prancl, Ph.D. is Professor of Sociology and Faculty Director of the Women's Institute at Russell Sage College. Her research interests focus on gender, family, work, and popular culture, and her publications include essays on the portrayal of gender in popular literature and articles on teaching pedagogy. Her first book, *Mothers Work: Confronting the Mommy Wars, Raising Children, and Working for Social Change* (2019), explores the institution of motherhood, mothering, and the mommy wars by sharing the voices of experts on the topic: the mothers themselves.

Laurie E. Naranch is Professor of Political Science & International Relations and Director of the Women's, Gender, and Sexuality Studies Program at Siena College, New York, USA. Her research is in the areas of political philosophy, political culture, feminist theory, craft, narrative, and aesthetics. Recent publications include "Could Old Be the New Cool?: Shifting Aesthetics of the Aging Body," *Zone Moda Journal* (2020) and "The Narratable Self: Adriana Cavarero and Sojourner Truth" in the journal *Hypatia* (2019). She is currently at work on materialisms in Italian philosophy, the indebted student, with larger projects about the philosophy and politics of craft as well as a book on the aging body and political theory.

Alana M. Nicastro is a civilian analyst to the United States Marine Corps, a longtime educator in the School of Communication at San Diego State University, and a national-level education consultant who brings together teams across departments, institutions, and workplace segments to help them achieve a deeper understanding of their work. Through facilitating conversations and innovations with change agents at all levels, Dr. Nicastro's work positively impacts performance to help organizations become more humane and empowering.

Gwendelyn S. Nisbett is an associate professor of public relations at the Mayborn School of Journalism, University of North Texas. Dr. Nisbett's research examines the intersection of mediated social influence, campaign communication, and popular culture. Her research incorporates a multi-methods approach to understanding the influence of fandom and celebrity in social and civic engagement. She has published in journals such as

Political Communication, *Health Communication*, and the *Atlantic Journal of Communication.*

Heather K. Olson Beal, Ph.D. is a Professor of Education Studies at Stephen F. Austin State University. She teaches courses in educational foundations, family and community engagement, and educational policy and advocacy. Her scholarship examines the issues of second language education, school choice, and the experiences of women and mothers in academia. She has three (now officially adult) children who inform her teaching and scholarly work and who bring her incalculable joy.

Newly Paul is an assistant professor of journalism at the Mayborn School of Journalism University at the University of North Texas in Denton. Dr. Paul's research areas include political communication, race and gender in politics, and media coverage of elections. She has taught principles of news, news reporting and writing, copyediting, political reporting, and minorities in media. Her research has won grants and awards, and has been published in top journals such as *Political Research Quarterly* and *Journalism and Mass Communication Quarterly.*

Seema Rivera is an Associate Professor of STEM Education in the Institute of STEM education and the Department of Education at Clarkson University. Her research examines identity and equity within secondary STEM education and in higher education. Her work has been published in journals like the *Cultural Studies of Science Education* and the *Journal of College Science Teaching*. She is also the Principal Investigator on the Noyce Scholarship Program at Clarkson, a program funded by the National Science Foundation.

Edith Ritt-Coulter is a Ph.D. candidate in the history department at the University of North Texas. She specializes in late 19th and early 20th century African American history focusing issues of body, place, and identity. She is currently working on her dissertation project entitled "Creating Black Space: Oklahoma City's African American Community During the Early Twentieth Century."

Sarah Royal is the co-host of *Enough Wicker: Intellectualizing The Golden Girls*, a scholarly podcast and website analyzing everyone and their grandmother's favorite 1980s television show. Royal is a celebrated author of many underground zines and novelty books, her most well-known being *The Book Bindery* and *Creative Cursing: A Mix 'N' Match Profanity Generator* respectively. By day, Royal works as a marketing communications professional for social good organizations. A native New Jerseyan, Royal currently lives in Brooklyn but has a predilection for Portland, Oregon.

Stephanie G. Schartel Dunn is an assistant professor and the W. Robert Corley Professor of Marketing in the Plaster College of Business at Missouri Southern State University. Dr. Schartel Dunn's research examines mediated social influence, consumer behavior, and attitude change. She has published in journals such as *Western Journal Communication*, *Social Marketing Quarterly*, and the *Howard Journal of Communication*.

Elizabeth L. Spradley, Ph.D. is an Associate Professor of Communication Studies at Stephen F. Austin State University, where she coordinates the Communication Studies program and basic courses. She serves on the editorial board for *The Intima: A Journal of Narrative Medicine* and research topics at the intersections of narrative, maternity, health, work/life, and crisis. Her publications include articles in *Journal of the Motherhood Initiative*, *Journal of Community Informatics*, *Journal of Leadership and Accountability*, and more and numerous book chapters centering around health, narrative, and pandemic/crisis communication.

David Staton is an Associate Professor at the University of Northern Colorado where he teaches in the Department of Journalism and Media Studies. His areas of research include visual communication, media ethics, and sports journalism. He has been involved in the production of three feature-length documentary films, which have been screened internationally, and the experimental documentary short, *Ghost Resort.*

Shelly M. Valdez is now retired from a decades-long career in education, organization consulting, and coaching teams through change. Dr. Valdez's multifaceted background includes developing and supporting collaborative change structures, conducting original research, teaching at the post-secondary level, as well as authoring and public speaking on a variety of subjects—most recently, on women's wellness and dynamic aging: rethinking aging from a time of decline to one of transition and vitality.

Martha (Marty) Whalen is a Research Assistant Professor at Clarkson University. She has worked in marketing, training and organizational development for companies (including Xerox and Dell EMC), as well as in research, teaching, curriculum development, and instructional design for academia. Marty's dissertation research explored faculty time management in online and blended/hybrid higher education.

www.ingramcontent.com/pod-product-compliance
Ingram Content Group UK Ltd.
Pitfield, Milton Keynes, MK11 3LW, UK
UKHW020839290926
15470UKWH00004B/1449

9 781666 901153